S0-CYH-679

## Teen Health Series

# Cosmetic and Reconstructive Surgery
# SOURCEBOOK

## *Second Edition*

## Health Reference Series

*Second Edition*

# Cosmetic and Reconstructive Surgery
## SOURCEBOOK

*Basic Consumer Information about Plastic Surgery
and Non-Surgical Appearance-Enhancing Procedures,
Including Facts about Botulinum Toxin, Collagen
Replacement, Dermabrasion, Chemical Peels, Eyelid
Surgery, Nose Reshaping, Lip Augmentation,
Liposuction, Breast Enlargement and Reduction,
Tummy Tucking, and Other Skin, Hair, Facial, and
Body Shaping Procedures*

*Along with Information about Reconstructive
Procedures for Congenital Disorders, Disfiguring
Diseases, Burns, and Traumatic Injuries, a Glossary
of Related Terms, and a Directory of Additional
Resources*

*Edited by*
**Karen Bellenir**

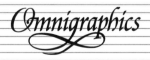

*Omnigraphics*

P.O. Box 31-1640 • Detroit, MI 48231-1640

Bibliographic Note

Because this page cannot legibly accommodate all the copyright notices, the Bibliographic Note portion of the Preface constitutes an extension of the copyright notice.

Edited by Karen Bellenir

*Health Reference Series*

Karen Bellenir, *Managing Editor*
David A. Cooke, M.D., *Medical Consultant*
Elizabeth Collins, *Research and Permissions Coordinator*
Cherry Stockdale, *Permissions Assistant*
EdIndex, Services for Publishers, *Indexers*

* * *

Omnigraphics, Inc.

Matthew P. Barbour, *Senior Vice President*
Kay Gill, *Vice President—Directories*
Kevin Hayes, *Operations Manager*
David P. Bianco, *Marketing Director*

* * *

Peter E. Ruffner, *Publisher*

Frederick G. Ruffner, Jr., *Chairman*

Copyright © 2007 Omnigraphics, Inc.

ISBN 978-0-7808-0951-1

Library of Congress Cataloging-in-Publication Data

Cosmetic and reconstructive surgery sourcebook : basic consumer information about plastic surgery and non-surgical appearance-enhancing procedures, including facts about botulinum toxin, collagen replacement, dermabrasion, chemical peels, eyelid surgery, nose reshaping, lip augmentation, liposuction, breast enlargement and reduction, tummy tucking, and other skin, hair, facial, and body shaping procedures; along with information about reconstructive procedures for congenital disorders, disfiguring diseases, burns, and traumatic injuries, a glossary of related terms, and a directory of additional resources / edited by Karen Bellenir.-- 2nd ed.
    p. cm.
  Rev. ed. of: Reconstructive and cosmetic surgery sourcebook. 1st ed. 2001.
  Summary: "Provides basic consumer health information about cosmetic surgery to enhance appearance, or correct defects due to congenital disorders, disease, or trauma. Includes index, glossary of related terms, and other resources"--Provided by publisher.
  Includes bibliographical references and index.
  ISBN-13: 978-0-7808-0951-2 (hardcover : alk. paper) 1. Surgery, Plastic. 2. Consumer education. I. Bellenir, Karen. II. Reconstructive and cosmetic surgery sourcebook.
  RD118.R365 2007
  617.9'5--dc22
                                                                    2007018893

The information in this publication was compiled from the sources cited and from other sources considered reliable. While every possible effort has been made to ensure reliability, the publisher will not assume liability for damages caused by inaccuracies in the data, and makes no warranty, express or implied, on the accuracy of the information contained herein.

This book is printed on acid-free paper meeting the ANSI Z39.48 Standard. The infinity symbol that appears above indicates that the paper in this book meets that standard.

Printed in the United States

# *Table of Contents*

Visit www.healthreferenceseries.com to view *A Contents Guide to the Health Reference Series*, a listing of more than 13,000 topics and the volumes in which they are covered.

## Part V: Reconstructive Procedures for Congenital Concerns

## Part VI: Disease-Related and Post-Traumatic Reconstructive Procedures

## Part VII: Additional Help and Information

# *Preface*

## About This Book

According to the American Society of Plastic Surgeons, nearly 11 million cosmetic surgery procedures were performed in 2006—up 7% from the previous year. Surgical procedures, led by breast augmentation, nose reshaping, and liposuction saw a two percent increase, while the number of minimally-invasive procedures—most popularly Botox® treatment, chemical peels, and laser hair removal—grew by eight percent. An additional 5.2 million procedures were performed for reconstructive reasons. Despite the popularity of these procedures, many people find they need assistance to develop realistic expectations, understand potential risks, find an appropriate surgeon, or evaluate product claims.

*Cosmetic and Reconstructive Surgery Sourcebook, Second Edition* provides updated information about both surgical and minimally-invasive procedures used to enhance appearance, diminish the cosmetic effects of aging, or improve the function of abnormal or injured body structures. It explains the criteria that make a person a good plastic surgery candidate and outlines specific procedures used to treat the skin, hair, face, neck, and body. The book concludes with a glossary of related terms and a directory of resources for additional help and information.

## How to Use This Book

This book is divided into parts and chapters. Parts focus on broad areas of interest. Chapters are devoted to single topics within a part.

*Part I: Understanding Plastic Surgery* provides basic information about cosmetic and reconstructive surgery. It describes the criteria that make a person a good candidate for appearance-altering procedures and explains how to evaluate whether or not expectations are realistic. It also summarizes the risks involved in both surgical and non-surgical procedures.

*Part II: Skin and Hair Procedures* describes age-related changes to the skin, including wrinkles and blemishes, and the tools used to combat them. It also describes skin resurfacing techniques, such as dermabrasion, chemical peels, and laser resurfacing. The use of permanent make up is discussed, and a separate chapter describes the procedures used in tattooing and tattoo removal. The part concludes with information about hair removal and hair restoration.

*Part III: Facial and Neck Surgical Procedures* discusses procedures used to alter the appearance of the eyes, nose, ears, forehead, cheeks, lips, chin, and neck. Individual chapters focus on specific procedures, such as blepharoplasty, rhinoplasty, otoplasty, and mentoplasty, and provide facts about how the procedures are done, what risks are involved, what results can be expected, and what to expect during recovery.

*Part IV: Body Shaping Procedures* provides information about surgical procedures used to modify the shape of the abdomen, hips, breasts, and arms. These include liposuction, breast enlargement and reduction, tummy tucks (abdominoplasty), and arm lifts. Individual chapters explain the procedures and their risks, outline the types of results that can be achieved, and describe the recovery process.

*Part V: Reconstructive Procedures for Congenital Concerns* describes the use of plastic surgery techniques in the treatment of birth defects such as birthmarks, cleft lip and palate, and deformities of the face, hands, and other body structures.

*Part VI: Disease-Related and Post-Traumatic Reconstructive Procedures* begins with information about how scars caused by surgery, accidents, or disease can be treated. It describes how mastectomy patients can benefit from plastic surgery techniques, and discusses how amputations, facial fractures, burns, and other injuries are treated.

*Part VII: Additional Help and Information* provides a glossary of terms related to cosmetic and reconstructive procedures and a directory of resources for more information about plastic surgery.

## Bibliographic Note

This volume contains documents and excerpts from publications issued by the following U.S. government agencies: Agency for Healthcare Research and Quality; Federal Citizen Information Center; National Women's Health Information Center; and the U.S. Food and Drug Administration.

In addition, this volume contains copyrighted documents from the following organizations and individuals: A.D.A.M., Inc.; American Academy of Dermatology; American Academy of Facial Plastic and Reconstructive Surgery; American Academy of Neurology; American Psychological Association; American Society for Aesthetic Plastic Surgery; American Society for Bariatric Surgery; American Society for Dermatologic Surgery; American Society for Laser Medicine and Surgery, Inc.; American Society for Surgery of the Hand; American Society of Anesthesiologists; American Society of Plastic Surgeons; Better Health Channel (Victoria, Australia); *BMJ (British Medical Journal)*; Canadian Society of Otolaryngology–Head and Neck Surgery; Ceatus Media Group LLC; Changes Plastic Surgery; Cleveland Clinic; Columbia University Department of Surgery; Enhancement Media; Facial Plastic Surgery Network; Imaginis Corporation; International Society of Hair Restoration Surgery; Johns Hopkins Cosmetic Center; Metropolitan Institute for Plastic Surgery; Sam P. Most, MD; Nemours Foundation; New Zealand Dermatological Society; Society of Permanent Cosmetic Professionals; University of Chicago Hospitals; University of Illinois Eye Center; University of Missouri Children's Hospital; University Oral Surgery; Washington University Physicians; and WoltersKluwer Health.

Full citation information is provided on the first page of each chapter. Every effort has been made to secure all necessary rights to reprint the copyrighted material. If any omissions have been made, please contact Omnigraphics to make corrections for future editions.

## Acknowledgements

In addition to the organizations, agencies, and individuals who have contributed to this *Sourcebook*, special thanks go to editorial assistants Nicole Salerno and Elizabeth Bellenir, research and permissions coordinator Liz Collins, and permissions assistant Cherry Stockdale.

## About the Health Reference Series

The *Health Reference Series* is designed to provide basic medical information for patients, families, caregivers, and the general public.

Each volume takes a particular topic and provides comprehensive coverage. This is especially important for people who may be dealing with a newly diagnosed disease or a chronic disorder in themselves or in a family member. People looking for preventive guidance, information about disease warning signs, medical statistics, and risk factors for health problems will also find answers to their questions in the *Health Reference Series*. The *Series*, however, is not intended to serve as a tool for diagnosing illness, in prescribing treatments, or as a substitute for the physician/patient relationship. All people concerned about medical symptoms or the possibility of disease are encouraged to seek professional care from an appropriate health care provider.

### A Note about Spelling and Style

*Health Reference Series* editors use *Stedman's Medical Dictionary* as an authority for questions related to the spelling of medical terms and the *Chicago Manual of Style* for questions related to grammatical structures, punctuation, and other editorial concerns. Consistent adherence is not always possible, however, because the individual volumes within the *Series* include many documents from a wide variety of different producers and copyright holders, and the editor's primary goal is to present material from each source as accurately as is possible following the terms specified by each document's producer. This sometimes means that information in different chapters or sections may follow other guidelines and alternate spelling authorities. For example, occasionally a copyright holder may require that eponymous terms be shown in possessive forms (Crohn's disease *vs.* Crohn disease) or that British spelling norms be retained (leukaemia *vs.* leukemia).

### Locating Information within the Health Reference Series

The *Health Reference Series* contains a wealth of information about a wide variety of medical topics. Ensuring easy access to all the fact sheets, research reports, in-depth discussions, and other material contained within the individual books of the *Series* remains one of our highest priorities. As the *Series* continues to grow in size and scope, however, locating the precise information needed by a reader may become more challenging.

A *Contents Guide to the Health Reference Series* was developed to direct readers to the specific volumes that address their concerns. It presents an extensive list of diseases, treatments, and other topics of general interest compiled from the Tables of Contents and major index headings. To access *A Contents Guide to the Health Reference Series*, visit www.healthreferenceseries.com.

## Medical Consultant

Medical consultation services are provided to the *Health Reference Series* editors by David A. Cooke, M.D. Dr. Cooke is a graduate of Brandeis University, and he received his M.D. degree from the University of Michigan. He completed residency training at the University of Wisconsin Hospital and Clinics. He is board-certified in Internal Medicine. Dr. Cooke currently works as part of the University of Michigan Health System and practices in Brighton, MI. In his free time, he enjoys writing, science fiction, and spending time with his family.

## Our Advisory Board

We would like to thank the following board members for providing guidance to the development of this *Series*:

- Dr. Lynda Baker,
  Associate Professor of Library and Information Science,
  Wayne State University, Detroit, MI

- Nancy Bulgarelli,
  William Beaumont Hospital Library, Royal Oak, MI

- Karen Imarisio,
  Bloomfield Township Public Library, Bloomfield Township, MI

- Karen Morgan,
  Mardigian Library, University of Michigan-Dearborn,
  Dearborn, MI

- Rosemary Orlando,
  St. Clair Shores Public Library, St. Clair Shores, MI

## Health Reference Series *Update Policy*

The inaugural book in the *Health Reference Series* was the first edition of *Cancer Sourcebook* published in 1989. Since then, the *Series* has been enthusiastically received by librarians and in the medical community. In order to maintain the standard of providing high-quality health information for the layperson the editorial staff at Omnigraphics felt it was necessary to implement a policy of updating volumes when warranted.

Medical researchers have been making tremendous strides, and it is the purpose of the *Health Reference Series* to stay current with the most recent advances. Each decision to update a volume is made on an individual basis. Some of the considerations include how much new information is available and the feedback we receive from people who use the books. If there is a topic you would like to see added to the update list, or an area of medical concern you feel has not been adequately addressed, please write to:

Editor
*Health Reference Series*
Omnigraphics, Inc.
P.O. Box 31-1640
Detroit, MI 48231
E-mail: editorial@omnigraphics.com

# Part One

# Understanding Plastic Surgery

# Chapter 1

# *Using Medicine to Improve Appearance*

A smaller nose. Bigger breasts. Slimmer thighs. Plumper lips. Less hair on the body. More hair on the head. Whether we're looking to tighten our tummies or lighten our laugh lines, America's fascination with youth and beauty has long fueled the development of medical products for cosmetic purposes. And if such "vanity drugs" can be shown to be safe and effective, the Food and Drug Administration (FDA) just may approve.

The ongoing fight to delay or reverse the aging process has dermatologists and cosmetic plastic surgeons responding with products like Restylane (hyaluronic acid), one of a handful of soft tissue fillers recently approved by the FDA to treat facial wrinkles. Restylane is an injectable gel that acts as a filler to remove the wrinkle, producing instantaneous results. Such products are not as invasive as face-lifts, eyelid surgery, and other reconstructive procedures. And they are more effective and last longer than creams, lotions and other topical products, whether over-the-counter or prescription. In addition, the fact that the treatments result in little or no downtime makes them more attractive to those seeking a quick fix. Without making a single incision, doctors can erase wrinkles, acne scars, and sun damage in a matter of minutes.

"This is a huge industry," says Jonathan K. Wilkin, M.D., a medical officer in the FDA's Division of Dermatologic and Dental Drug

"Science Meets Beauty: Using Medicine to Improve Appearances," by Carol Rados, in *FDA Consumer magazine,* U.S. Food and Drug Administration, March–April 2004.

Products. "The way people try to move the clock back is through the skin." Basically, he says, through various products and procedures, "they are addressing the effects of gravity on the skin over time."

## Aging Skin 101

An increased understanding of the structure and function of the skin is helping to drive the development of products that reduce the visible signs of facial aging, according to the American Academy of Dermatology (AAD).

With aging, all skin cells begin to produce excess amounts of free radicals—unstable oxygen molecules that, under ideal circumstances, are removed by naturally occurring antioxidants within the skin's cells. In aging skin cells, antioxidants are in short supply. The free radicals generated are left unchecked and cause damage to cell membranes, proteins, and DNA. These free radicals eventually break down a protein substance in connective tissue (collagen) and release chemicals that cause inflammation in the skin. It is a combination of these cellular and molecular events that leads to skin aging and the formation of wrinkles, the AAD says.

Considerable research has been done to understand the aging process, and studies now show that products containing bioactive ingredients (those that interact with living tissues or systems) can benefit sun-damaged, discolored, and aging skin, giving consumers new choices for restoring their overall appearance. But why is the FDA reviewing products that simply make people look and feel good when typically the agency evaluates disease-fighting treatments?

"If something that is being implanted into the body could have health consequences, we're concerned about it," says Stephen P. Rhodes, M.S., chief of the FDA's Plastic and Reconstructive Surgery Devices Branch. "Wrinkle fillers affect the structure of the face and could have such health consequences."

## Facing Facts

Under the Federal Food, Drug and Cosmetic Act, the FDA legally defines products by their intended uses. Drugs are defined as products intended for treating or preventing disease and affecting the structure or any function of the body. A medical device is a product that also is intended to affect the structure or function of the body, but which does not achieve its primary intended purposes through the chemical action of a drug—nor is it dependent on being metabolized.

The hyaluronic acid in Restylane, although biosynthetically produced (formed of chemical compounds by the enzyme action of living organisms), is almost identical to that in all living organisms. Hyaluronic acid is a structural component of skin that creates volume and shape. Concentrations of hyaluronic acid throughout the body decline with age, causing undesirable changes in the skin. Restylane binds to water and provides volume to easily fill in larger folds of skin left by tissue loss around the mouth and cheeks. "This makes it a structural action," says Rhodes, "much like a chin implant."

In contrast, cosmetics are defined as substances that cleanse, beautify, promote attractiveness, or alter the appearance, without affecting the body's structure or function. This definition includes skin-care products such as creams, lotions, powders and sprays, perfume, lipstick, fingernail polish, and more.

Different laws and regulations apply to each type of product. Some products must comply with the requirements for both cosmetics and drugs. This happens when a product has two intended uses, such as an antidandruff shampoo. An antidandruff shampoo is a cosmetic and a drug because it is intended to treat dandruff (which affects the follicles where the hair is formed) and clean hair.

Warning letters issued by the FDA recently to firms that marketed hair care products with claims such as restoration of hair growth and hair loss prevention illustrate an important distinction between the legal definitions of cosmetics and drugs. Warning letters officially inform companies that they may be engaged in illegal activities, and instruct manufacturers on how to bring their products into compliance with the law. Hair growers and hair loss prevention products, because of their mechanism of action, are considered drugs, not cosmetics, and these firms were not meeting the legal requirements for marketing a drug.

Unlike drugs and medical devices, neither cosmetic products nor cosmetic ingredients are reviewed or approved by the FDA before they are sold to the public. The agency only acts against cosmetic products found to cause harm after they are on the market.

## Cosmetics or Drugs?

Much confusion exists about the status of cosmetic products having medicinal or drug-like benefits, says Linda Katz, M.D., M.P.H., director of the FDA's Office of Cosmetics and Colors. Although the FDA does not consider the term "cosmeceutical" to be a valid product class, Katz says it is used throughout the cosmetic industry to describe products that are marketed as cosmetics but that have drug-like effects. Tretinoin (retinoic acid), the biologically active form of vitamin A, for example, is not prohibited from use in cosmetics. However, when it is used topically for treating mild to moderate acne, sun-damaged skin, and other skin conditions, it is recognized by the FDA as a drug. This is because it acts deep at the skin's cellular level by increasing collagen.

According to the AAD, the answer to whether or not cosmeceuticals really work lies in the ingredients and how they interact with the biological mechanisms that occur in aging skin. The regulatory question the FDA faces when considering such products, Katz says, "is whether or not a manufacturer is making a structure or function claim."

The FDA uses different standards when evaluating the risks and benefits of products used for cosmetic treatments than for therapeutic uses of products. Steven K. Galson, M.D., M.P.H., acting director for the FDA's Center for Drug Evaluation and Research, adds that products like tretinoin and Restylane that are not indicated for serious or life-threatening conditions are subject to close examination by the agency because of the benefit-to-risk ratio.

"Because these products are for cosmetic purposes, they must be extraordinarily safe," Galson says. This means that the FDA may allow someone to incur a greater risk from products that treat medical conditions, rather than from those that are intended for cosmetic purposes. "We generally won't tolerate much risk for a drug whose primary use is cosmetic," he says.

## Welcome Side Effects

Many cosmetic treatments are the result of common disease therapies whose unexpected side effects were pleasant surprises. Vaniqa (eflornithine hydrochloride), the first prescription drug for removing unwanted hair, is a topically applied version of a drug that was originally developed to treat African sleeping sickness. Similarly, minoxidil originally had been prescribed as an oral tablet to treat high blood pressure. As a result of side effects that included hair growth and reversal of male baldness, Rogaine (2 percent minoxidil) was the first drug approved by the FDA for the treatment of hair loss (androgenetic alopecia).

"There's a lot of serendipity in drug development," says the FDA's Wilkin. A pill to help smokers quit, for example, evolved out of the unexpected observation that a drug intended to treat depression also seemed to take away the desire to smoke. Bupropion was first marketed in 1989 by GlaxoSmithKline as an antidepressant under the name Wellbutrin. After doctors noticed that patients being treated with Wellbutrin gave up smoking spontaneously, studies were done to show that the product could help smokers quit, as well. As a result, the slow-release form of bupropion, marketed as Zyban, was approved by the FDA in 1997 as an aid to smoking cessation treatment.

Some pharmaceutical companies, however, apparently aren't ready to enter the vanity drugs arena. Patrick Davish, the global product communications spokesman for Merck & Co. Inc., says that the drug company has no "cosmetic" drugs in its product pipeline at this time.

"The fact that we don't participate in that market right now—I'm not sure that's reflective of any particular deliberation or decision," he says. "That's just not where the science has taken us."

Before electing to have a cosmetic procedure:

- Discuss it with a physician who can refer you to a specialist in the fields of dermatology and aesthetic plastic surgery.

- Begin with a consultation to find the right doctor, and select one who is qualified to do the procedure you want.

- Make sure the doctor you choose is certified by an appropriate medical board.

- Have realistic expectations about the benefits you want to achieve.

- Compare fees—insurance does not usually cover elective procedures.

## Saving Face

According to the American Society for Aesthetic Plastic Surgery (ASAPS), nearly 7 million Americans underwent surgical and nonsurgical cosmetic procedures in 2002. Laura Bradbard was one of them.

Despite the sudden explosion of such "lunchtime" techniques as Restylane for erasing wrinkles, and Botox (botulinum toxin type A) for smoothing out frown lines, Bradbard, of Gaithersburg, Maryland, opted for a longer-lasting reconstructive facelift that included a chin implant, eyelid surgery, and surprisingly, only a few days of pain-free recovery.

"None of this was medically necessary," admits Bradbard, a 48-year-old FDA press officer, "but I had been feeling worn out and tired. What I saw in the mirror was sad." Bradbard says she didn't get a facelift

7

to look younger; she only wanted her face to look more balanced. In the end, she says, "My doctor gave me a chin that geometrically fit my face," and a look that she says makes her feel better about herself.

Like Bradbard, others are spending a lot of money to look good. "With patients living 90-plus years, today's anti-aging modalities offer people noninvasive procedures that mimic true facelifts," says Craig R. Dufresne, M.D., a plastic and reconstructive surgeon in Chevy Chase, Maryland, who performed Bradbard's surgery. However, Dufresne says he suggested reconstructive surgery for Bradbard because "she wanted to deal with structural changes to restore facial balance," which was more than the chemical action of a drug could produce. "And skin product application (such as wrinkle fillers) following a facelift," adds Dufresne, "will actually allow the facelift or any other reconstructive procedure to last longer and make a great result even better."

## *Seeking Professional Advice*

Since it is often difficult for people to determine the validity of claims made about topical products and to decide among the overwhelming number of anti-aging procedures, how do people know what's right for them?

"A good place to start is with a dermatologist," says Arielle N.B. Kauvar, M.D., clinical associate professor of dermatology at the New York University School of Medicine. "Dermatologists are trained in the health, function and disease state of the skin, and people could save time, money and confusion by seeking the advice of a dermatologist rather than guessing what might work for them."

Kauvar says a dermatologist's recommendations can help consumers make informed decisions. "People shouldn't hunt and peck for products," she adds. "Not knowing what type of skin you have is why so many people try unnecessary products that can often do more harm than good."

An expert in laser procedures, Kauvar says that, in the past, techniques for improving aging skin required invasive laser or surgical procedures, which produced open wounds and required long recovery times. Today, she says, people can choose from a variety of non-ablative (non-wounding) laser treatments that are designed to reverse, improve or erase the early signs of aging, take very little time to perform, and have a minimal, if any, recovery time.

While Bradbard wasn't interested in removing wrinkles at the time of her facelift, given what she knows about new technologies and drug delivery systems today, she says, "I would consider both non-invasive procedures and another facelift down the road, depending on how much my skin changes. I would ask my doctor what would give me the best results with the longest-lasting effects."

## Buyer Beware

Anti-aging products that promise to diminish wrinkles and fine lines are found on many store shelves. However, dermatologists recommend that people consider only those procedures and products that have proven, over time, to be most effective at reversing the aging process. Most doctors agree that the leading product to prevent premature wrinkles and sun damage is sunscreen. A broad-spectrum sunscreen that protects the skin from both UVA and UVB rays, with a sun protection factor (SPF) of 15 or higher, can prevent the skin from looking older than it is.

According to the ASAPS, it's important to realize that although certain products and procedures are effective, they are also limited by the skin's normal aging process. A product that has been deemed effective for erasing wrinkles doesn't necessarily erase wrinkles—there are lots of variables that determine its effectiveness.

For example, the active ingredient in a drug must be delivered to the skin at a therapeutic concentration and remain in the skin long enough to have an effect. Also, because the composition of a man's body differs from a woman's, products or procedures can have different effects. The facial area in men contains hair, for example, and their skin is thicker. This means the blood supply is greater—and so is the risk of bleeding—but it also could mean better healing.

And cosmetic procedures come with risks. If a procedure is performed poorly, the physical and emotional scars could be carried for life. Understand the risks and side effects that may be involved.

"My wanting to improve my appearance is like my husband's desire to restore a vintage automobile," says Bradbard. "We both want something to look good for as long as it can."

# Chapter 2

# *Frequently Asked Questions about Plastic Surgery*

Here are the answers to some of the most frequently asked questions about plastic surgery.

When reviewing information about specific plastic surgery procedures, it is important to understand that the circumstances and experience of every individual are unique. If you are considering plastic surgery, please ask your plastic surgeon for further information about the particular procedure and what you can expect.

### What is plastic surgery?

Plastic surgery is a surgical specialty dedicated to reconstruction of facial and body defects due to birth disorders, trauma, burns, and disease. The art and science of plastic surgery is also involved with the enhancement of the appearance of a person through such operations as facelift, rhinoplasty, breast augmentation, and liposuction.

### Why the "plastic" in plastic surgery?

The word "plastic" comes from the Greek word *plastikos*, meaning "to mold or shape." Many of the first plastic surgeries were developed to close a difficult wound or replace tissue lost due to injury or cancer. These procedures often involved the formation of a skin flap to reshape or mold the defect so as to approximate the original shape.

## What is the difference between cosmetic and reconstructive surgery?

Cosmetic surgery is performed to reshape normal structures of the body in order to improve the patient's appearance and self-esteem. Cosmetic surgery is usually not covered by health insurance because it is elective.

Reconstructive surgery is performed on abnormal structures of the body, caused by congenital defects, developmental abnormalities, trauma, infection, tumors, or disease. It is generally performed to improve function, but may also be done to approximate a normal appearance. Reconstructive surgery is generally covered by most health insurance policies although coverage for specific procedures and levels of coverage may vary greatly.

There are a number of "gray areas" in coverage for plastic surgery that sometimes require special consideration by an insurance carrier. These areas usually involved surgical operations which may be reconstructive or cosmetic, depending on each patient's situation. For example, eyelid surgery (blepharoplasty)—a procedure normally performed to achieve cosmetic improvement may be covered if the eyelids are drooping severely and obscuring a patient's vision.

## What is recovery from plastic surgery like? Will I be able to tolerate the pain post-operatively?

Each patient will tolerate pain post-operatively in a different way, and we consider this. While some patients may describe the pain as an ache, others experience greater discomfort. Appropriate pain medications are prescribed for the postoperative patients, and these help minimize discomfort. Most facial cosmetic operations have minimal discomfort post-operatively. Liposuction is slightly more uncomfortable, and operations that require elevation or tightening of the muscles—such as an abdominoplasty or breast augmentation have discomfort equal to that of a C-section.

## How long is the recuperative period and when can I return to work?

The length of time it takes to recuperate after plastic surgery varies depending on the procedure performed and the person operated on. Most patients will require assistance for the first two days. Then most patients are able to care for themselves, but may still need assistance if they have small children to care for. The specific lengths of disability are outlined below by procedure. These are approximations, and do not include return to exercise.

- **Eyelid surgery:** Usually can get around independently by the second day. With the use of sunglasses, may feel comfortable going to the store by day 3–4, and with makeup could return to work by 5–7 days.

- **Facelift surgery:** Usually can get around independently by the second day. Usually do not feel comfortable going out in public for 5–7 days. Requires 10–14 days before returning to work if in the public eye.

- **Breast surgery:** Usually can get around independently by the second day. May return to work at 5–7 days if not required to lift more than 15 pounds.

- **Liposuction:** Usually can get around independently by the second day, earlier if smaller number of areas treated. One can return to work and normal activities in 5–7 days.

- **Abdominoplasty:** Patients may take between 2–4 days before getting around independently. The recovery is almost identical to C-section. One can return to a desk job at 5–7 days, other jobs 10–14 days.

### When can I resume regular exercise?

The time a patient resumes regular exercises varies based on the operation performed. All patients are encouraged to start a slow walking routine on the second postoperative day. Regular aerobic and more vigorous activities are not allowed during the first two weeks in order to decrease the risks of bleeding, swelling, and bruising. Weight lifting and contact sports are allowed at one month in most cases.

### What should you know about the safety of outpatient plastic surgery?

When considering plastic surgery, it's natural to focus more on the expected result than on the surgical process. However, to be fully informed, it's important to learn about the safety of the procedure as well as the expected outcome. Although thousands of people have plastic surgery every year without complications, no surgical procedure is risk-free. To maximize safety, ensure that:

- Your surgeon is adequately trained and is board certified by the American Board of Plastic Surgery;

- The facility where your surgery will be performed conforms to strict safety standards;

- Your surgeon is informed of any drugs you are taking and your full medical history, especially if you have had any circulation disorders, heart or lung ailments or problems with blood clots;

- The surgical facility will use skilled, licensed personnel to administer and monitor your anesthesia and your recovery immediately following the procedure;

- Extra safety measures are taken if you are having a more extensive liposuction procedure.

The American Society of Plastic Surgeons (ASPS), an organization of board-certified plastic surgeons who are dedicated to the highest standards of patient care, has prepared this document to help you get the safety information you need. It contains recommendations developed by the society's expert task forces, whose members have consulted the most recent research available. If you have questions about these guidelines or any specific concerns not covered in this document, talk with your board-certified plastic surgeon. Only ASPS members are entitled to display the logo above.

### *How can I be sure that my surgeon has adequate training?*

Good credentials can't guarantee a successful outcome; however, they can significantly increase the likelihood of it. Patients are advised to find a doctor who is certified by the American Board of Plastic Surgery (ABPS), the only board recognized by the American Board of Medical Specialties to certify a surgeon in plastic surgery of the face and of the entire body. Certification by the ABPS is "the gold standard" for plastic surgeons because it signifies that the surgeon has had formal training in an accredited plastic surgery residency program. If your surgeon is ABPS-certified, you can be assured that your doctor:

- Has completed at least five years of surgical residency training after medical school, including at least two years in plastic surgery;

- Has passed comprehensive cosmetic and reconstructive surgery exams;

- Is qualified to perform cosmetic and reconstructive procedures—everything from liposuction and facelifts to intricate wound repair.

To verify a surgeon's certification status, contact the American Board of Plastic Surgery at 215-587-9322 or visit the board's website at www.abplsurg.org or the American Board of Medical Specialties at www.abms.org or by phoning 800-776-2378.

### *How can I determine if my plastic surgeon's surgical facility meets acceptable safety standards?*

The American Society of Plastic Surgeons and the American Society for Aesthetic Plastic Surgery have issued a statement to their members that by July 1, 2002 all plastic surgery performed under anesthesia, other than minor local anesthesia and/or minimal oral tranquilization, must be performed in a surgical facility that meets at least one of the following criteria:

- Accredited by a national or state recognized accrediting agency/organization such as the American Association for Accreditation of Ambulatory Surgery Facilities (AAAASF), Accreditation Association for Ambulatory Health Care (AAAHC), or Joint Commission on Accreditation of Healthcare Organizations (JCAHO)

- Certified to participate in the Medicare program under Title XVIII

- Licensed by the state in which the facility is located

Patients should ensure that the facility is accredited or is in the process of being accredited. To find out about a facility's accreditation status, contact the AAAASF at 888-545-5222 or www.aaaasf.org the AAAHC at 847-853-6060 or www.aaahc.org the JCAHO at 630-792-5005 or www.jcaho.org.

Plastic surgery procedures performed in accredited surgical facilities by board-certified plastic surgeons have an excellent safety record. A 1997 survey[1] based on more than 400,000 operations performed in accredited facilities found that:

- The rate of serious complications was less than half of 1 percent.

- The mortality rate was extremely low—only one in 57,000 cases.

- The overall risk of serious complications in an accredited office surgical facility is comparable with the risk in a freestanding surgical center or hospital ambulatory surgical facility.

***Why is it so important for my plastic surgeon to know detailed information about my personal and family health history, even if I am only having a simple cosmetic procedure?***

There is always risk with any surgical procedure. However, as a patient, you can play an important role in reducing your risk by providing a full and complete health history to your surgeon.

Although rare, one of the most serious complications associated with surgery is the development of blood clots in the large veins of the abdomen and legs. This complication can lead to a potentially fatal pulmonary embolism (blocked lung artery). Therefore, it is extremely important to tell your plastic surgeon if you or any of your family members have a history of blood clots or if you have had a family member who died suddenly, shortly after surgery or childbirth.

You will also be evaluated for other factors that may increase the risk of blood clots. These include:

- Being extremely overweight;
- Having recent traumatic injury;
- Any disorder of the heart, lungs, or central nervous system;
- A history of cancer, recurrent severe infection, or genetic problems that affect blood clotting.

For women, additional risk factors include:

- Taking oral contraceptives or having recently ceased taking them;
- Undergoing hormone-replacement therapy.

Safety measures to prevent blood clots will be determined by your individual degree of risk. If you are considered low risk, your doctor may simply ensure that you are positioned on the operating table in a way that allows for adequate blood circulation to the legs. If you are of moderate or high risk for developing blood clots, you may also be advised to wear elastic stockings before, during and after your procedure, or to take special anti-clotting medications. Compression devices on the legs may be used during surgery to support your normal circulation.

### *How can I be sure that the anesthesia care I receive in my plastic surgeon's surgical facility is adequate?*

Anesthesia care in an accredited or licensed facility has reached a level of sophistication that is absolutely comparable to the care received in the hospital. For maximum safety, ASPS recommends that:

- Any planned anesthesia should be administered by skilled, licensed personnel acting under the direction of an anesthesiologist or the operating surgeon.

- Before any type of anesthesia is used, the surgeon or anesthetist must take a full medical history. A physical examination and appropriate lab tests may also be performed. Your surgeon needs to know if you have any serious medical problems or have had previous adverse reaction to any other type of anesthesia. Also, you must let the anesthetist know about any medications you are taking (including herbal supplements), any known drug allergies, when you last ate and whether you smoke cigarettes or use alcohol or illegal drugs.

- You should be assured that you will receive individual monitoring by skilled, licensed personnel before, during and after the procedure. Staff who are familiar with the warning signs of cardiac or respiratory distress and are trained in advanced cardiac life support (ACLS), should be on hand to monitor your procedure and recovery following your surgery.

- If you are told that you will be kept overnight at the surgical facility while you recuperate, make sure that the facility is accredited by a recognized agency. In an accredited facility you will receive around-the-clock care and monitoring by two or more skilled and licensed staff members with at least one trained in ACLS. You will also be assured that the facility has the necessary equipment and medications to handle complications that may arise and an emergency plan in case you need to be transferred to the hospital.

### *To achieve the cosmetic results I want, my plastic surgeon has recommended "large-volume" liposuction. What types of safety measures should I expect my surgeon to take?*

Due to recent advances in technique and technology, serious medical complications in liposuction are quite rare. However, the risk of complications increases with the number of areas treated and the amount of fat removed. A liposuction procedure is classified as "large volume" when 11 pounds (5,000 cc) or more of fat and fluid are removed.

Factors that may increase the risk of complication are:

- Excessive amounts of local anesthesia or excessive amounts of fluid administered intravenously or within the tissues at the surgical site;

- Multiple, unrelated procedures performed during the same surgery;

- Being in poor health prior to surgery;

- Having a personal or family history of blood clots of the legs or a blocked lung artery;

- Having a personal or family history of breathing or bronchial disorders or other lung problems;

- For women: Current use of oral contraceptives.

For maximum safety, a patient planning to have either large-volume liposuction or ultrasound-assisted liposuction (known as UAL) should be aware of the following:

- Large-volume liposuction requires specialized knowledge. Therefore, it's important for your surgeon to have additional training specifically in UAL or large-volume liposuction.

- Your surgeon should keep track of the amount of fluid that is infused into your body and the amount that is withdrawn from your body. The surgeon should also have systems to record intravenous fluid, the amount of fat removed and urinary output.

- Extended postoperative monitoring of vital signs and urinary output is critical following large-volume liposuction. An overnight stay in a hospital or other overnight-stay-accredited facility may be required.

ASPS believes that in the hands of an appropriately trained specialist, liposuction is a generally safe procedure. Still, ASPS is collecting additional data on the safety and effectiveness of liposuction. The Liposuction Outcomes Study and will yield valuable data in the near future.

## *Safety Is a Team Effort*

Quality patient care, safety, and successful surgical outcomes are the result of the patient, the surgeon and the surgical staff working together. The ASPS has supported this concept by establishing task forces on liposuction, deep vein thrombosis prophylaxis, and outpatient surgical safety. These professional groups have thoroughly investigated the surgical techniques, equipment, and medications commonly used in outpatient plastic surgery and have set safety guidelines for use by all plastic surgeons, their staffs and their facilities. The task forces have also supplied the patient-safety information for this document.

As the ASPS continues to support the safety research being conducted by its Educational Foundation and the National Endowment for Plastic Surgery, patients are encouraged to learn everything they can about the procedures they are considering and to ask a lot of questions. Your concerns about safety should be discussed in detail with your plastic surgeon. This will help promote a safe outpatient surgery experience as well as fulfilling your surgical expectations.

1.  Morello, D.C., Colon, G.A., Fredericks, S., Iverson, R., Singer, R. Patient safety in accredited office surgical facilities. *Plast. Reconstr. Surg.* 99: 1496, 1997.

# Chapter 3

# *If You're Thinking about Cosmetic Surgery*

If you are considering cosmetic surgery, you must be honest with yourself. Why do you want surgery and, what do you expect surgery to do for you? According to the American Society of Plastic Surgeons (ASPS), there are two categories of patients who are good candidates for surgery. The first includes patients with a strong self-image, who are bothered by a physical characteristic that they'd like to improve or change. The second category includes patients who have a physical defect or cosmetic flaw that has diminished their self-esteem over time. It's important to remember that cosmetic surgery can create both physical changes and changes in self-esteem. If you are seeking surgery with the hope of influencing a change in someone other than yourself, you might end up disappointed.

## *ASPS List of Inappropriate Candidates for Surgery*

- Patients in crisis, such as those who are going through divorce, the death of a spouse, or the loss of a job. These patients may be seeking to achieve goals that cannot be obtained through an

---

This chapter begins with text excerpted from "Loving Your Body Inside and Out," National Women's Health Information Center (NWHIC; www.4woman.gov), January 2006. Text under the heading "Safety Considerations" is from "Safety," NWHIC, August 2004. Text under the heading "How to Choose a Cosmetic Surgeon" is excerpted from "Rolling Back the Hands of Time: The Facts on Plastic Surgery," *Consumer Focus: The Facts on Plastic Surgery*, Federal Citizen Information Center, May 2000.

appearance change; goals that relate to overcoming crisis through an unrelated change in appearance is not the solution. Rather, a patient must first work through the crisis.

- Patients with unrealistic expectations, such as those who insist on having a celebrity's nose, with the hope that they may acquire a celebrity lifestyle; patients who want to be restored to their original "perfection" following a severe accident or a serious illness; or patients who wish to find the youth of many decades past.

- Impossible-to-please patients, such as individuals who consult with surgeon after surgeon, seeking the answers they want to hear. These patients hope for a cure to a problem, which is not primarily, or not at all physical.

- Patients who are obsessed with a very minor defect, and may believe that once their defect is fixed, life will be perfect. Born perfectionists may be suitable candidates for surgery, as long as they are realistic enough to understand that surgical results may not precisely match their goals.

- Patients who have a mental illness, and exhibit delusional or paranoid behavior, may also be poor candidates for surgery. Surgery may be appropriate in these cases if it is determined that the patient's goals for surgery are not related to the psychosis. In these cases, a plastic surgeon may work closely with the patient's psychiatrist.

- Because the changes resulting from cosmetic surgery are often dramatic and permanent, it's important that you have a clear understanding of how surgery might make you feel—long before a procedure is scheduled.

## Body Dysmorphic Disorder (BDD)

Body dysmorphic disorder (BDD) is a serious illness when a person is preoccupied with minor or imaginary physical flaws, usually of the skin, hair, and nose. A person with BDD tends to have cosmetic surgery, and even if the surgeries are successful, does not think they are and is unhappy with the outcomes.

### Symptoms of BDD

Being preoccupied with minor or imaginary physical flaws, usually of the skin, hair, and nose, such as acne, scarring, facial lines, marks, pale skin, thinning hair, excessive body hair, large nose, or crooked nose.

Having a lot of anxiety and stress about the perceived flaw and spending a lot of time focusing on it, such as frequently picking at skin, excessively checking appearance in a mirror, hiding the imperfection, comparing appearance with others, excessively grooming, seeking reassurance from others about how they look, and getting cosmetic surgery.

Getting cosmetic surgery can make BDD worse. They are often not happy with the outcome of the surgery. If they are, they may start to focus attention on another body area and become preoccupied trying to fix the new "defect." In this case, some patients with BDD become angry at the surgeon for making their appearance worse and may even become violent towards the surgeon.

### Treatment for BDD

- Medications. Serotonin reuptake inhibitors (SSRIs) are antidepressants that decrease the obsessive and compulsive behaviors.

- Cognitive behavioral therapy. This is a type of therapy with several steps:
  - The therapist asks the patient to enter social situations without covering up her "defect."
  - The therapist helps the patient stop doing the compulsive behaviors to check the defect or cover it up. This may include removing mirrors, covering skin areas that the patient picks, or not using make-up.
  - The therapist helps the patient change their false beliefs about their appearance.

## Safety Considerations

If you're thinking about getting cosmetic surgery, it's your job to become an informed consumer. Selecting a qualified doctor, with a lot of training and experience in the procedure you'd like to get, is essential.

Ask the right questions to get the best treatment:

- What state is the doctor licensed to practice surgery?

- Is the doctor board certified? With which board? The doctor should be certified by the American Board of Plastic Surgery.

- What training did the surgeon have after medical school? Was it plastic surgery?

- How many surgeries of this type does the doctor perform each year?

- How many years has the doctor performed this type of surgery?

- What hospital can the doctor admit patients or work in? You'll want to know in case of an emergency. You can also check with the hospital for the surgeon's credentials.

- If the doctor operates in his or her office or ambulatory health care facility, is it accredited? Check with the American Association for Accreditation of Ambulatory Surgery Facilities or Accreditation Association for Ambulatory Health Care, Inc. to find out. It can mean a higher standard of care.

- Does the doctor have life-saving equipment and monitoring devices?

- Who administers the anesthesia? Ideally, this person is a board-certified anesthesiologist or certified registered nurse anesthetist.

- What are the risks of the procedure? How often do they happen? What does the doctor do if they happen?

- What is the expected recovery for the procedure you're having?

- Check with the state medical board for complaints or malpractice suits against the doctor.

### Check Out Your Doctor's Credentials

If you're thinking about having your surgery in the doctor's office, there are advantages and disadvantages. The office might be convenient, private, and have more amenities than a hospital or ambulatory care center (non-emergency, outpatient facility). But it may not be safe. Don't assume that the doctor has the right credentials or the right equipment to keep you safe in the office.

In many states, any doctor with a valid medical license who's in private practice can legally perform surgery. So some doctors are doing surgery outside of their specialty, like an eye doctor performing breast implant surgery. Depending on the state, doctors in private practice don't need to meet the same legal requirements as a hospital or accredited ambulatory care center for surgery or anesthesia services.

It's also important that if you choose to go to an ambulatory care center, that it's accredited. Contact these organizations to find out your doctor's education, licensure, and board certification in addition to the doctor's or ambulatory care center's accreditation:

### Accreditation Association for Ambulatory Health Care, Inc. (AAAHC)
Accredits physician offices with surgical facilities.
847-853-6060
www.aaahc.org

### American Association for Accreditation of Ambulatory Surgery Facilities (AAAASF)
Certifies ambulatory surgery facilities and provides practice guidelines for surgeons working in ambulatory surgical facilities.
888-545-5222
www.aaaasf.org

### American Society of Plastic Surgeons (ASPS)/ The American Board of Plastic Surgery (ABPS)
All of the surgeons listed through this service are ASPS members who are board-certified by the American Board of Plastic Surgery. They have graduated from an accredited medical school and completed at least five years of surgical residency, usually three years of general surgery and two years of plastic surgery.
888-4-PLASTIC
www.plasticsurgery.org/find_a_plastic_surgeon

### Federation of State Medical Boards/Federated Credentials Verification Service (FCVS)
FCVS verifies medical education, postgraduate training, licensure examination history, board action history, and identity.
817-868-4000
http://www.fsmb.org

## How to Choose a Cosmetic Surgeon

With the growing popularity of plastic surgery, and the increase in number of physicians performing cosmetic procedures every year, it's important you understand the credentials of the person you choose to be your plastic surgeon.

### *Step I: Develop A List of Candidates' Names*

- Seek recommendations from a family member or friend.
- Seek recommendations from your family doctor or nurse.
- Verify the surgeon has completed residency in Plastic Surgery.
- Check if the surgeon is board-certified by the American Board of Plastic Surgery.
- Inquire about any privileges the surgeon may have to do your specific cosmetic procedure at an accredited hospital.

### *Step II: Check All Credentials*

- Once a list of names is compiled, check credentials by contacting hospitals (verify official approval of privileges), professional societies, and even the surgeon's office to verify the type of training and experience the surgeon has had.

### *Step III: The Consultation*

- Once your list is narrowed down, consider a consultation with 2–3 candidates to discuss their opinions on which surgery is best suited for you, type of anesthesia to be used, post-surgical protocol, and their fees. If the procedure is to be performed on an outpatient basis, it is important to verify the location is an accredited operating facility. Accredited facilities have been reviewed by an independent organization and means the facility meets national health and safety standards.

### *Your Choice*

Now it's time to choose the surgeon that's right for you.

- If you've obtained your surgeon's name from a good source, checked his or her credentials, are satisfied with your initial consultation, and have realistic expectations for the surgery, chances are very good that you'll be happy with the outcome of your plastic surgery.

Chapter 4

# Is Plastic Surgery the Right Choice for Teens?

When you hear of plastic surgery, what do you think of? A Hollywood star trying to delay the effects of aging? Somebody's cute "new" nose that cost quite a few allowances? People who want to change the size of their stomachs, breasts, or other body parts because they see it done so easily on TV?

Those are common images of plastic surgery, but what about the 4-year-old boy who has his chin rebuilt after a dog bit him? Or the young woman who has the birthmark on her forehead lightened with a laser?

### What is plastic surgery?

Just because the name includes the word "plastic" doesn't mean patients who have this surgery end up with a face full of fake stuff. The name isn't taken from the synthetic substance but from the Greek word *plastikos*, which means to form or mold (and which gives plastic its name as well).

Plastic surgery is a special type of surgery that involves both a person's appearance and ability to function. Plastic surgeons strive

From "Plastic Surgery," reviewed by Paul H. Izenberg, M.D., October 2004; this information was provided by TeensHealth, one of the largest resources online for medically reviewed health information written for parents, kids, and teens. For more articles like this one, visit www.TeensHealth.org, or www.KidsHealth .org. © 2004 The Nemours Foundation.

to improve patients' appearance, self-image, and confidence through both reconstructive and cosmetic procedures.

Reconstructive procedures correct defects on the face or body. These include physical birth defects like cleft lips and palates and ear deformities, traumatic injuries like those from dog bites or burns, or the aftermath of disease treatments like rebuilding a woman's breast after surgery for breast cancer.

Cosmetic (also called aesthetic) procedures alter a part of the body that the person is not satisfied with. Common cosmetic procedures include making the breasts larger (augmentation mammoplasty) or smaller (reduction mammoplasty), reshaping the nose (rhinoplasty), and removing pockets of fat from specific spots on the body (liposuction). Some cosmetic procedures aren't even surgical in the way that most people think of surgery—that is, cutting and stitching. For example, the use of special lasers to remove unwanted hair and injections or sanding skin to improve severe scarring are two such treatments.

### Why do teens get plastic surgery?

Most teens don't, of course—but some do. Interestingly, the American Society of Plastic Surgeons (ASPS) reports a difference in the reasons teens give for having plastic surgery and the reasons adults do: Teens view plastic surgery as a way to fit in and look acceptable to friends and peers. Adults, on the other hand, frequently see plastic surgery as a way to stand out from the crowd.

The number of teens who choose to get plastic surgery is on the rise. According to the ASPS, 335,000 people 18 years and younger had plastic surgery in 2003, up from about 306,000 in 2000.

Some people turn to plastic surgery to correct a physical defect or to alter a part of the body that makes them feel uncomfortable. For example, guys with a condition called gynecomastia (excess breast tissue) that doesn't go away with time or weight loss may opt for reduction surgery. A girl or guy with a birthmark may turn to laser treatment to lessen its appearance.

Other people decide they want a cosmetic change to feel better about the way they look. Teens who have cosmetic procedures—such as otoplasty (surgery to pin back ears that stick out) or dermabrasion (a procedure that can help smooth or camouflage severe acne scars)—often say that having the surgery gives them greater confidence and boosts their self-esteem.

The most common procedures teens choose include nose reshaping, ear reshaping, acne and acne scar treatment, and breast reduction.

## *Is plastic surgery the right choice?*

Reconstructive surgery helps repair significant defects or problems. But what about having cosmetic surgery just to change your appearance? Is it a good idea for teens? It can be. But as with everything, there are right and wrong reasons. And there are no quick fixes.

Unlike on TV, cosmetic surgery is unlikely to change your life—or even get you a date to the prom. Shows like *I Want a Famous Face* are actually far from reality. In fact, it's impossible for a surgeon to make one person look exactly like another: You and Brad Pitt probably have very different bone structures.

In reality, most board-certified plastic surgeons spend a lot of time interviewing teens who want plastic surgery to decide if they are good candidates for the surgery. Some doctors won't perform certain procedures (like rhinoplasty) on a teen until they are sure that person is old enough and has finished growing. For rhinoplasty, that means about 14 or 15 for girls and a little older for guys.

Girls who want to enlarge their breasts for cosmetic reasons usually must be at least 18 because saline implants are only approved for women 18 and older. In some cases, though, such as when there's a tremendous size difference between the breasts or one breast has failed to grow at all, a plastic surgeon may get involved earlier.

Doctors also want to know that teens are emotionally mature enough to handle the surgery and that they're doing it for the right reasons. Many plastic surgery procedures are just that—surgery. They involve anesthesia, wound healing, and other serious risks. Doctors who perform these procedures want to know that their patients are capable of understanding and handling the stress of surgery.

Here are a few things to think about if you're considering plastic surgery:

- Almost all teens (and many adults) are self-conscious about their bodies. Almost everyone wishes there were a thing or two that could be changed. A lot of this self-consciousness goes away with time. And ask yourself if you're considering plastic surgery only for yourself or whether it's to please someone else.

- A person's body continues to change through the teen years. Body parts that might appear too large or too small now can become more proportionate over time. Sometimes, for example, what seems like a big nose looks more the right size as the rest of the person's face catches up during growth.

- Getting in good shape through appropriate weight control and exercise can do great things for a person's looks without surgery. In fact, it's never a good idea to choose plastic surgery as a first option for something like weight loss that can be corrected in a nonsurgical manner. Sure, gastric bypass or liposuction may seem like quick and easy fixes compared with sticking to a diet. Both of these procedures, however, carry far greater risks than dieting, and doctors should reserve them for extreme cases when all other options have failed.

- Some people's emotions have a really big effect on how they think they look. People who are depressed, extremely self-critical, or have a distorted view of what they really look like sometimes think that changing their looks will solve their problems. In these cases, it won't. Working out the emotional problem with the help of a trained therapist is a better bet. In fact, many doctors won't perform plastic surgery on teens who are depressed or have other mental health problems until these problems are treated first.

### *What's involved?*

If you're considering plastic surgery, talk it over with your parents. If you're serious and your parents agree, the next step is meeting with a plastic surgeon to help you learn what to expect before, during, and after the procedure—as well as any possible complications or downsides to the surgery. Depending on the procedure, you may feel some pain as you recover, and temporary swelling or bruising can make you look less like yourself for a while.

Procedures and healing times vary, so you'll want to do your research into what's involved in your particular procedure and whether the surgery is reconstructive or cosmetic. It's a good idea to choose a doctor who is certified by the American Board of Plastic Surgery.

Cost will likely be a factor, too. Elective plastic surgery procedures can be expensive. Although medical insurance covers many reconstructive surgeries, the cost of cosmetic procedures almost always comes straight out of the patient's pocket. Your parents can find out what your insurance plan will and won't cover. For example, breast enlargement surgery is considered a purely cosmetic procedure and is rarely covered by insurance. But breast reduction surgery may be covered by some plans because large breasts can cause physical discomfort and even pain for many girls.

Plastic surgery isn't something to rush into. If you're thinking about plastic surgery, find out as much as you can about the specific procedure you're considering and talk it over with doctors and your parents. Once you have the facts, you can decide whether the surgery is right for you.

# Chapter 5

# *Understanding the Risks Associated with Cosmetic Procedures*

Below is a basic guide to the risks involved in both surgical and non-surgical cosmetic procedures.

## *Cosmetic Procedures: Surgical*

**Breast augmentation:** Breasts are enlarged by placing an implant behind each breast.

*Risks*

- implants can rupture, leak, and deflate
- infection
- hardening of scar tissue around implant, causing breast firmness, pain, distorted shape, or implant movement
- bleeding
- pain
- nipples may get more or less sensitive
- numbness near incision
- blood collection around implant/incision

---

From "Cosmetic Procedures," National Women's Health Information Center (www.4woman.gov), August 2004.

33

- calcium deposits around implant
- harder to find breast lumps

**Breast lift:** Extra skin is removed from the breast to raise and re-shape breast.

*Risks*

- scarring
- skin loss
- infection
- loss of feeling in nipples or breast
- nipples put in the wrong place
- breasts not symmetrical

**Breast reduction:** Fat, tissue, and skin is removed from breast.

*Risks*

- if nipples and areola are detached, may lose sensation and de-creased ability to breastfeed
- bleeding
- infection
- scarring
- harder to find breast lumps
- poor shape, size, or position of nipples or breasts

**Eyelid surgery:** Extra fat, skin, and muscle in the upper or lower eyelid is removed to correct "droopy" eyelids.

*Risks*

- blurred or double vision
- infection
- bleeding under the skin
- swelling
- dry eyes

- whiteheads
- can't close eye completely
- pulling of lower lids
- blindness

**Facelift:** Extra fat is removed, muscles are tightened, and skin is rewrapped around the face and neck to improve sagging facial skin, jowls, and loose neck skin.

*Risks*

- infection
- bleeding under skin
- scarring
- irregular earlobes
- nerve damage causing numbness or inability to move your face
- hair loss
- skin damage

**Facial implant:** Implants are used to change the nose, jaws, cheeks, or chin.

*Risks*

- infection
- feeling of tightness or scarring around implant
- shifting of implant

**Forehead lift:** Extra skin and muscles that cause wrinkles are removed, eyebrows are lifted, and forehead skin is tightened.

*Risks*

- infection
- scarring
- bleeding under skin
- eye dryness or irritation

- impaired eyelid function
- loss of feeling in eyelid skin
- injury to facial nerve causing loss of motion or muscle weakness

**Lip augmentation:** Material is injected or implanted into the lips to create fuller lips and reduce wrinkles around the mouth.

*Risks*

- infection
- bleeding
- lip asymmetry
- lumping
- scarring

**Liposuction:** Excess fat from a targeted area is removed with a vacuum to shape the body.

*Risks*

- baggy skin
- skin may change color and fall off
- fluid retention
- shock
- infection
- burning
- fat clots in the lungs
- pain
- damage to organs if punctured
- numbness at the surgery site
- heart problems
- kidney problems
- disability
- death

**Nose surgery:** Nose is reshaped by resculpting the bone and cartilage in the nose.

*Risks*

- infection
- bursting blood vessels
- red spots
- bleeding under the skin
- scarring

**Tummy tuck:** Extra fat and skin in the abdomen is removed, and muscles are tightened to flatten tummy.

*Risks*

- blood clots
- infection
- bleeding
- scarring
- fluid accumulation under the skin

## Cosmetic Procedures: Non-Surgical

**Botox injection:** Botox is injected into a facial muscle to paralyze it, so lines don't form when a person frowns or squints.

*Risks*

- face pain
- muscle weakness
- flu-like symptoms
- headaches
- loss of facial expression
- droopy eyelids
- asymmetric smile
- drooling

**Collagen/fat injection:** Collagen from a cow or fat from your thigh or abdomen is injected into facial wrinkles, pits, or scars.

*Risks*

- trigger an autoimmune disease
- contour problems
- hives
- rash
- swelling
- flu-like symptoms

**Dermabrasion:** A small, spinning wheel or brush with a roughened surface removes the upper layers of facial skin. A new layer of skin appears during healing, giving the face a smoother appearance. Used to treat facial scars, heavy wrinkles, and problems like rosacea.

*Risks*

- abnormal color changes
- whiteheads
- infection
- allergic reaction
- fever blisters
- cold sores
- thickened skin

**Hyaluronic acid injection:** This gel is injected into your face to smooth lines, wrinkles, and scars on the skin.

*Risks*

- swelling
- infection
- redness
- tenderness
- acne
- lumps

- tissue hardening
- risks unknown if used in combination with collagen

**Laser hair removal:** Laser light is passed over the skin to remove hair.

*Risks*

- hair regrowth
- scarring
- change in skin color

**Laser skin resurfacing:** Laser light is used to remove wrinkles, lines, age spots, scars, moles, tattoos, and warts from the surface of the skin.

*Risks*

- burns
- scarring
- change in skin color
- infection
- herpes flare-up (fever, facial pain, and flu-like symptoms)

**Sclerotherapy:** A solution is injected into spider and varicose leg veins (small purple and red blood vessels) to remove the veins.

*Risks*

- blood clots
- color changes in the skin
- vein removal may not be permanent
- scarring

**Chemical peel:** A solution is put onto the face (or parts of the face) that causes the skin to blister and peel off. It is replaced with new skin.

*Risks*

- whiteheads

- infection
- raised scarring
- allergic reaction
- cold sores
- color changes or blotchiness
- heart problems

**Tooth whiteners (peroxide agents):** Depending on the product, either you or the dentist applies peroxide using strips; a mouth guard with gel; or a tray inside your mouth around your teeth.

*Risks*

- if not customized for you by a dentist or dental hygienist, there may be unknown ingredients and unknown results

# Chapter 6

# *Risks of Erasing Wrinkles*

Many times when one looks back, it is easy to say "it seemed like a good idea at the time." After all, Botox (botulinum toxin type A), has been shown to help erase skin wrinkles. The results have been great. So when a friend offers to get some of it for you, perhaps at much less cost, and even inject it for you, well, that seems like a deal that's too good to be true. Sometimes it is.

*Caveat emptor* in Latin means "let the buyer beware." This might be a good subtitle of the article by Dr. Souayah and coauthors in *Neurology* (Souayah N, Karim H, Kamin SS, McArdle J, Marcus S. Severe botulism after focal injection of botulinum toxin. *Neurology* 2006;67: 1855–1856). The article tells what happens when someone was treated with an inappropriate preparation of botulinum toxin, apparently by a friend. The results were disastrous.

A 34-year-old woman received botulinum toxin injections for cosmetic purposes. However, the preparation was not the FDA-approved botulinum toxin type A (brand name Botox). The injected substance was apparently research-grade toxin and was bought on the internet. Two days after the injection, the woman developed progressive shortness of breath, swallowing difficulties, double vision, and generalized weakness. By the time she was examined by a neurologist, she was totally paralyzed with the exception of a little movement of her left big

From "Risks of Erasing Wrinkles: Buyer Beware!" by Richard Barbano, MD, PhD, FAAN, in *Neurology*, 2006:67:E17–E18. © 2006 American Academy of Neurology; reprinted with permission.

toe. An attempt to limit the paralysis with serum against the toxin was too late and did not help.

Electrical studies of various arm and leg muscles showed them to be totally inactive. Tests showed that the woman had extremely high levels of botulinum toxin in her blood. In fact, the authors of the article estimate that she had been given over 2,000 to 5,000 times the usual amount given for cosmetic purposes.

Botulinum toxin works by interrupting the connections between nerves and muscles. Recovery occurs only when more of the protein that has been inactivated by the toxin is made. The patient was treated in the intensive care unit for any developing problems while waiting for recovery, which was slow. By 3 weeks, she could only shrug her shoulders and move her eyes. By 5 weeks, she could answer with a yes or no. The last time she was evaluated, 10 months after she was hospitalized, she still had problems with muscle pain and weakness and had some shortness of breath.

Apparently, a second person also received injections at the same time. The authors do not give information about the second person, but hopefully he or she recovered as well as the person described in the article. Although having continued problems with muscle pain and weakness does not sound like a "good" recovery, it must be remembered that botulism has claimed many lives over the last hundred years. Even now, deaths occur.

Botulinum toxin is one of the most poisonous substances known. But when that same toxin is carefully isolated and purified, it can be used as a powerful and effective medication.

Botulinum toxin was first introduced as a clinical tool in the 1980s, and its use has skyrocketed as doctors have applied it to an increasing number of medical conditions. It has revolutionized the treatment of a condition called dystonia. This movement disorder causes involuntary contractions of muscles acting in opposite directions, which results in odd postures and twisting, writhing movements of the neck, trunk, hands, or legs. With periodic injections of botulinum toxin into the muscles most affected, countless patients have been relieved of their symptoms.

Perhaps there is a general misunderstanding that anything that can be used for cosmetic purposes must be easy to use and safe. But just like cosmetic surgery, professional training is a must.

All medications have potential side effects. However, patients need to be aware that when appropriately used by trained doctors, botulinum toxin has a remarkable safety record. The important point is that it should be administered only by someone with considerable experience with the medication. It also must be emphasized that the botulinum toxin used in this sad case was not the commercial product found in pharmacies and administered by doctors. This was a research-grade product never meant for medical use in humans. And that is another lesson to be learned from this story, one that has a parallel in a warning of innumerable mothers to innumerable children. Don't take candy from strangers, and don't use a medication unless you know where it came from.

## What is botulism?

Botulism is a poisoning from one of the most powerful toxins known. It is produced by a family of bacteria, the *Clostridia*. This poison, called botulinum toxin, is a protein that interferes with the normal flow of signals from certain nerves to muscles and glands. If enough toxin is present, it can cause a serious or even fatal illness.

## What causes botulism?

The spores of *Clostridia* bacteria are found in the soil, and the bacteria grow in many places. However, it is in conditions where there is little oxygen that they multiply rapidly and are most likely to be harmful to people. There are three common ways to get botulism:

- Food-borne botulism occurs by ingesting the toxin itself by eating foods that have not been properly sterilized.

- Infant botulism occurs by eating the bacteria or spores.

- Wound botulism occurs by infection of cuts and wounds by contaminated soil.

## Who is likely to get botulism?

There are somewhat over 100 cases of botulism reported each year in the United States. The largest number of these cases is reported in infants. Infant botulism results from eating bacteria or spores, which then grow in the gastrointestinal tract. After multiplying in the gut, the poison is produced and then absorbed. This mostly occurs in infants less than 6 months old who do not yet have the usual bacteria in their intestines. About a quarter of all cases are adult food-borne. These occur mostly after people eat improperly sterilized or contaminated home-preserved food, although any source can be contaminated. So people who eat improperly prepared foods are at risk. The small

43

number of remaining cases of botulism is from infected wounds, since the bacteria live in the soil.

### What are the symptoms of botulism?

Botulinum toxin is taken in by certain nerve cells (neurons). The particular neurons that take up the toxin are those that use a specific neurotransmitter, called acetylcholine. (Neurotransmitters are substances that help messages pass between neurons and their targets, such as a muscle or gland.) These neurons control muscle movements and certain secreting glands, such as saliva and tears. Therefore, the symptoms of poisoning are dry eyes, dry mouth, and muscle weakness. The muscle weakness includes the face, limbs, and even the digestive tract, leading to constipation. Double vision and difficulty speaking and swallowing are common. Weakness of the diaphragm and rib muscles leads to difficulty breathing, and sometimes patients need to be put on a respirator. Infant botulism is usually suspected when young infants develop constipation, poor feeding, and floppy heads.

*Signs of Botulism*

- Difficulty swallowing
- Difficulty speaking
- Double vision
- Arm, leg, and trunk weakness
- Difficulty breathing
- Constipation
- Dry mouth
- Dry eyes

### Can botulism be prevented?

Destroying the spores requires moist heat of 120° C (220° F) for 30 minutes. However, the toxin can be easily inactivated by boiling for 10 minutes or heating to 80° C (180° F) for 30 minutes. If you enjoy home canning, make sure to use the proper methods for sterilizing and sealing. Do not eat canned or bottled food where the seal has been broken. Acidic foods (such as tomatoes) and acidic conditions seem to make it more difficult for the spores to become active bacteria.

### Is there any treatment?

A specific antiserum is available to counteract the toxin. However, this must be used before the toxin enters the neuron. Whatever amount enters the neuron will not be able to be "neutralized" by the antiserum, and some weakness will develop. Patients must go immediately to a hospital, since difficulty breathing can develop rapidly. When such breathing difficulties are severe, patients need to go on a respirator. Luckily, the toxin is eventually destroyed by the body, and with intensive care, most patients can make a full recovery.

### What about medical uses?

When the toxin is carefully purified, it can be used as a powerful medical tool. By taking advantage of the fact that the toxin lessens muscle activity, we can use it to treat a number of medical conditions where muscle overactivity is a problem. The doctor must be careful with the amount used and where it is placed (it is given by injection with a needle rather than taken by mouth). However, manufactured product is carefully measured in each vial and when used correctly has a very good safety record.

Botulinum toxin under the brand Botox has received approval from the Food and Drug Administration for cosmetic (nonmedical) uses as well. The major use is in treating wrinkles and facial lines that result from overactive pulling of the small muscles under the skin. It has proven to be an additional choice to the traditional "face lift."

# Chapter 7

# *Questions to Ask before Surgery*

This information is for patients who are facing surgery that is not an emergency. Some of the questions in this chapter may help you and your family understand more about your surgery, whether it has to be done right away or can be done later. Your doctor or nurse also can help you understand what is being done and why. Don't be afraid to ask questions.

## *Care about Your Health: Help Make the Decisions*

Are you facing surgery? You are not alone. Every year, more than 15 million Americans have surgery.

Most operations are not emergencies and are considered elective surgery. This means that you have time to learn about your operation to be sure it is the best treatment for you. You also have time to work with your surgeon to make the surgery as safe as possible. Be active in your health care to have quality care.

Your regular doctor is your primary care doctor. He or she may be the doctor who suggests that you have surgery and may refer you to a surgeon. You may also want to find another surgeon to get a second opinion, to confirm if surgery is the right treatment for you. You might want to ask friends or coworkers for the names of surgeons they have used.

This chapter gives you some questions to ask your primary care doctor and surgeon before you have surgery. It also gives the reasons

"Having Surgery? What You Need to Know," Agency for Healthcare Research and Quality (www.ahrq.gov), AHRQ Pub. No. 05(06)-00754A, October 2005.

for asking these questions. The answers will help you make the best decisions. Throughout the chapter there are tips about where you can get more information on surgery.

Your doctors should welcome questions. If you do not understand the answers, ask the doctor to explain them clearly. Bring a friend or relative along to help you talk with the doctor. Research shows that patients who are well informed about their treatment are more satisfied with their results.

## Get the Basic Facts

### Why do I need an operation?

There are many reasons to have surgery. Some operations can relieve or prevent pain. Others can reduce a symptom of a problem or improve some body function. Some surgeries are done to find a problem. Surgery can also save your life. Your doctor will tell you the purpose of the procedure. Make sure you understand how the proposed operation will help fix your medical problem. For example, if something is going to be repaired or removed, find out why it needs to be done.

### What operation are you recommending?

Ask your surgeon to explain the surgery and how it is done. Your surgeon can draw a picture or a diagram and explain the steps in the surgery.

Is there more than one way of doing the operation? One way may require more extensive surgery than another. Some operations that once needed large incisions (cuts in the body) can now be done using much smaller incisions (laparoscopic surgery—performing the surgery with a small camera and tools, only using a few small incisions instead of a big one, which usually quickens healing time). Some surgeries require that you stay in the hospital for one or more days. Others let you come in and go home on the same day. Ask why your surgeon wants to do the operation one way over another.

### Are there alternatives to surgery?

Sometimes, surgery is not the only answer to a medical problem. Medicines or treatments other than surgery, such as a change in diet or special exercises, might help you just as well—or more. Ask your surgeon or primary care doctor about the benefits and risks of these other choices. You need to know as much as possible about these benefits and risks to make the best decision.

One alternative to surgery may be watchful waiting. During a watchful wait, your doctor and you check to see if your problem gets better or worse over time. If it gets worse, you may need surgery right away. If it gets better, you may be able to wait to have surgery or not have it at all.

### How much will the operation cost?

Even if you have health insurance, there may be some costs for you to pay. This may depend on your choice of surgeon or hospital. Ask what your surgeon's fee is and what it covers. Surgical fees often also include some visits after the operation. You also will get a bill from the hospital for your care and from the other doctors who gave you care during your surgery.

Before you have the operation, call your insurance company. They can tell you how much of the costs your insurance will pay and what share you will have to pay. If you are covered by Medicare, call 800-MEDICARE (800-633-4227) to find out your share of surgery costs.

## Learn about the Benefits and Risks

### What are the benefits of having the operation?

Ask your surgeon what you will gain by having the operation. For example, a hip replacement may mean that you can walk again with ease.

Ask how long the benefits will last. For some procedures, it is not unusual for the benefits to last for a short time only. You may need a second operation at a later date. For other procedures, the benefits may last a lifetime.

When finding out about the benefits of the operation, be realistic. Sometimes patients expect too much and are disappointed with the outcome or results. Ask your doctor if there is anything you can read to help you understand the procedure and its likely results.

### What are the risks of having the operation?

All operations have some risk. This is why you need to weigh the benefits of the operation against the risks of complications or side effects.

Complications are unplanned events linked to the operation. Typical complications are infection, too much bleeding, reaction to anesthesia,

49

or accidental injury. Some people have a greater risk of complications because of other medical conditions. There also may be side effects after the operation. Often, your surgeon can tell you what side effects to expect. For example, there may be swelling and some soreness around the incision.

There is almost always some pain with surgery. Ask your surgeon how much pain there will be and what the doctors and nurses will do to help stop the pain. Controlling the pain will help you to be more comfortable while you heal. Controlling the pain will also help you get well faster and improve the results of your operation.

### What if I don't have this operation?

Based on what you learn about the benefits and risks of the operation, you might decide not to have it. Ask your surgeon what you will gain—or lose—by not having the operation now. Could you be in more pain? Could your condition get worse? Could the problem go away?

## Learn How to Get More Information

### Where can I get a second opinion?

Getting a second opinion from another doctor is a very good way to make sure that having the operation is the best choice for you. You can ask your primary care doctor for the name of another surgeon who could review your medical file. If you consult another doctor, make sure to get your records from the first doctor so that your tests do not have to be repeated.

Many health insurance plans ask patients to get a second opinion before they have certain operations that are not for an emergency. If your plan does not require a second opinion, you may still ask to have one. Check with your insurance company to see if they will pay for a second opinion. You should discuss your insurance questions with your health insurance company or your employee benefits office. If you are eligible for Medicare, they will pay for a second opinion.

## Find Out More About Your Operation

### What kind of anesthesia will I need?

Anesthesia is used so that surgery can be performed without unnecessary pain. Your surgeon can tell you whether the operation calls for local, regional, or general anesthesia and why this form of anesthesia is best for your procedure.

Local anesthesia numbs only a part of your body and only for a short period of time. For example, when you go to the dentist, you may get a local anesthetic called Novocain. It numbs the gum area around a tooth. Not all procedures done with local anesthesia are painless. Regional anesthesia numbs a larger portion of your body—for example, the lower part of your body—for a few hours. In most cases, you will be awake during the operation with regional anesthesia. General anesthesia numbs your entire body. You will be asleep during the whole operation if you have general anesthesia.

Anesthesia is quite safe for most patients. It is usually given by a specialized doctor (anesthesiologist) or nurse (nurse anesthetist). Both are highly skilled and have been trained to give anesthesia. If you decide to have an operation, ask to meet with the person who will give you anesthesia. It is okay to ask what his or her qualifications are. Ask what the side effects and risks of having anesthesia are in your case. Be sure to tell him or her what medical problems you have—including allergies and what medicines you have been taking. These medicines may affect your response to the anesthesia. Be sure to include both prescription and over-the-counter medicines, like vitamins and supplements.

### How long will it take me to recover?

Your surgeon can tell you how you might feel and what you will be able to do—or not do—the first few days, weeks, or months after surgery. Ask how long you will be in the hospital. Find out what kind of supplies, equipment, and help you will need when you go home. Knowing what to expect can help you get better faster.

Ask how long it will be before you can go back to work or start regular exercise again. You do not want to do anything that will slow your recovery. For example, lifting a 10-pound bag of potatoes may not seem to be "too much" a week after your operation, but it could be. You should follow your surgeon's advice to make sure you recover fully as soon as possible.

## Making Sure Your Surgery Is Safe

Check with your insurance company to find out if you may choose a surgeon or hospital or if you must use ones selected by the insurer. Ask your doctor about which hospital has the best care and results

51

for your condition if you have more than one hospital to choose from. Studies show that for some types of surgery, numbers count—using a surgeon or hospital that does more of a particular type of surgery can improve your chance of a good result.

If you do have a choice of surgeon or hospital, ask the surgeon the following questions:

**What are your qualifications?** You will want to know that your surgeon is experienced and qualified to perform the operation. Many surgeons have taken special training and passed exams given by a national board of surgeons. Ask if your surgeon is "board certified" in surgery. Some surgeons also have the letters F.A.C.S. after their name. This means they are Fellows of the American College of Surgeons and have passed another review by surgeons of their surgical skills.

**How much experience do you have doing this operation?** One way to reduce the risks of surgery is to choose a surgeon who has been well trained to do the surgery and has plenty of experience doing it. You can ask your surgeon about his or her recent record of successes and complications with this surgery. If it is easier for you, you can discuss the surgeon's qualifications with your primary care doctor.

**At which hospital will the operation be done?** Most surgeons work at one or two local hospitals. Find out where your surgery will be done and how often the same operation is done there. Research shows that patients often do better when they have surgery in hospitals with more experience in the operation. Ask your doctor about the success rate at the hospitals you can choose between. The success rate is the number of patients who improve divided by all patients having that operation at a hospital. If your surgeon suggests using a hospital with a lower success rate for your surgery, find out why.

**Ask the surgeon how long you will be in the hospital:** Until recently, most patients who had surgery stayed in the hospital overnight for one or more days. Today, many patients have surgery done as an outpatient in a doctor's office, a special surgical center, or a day surgery unit of a hospital. These patients have an operation and go home the same day. Outpatient surgery is less expensive because you do not have to pay for staying in a hospital room.

Ask whether your operation will be done in the hospital or in an outpatient setting, and ask which of these is the usual way the surgery is done. If your doctor recommends that you stay overnight in the hospital (have inpatient surgery) for an operation that is usually done as outpatient surgery—or recommends outpatient surgery that is usually done as inpatient surgery—ask why. You want to be in the right place for your operation.

**Have the surgeon mark the site he or she will operate on:** Rarely, surgeons will make a mistake and operate on the wrong part of the body. A number of groups of surgeons now urge their members to use a marking pen to show the place that they will operate on. The surgeons do this by writing directly on the patient's skin on the day of surgery. Don't be afraid to ask your surgeon to do this to make your surgery safer.

## For More Information

Here are some places you can get more information.

**Surgery:** The American College of Surgeons (ACS) has free pamphlets on "When You Need an Operation." For copies, write to the ACS, Office of Public Information, 633 N. St. Clair Street, Chicago, IL 60611, or call 312-202-5000 (toll free: 800-621-4111). This group has pamphlets that give general information about surgery and other pamphlets that describe specific surgical procedures. These pamphlets are also available on the ACS website at http://www.facs.org/public_info/ppserv.html.

**Second opinion:** For the free brochure "Getting a Second Opinion Before Surgery: Your Choices and Medicare Coverage," write to Centers for Medicare & Medicaid Services (CMS), Room 555, East High Rise Building, 6325 Security Boulevard, Baltimore, MD 21207. Ask for Publication No. CMS 02173. The brochure can also be found on the CMS website at http://www.medicare.gov.Publications/home.asp.

For the name of a specialist in your area who can give you a second opinion, ask your primary care doctor or surgeon, the local medical society, or your health insurance company. Medicare beneficiaries may also obtain information from the U.S. Department of Health and Human Services' Medicare hotline; call toll-free 800-633-4227.

**Anesthesia:** Free booklets on what you should know about anesthesia are available from the American Society of Anesthesiologists

(ASA) or the American Association of Nurse Anesthetists (AANA). For copies, write to ASA at 520 North Northwest Highway, Park Ridge, IL 60068, or call 847-825-5586; or write to AANA at 222 S. Prospect Avenue, Park Ridge, IL 60068-4001, or call 708-692-7050.

**General:** For almost every disease, there is a national or local association or society that publishes patient information. Check your local telephone directory. There are also organized groups of patients with certain illnesses that may be able to provide information about a condition, alternative treatments, and experiences with local doctors and hospitals. Ask your hospital or doctors if they know of any patient groups related to your condition. Also, your local public library has medical reference materials about health care treatments. Many libraries now have Health Information Centers, special sections with books and pamphlets on health and disease. Your librarian also can help you find trusted sources of medical information on the internet. One such site is Healthfinder (http://www.healthfinder.gov).

# Chapter 8

# *An Introduction to Anesthesia*

## *Anesthesia for Ambulatory Surgery*

Today the majority of patients who undergo surgery or diagnostic tests do not need to stay overnight in the hospital. In most cases, you will be well enough to complete your recovery at home.

Ambulatory (or outpatient) anesthesia and surgical care has proven to be safe, convenient and cost-effective, and can be performed in a variety of facilities. You may have your procedure done in a hospital, a freestanding surgery center or, in some cases, a surgeon's office. Your anesthesia care will be given or supervised by an anesthesiologist.

### *What is ambulatory anesthesia?*

Ambulatory anesthesia is tailored to meet the needs of ambulatory surgery so you can go home soon after your operation. Short-acting anesthetic drugs and specialized anesthetic techniques as well as care specifically focused on the needs of the ambulatory patient are used to make your experience safe and pleasant. In general, if you are in reasonably good health, you are a candidate for ambulatory anesthesia and

This chapter includes "Anesthesia for Ambulatory Surgery," © 2003 and "Sedation Analgesia," © 2001. Both are reprinted with permission of the American Society of Anesthesiologists, 520 N. Northwest Highway, Park Ridge, Illinois 60068-2573. For additional information, visit http://www.asahq.org/ patienteducation.

surgery. Because each patient is unique, your anesthesiologist will carefully evaluate you and your health status to determine if you should undergo ambulatory anesthesia.

After your early recovery from anesthesia, you usually will return directly home. In most cases, family and friends can provide all the needed assistance. If you do not have family members to help at home, you may require additional help. Some ambulatory facilities offer special post-surgical recovery facilities or extended services with nurses who visit you at home. Appropriate pain management will be included as part of your discharge planning.

## How will I meet my anesthesiologist?

Your anesthesiologist or an associate will interview you before your anesthesia to gather the information needed to evaluate your general health. This interview may be a telephone call, a visit to the facility, or a visit in the office. Laboratory tests may be ordered, and other medical, surgical and anesthetic records will be reviewed. You may be asked to fill out a questionnaire about your previous anesthetic experiences and medical conditions, allergies, medications, or herbal products. If you have particular concerns, you should discuss them with the anesthesiologist.

## What types of anesthesia are available?

There are several types of anesthetic techniques available for your surgery ranging from local anesthesia to general anesthesia. The anesthetic technique recommended will depend on several factors. In some cases, the surgical procedure will dictate what kind of anesthesia will be needed. Based on your medical history, a type of anesthetic may have an additional margin of safety. As an outpatient, some techniques may allow you to recover more quickly with fewer side effects. Your preferences also will be incorporated in the selection of the best anesthetic plan for your procedure.

There are four anesthetic options:

- **General anesthesia:** This anesthetic choice produces unconsciousness so that you will not feel, see, or hear anything during the surgical procedure. The anesthetic medications are given to you through an intravenous line or through an anesthesia mask.

- **Regional anesthesia:** This technique produces numbness with the injection of local anesthesia around nerves in a region of the body corresponding to the surgical procedure. Epidural or spinal blocks anesthetize the abdomen and both lower extremities. Other nerve blocks may be done with the nerves in the arms or legs to anesthetize individual extremities. With regional anesthesia, medications can be given that will make you comfortable, drowsy, and blur your memory.

- **Monitored anesthesia care:** With this approach, you usually receive pain medication and sedatives through your intravenous line from your anesthesiologist. The surgeon or anesthesiologist also will inject local anesthesia into the skin, which will provide additional pain control during and after the procedure. While you are sedated, your anesthesiologist will monitor your vital body functions.

- **Local anesthesia:** The surgeon will inject local anesthetic to provide numbness at the surgical site. In this case, there may be no anesthesia team member with you.

Before receiving any sedatives or anesthetics, you will meet your anesthesiologist to discuss the most appropriate anesthetic plan. Your anesthesiologist will discuss the risks and benefits associated with the different anesthetic options. Occasionally it is not possible to keep you comfortable with regional, monitored, or local anesthesia, and general anesthesia may be needed. Although uncommon, complications or side effects can occur with each anesthetic option even though you are monitored carefully and your anesthesiologist takes special precautions to avoid them. With this information, you will together determine the type of anesthesia best suited for you.

### What about eating or drinking before my anesthesia?

As a general rule, you should not eat or drink anything after midnight before your surgery. Under some circumstances, you may be given permission by your anesthesiologist to drink clear liquids up to a few hours before your anesthesia. If you smoke, please refrain.

### Will I need someone to take me home?

Yes, you must make arrangements for a responsible adult to take you home after your anesthetic or sedation. You will not be allowed to leave alone or drive yourself home. It is strongly suggested that you have someone stay with you during the first 24 hours. If you have local anesthesia only, with no sedation, it may be possible to go home without someone to accompany you. Check with your doctor first.

These instructions are important for your safety. If you do not follow your physician's instructions about not eating and having an adult take you home, your surgery may be canceled.

### Should I take my usual medicines?

Some medications should be taken and others should not. It is important to discuss this with your anesthesiologist. Do not interrupt medications unless your anesthesiologist or surgeon recommends it.

### What should I wear?

If at all possible, wear loose-fitting clothes that are easy to put on and will fit over bulky bandages or surgical dressings. Leave your jewelry and valuables at home.

### What happens before my surgery?

Most commonly, you will meet the anesthesiologist who will care for you on the day of your surgery before you go into the operating room. Your anesthesiologist will then review your medical and anesthesia history and the results of any laboratory tests and will answer any further questions you may have.

Nurses will record your vital signs, and your anesthesiologist and surgeon will visit with you, completing any evaluations and laboratory tests. Intravenous fluids will be started and preoperative medications given, if needed. Once in the operating room, monitoring devices will be attached such as a blood pressure cuff, EKG (electrocardiogram), and other devices for your safety. At this point, you will be ready for anesthesia.

### What happens during my surgery?

Your anesthesiologist is personally responsible for your comfort and well-being. Your anesthesiologist leads the anesthesia care team to monitor as well as manage your vital body functions during your surgery. Your anesthesiologist is also responsible for managing medical problems that might arise related to surgery as well as any chronic medical conditions you may have, such as asthma, diabetes, high blood pressure, or heart problems. A member of your anesthesia team will be with you throughout your procedure.

### What can I expect after the operation until I go home?

After surgery, you will be taken to the postanesthesia care unit, often called the recovery room. Your anesthesiologist will direct the monitoring and medications needed for your safe recovery. For about the first 30 minutes, you will be watched closely by specially trained nurses. During this period, you may be given extra oxygen, and your breathing and heart functions will be observed closely.

In some facilities, you may then be moved to another area where you will continue to recover, and family or friends may be allowed to be with you. Here you may be offered something to drink, and you will be assisted in getting up.

### Will I have any side effects?

The amount of discomfort you experience will depend on a number of factors, especially the type of surgery. Your doctors and nurses can relieve pain after your surgery with medicines given by mouth, injection, or by numbing the area around the incision. Your discomfort should be tolerable, but do not expect to be totally pain-free.

Nausea or vomiting may be related to anesthesia, the type of surgical procedure or postoperative pain medications. Although less of a problem today because of improved anesthetic agents and techniques, these side effects continue to occur for some patients.

Medications to minimize postoperative pain, nausea, and vomiting are often given by your anesthesiologist during the surgical procedure and in recovery.

### When will I be able to go home?

This will depend on the policy of the surgery center, the type of surgery, and the anesthesia used. Most patients are ready to go home between one and four hours after surgery. Your anesthesiologist will be able to give you a more specific time estimate. Occasionally, it is necessary to stay overnight. All ambulatory surgical facilities have arrangements with a hospital if this is medically necessary.

### What instructions will I receive?

Both written and verbal instructions will be given. Most facilities have both general instructions and instructions that apply specifically to your surgery. In general, for 24 hours after your anesthesia:

59

- Do not drink alcoholic beverages or use nonprescription medications.

- Do not drive a car or operate dangerous machinery.

- Do not make important decisions.

You will be given telephone numbers to call if you have any concerns or if you need emergency help after you go home.

## What can I expect with my recovery at home?

Be prepared to go home and finish your recovery there. Patients often experience drowsiness and minor aftereffects following ambulatory anesthesia, including muscle aches, sore throat, and occasional dizziness or headaches. Nausea also may be present, but vomiting is less common. These side effects usually decline rapidly in the hours following surgery, but it may take several days before they are gone completely. The majority of patients do not feel up to their typical activities the next day, usually due to general tiredness or surgical discomfort. Plan to take it easy for a few days until you feel back to normal. Know that a period of recovery at home is common and to be expected.

## Special Considerations for Children

Anesthesia can be safely administered to children in a hospital, a freestanding ambulatory center, or a suitably equipped physician's office. Many procedures for children are often done in such outpatient settings. Children benefit from the early return to comfortable and familiar surroundings. Parents benefit because of less time away from other family members and less interruption in their work schedules.

In some facilities, there may be programs to help prepare you and your child for ambulatory surgery and anesthesia. In these programs, you may visit the facility, see equipment that will be used and ask questions regarding anesthesia, surgery, and recovery.

On the day of surgery, your child should not eat solid food. The anesthesiologist may allow liquids to be given. Parents should plan to stay in the facility during their child's procedure and to make every attempt to have siblings stay home.

Upon arrival at the surgical facility, a nurse will check vital signs and orient you and your child. The anesthesiologist will conduct a preoperative interview and physical exam and discuss the anesthetic plan. For most children, general anesthesia is the preferred form of anesthesia. Anesthesia may begin with intravenous medication, or with breathing anesthetic through a facemask, and then, an intravenous line may be placed after your child is asleep. This may be supplemented by local anesthesia injected by the surgeon or anesthesiologist to control postoperative pain. After surgery, your child will awaken in a recovery area where a nurse will check vital signs, the surgical site, and pain control.

Before going home, your child may be offered something to drink. Parents will receive detailed instructions regarding post-anesthetic and post-surgical care. All questions should be answered and you should feel comfortable taking your child home from the facility.

### Follow-Up

Be sure to follow the instructions given to you while at the surgical facility. These instructions are important to permit the fastest, safest, and most pleasant recovery possible. If you have any questions, please feel free to call your anesthesiologist.

Sometime after your ambulatory anesthesia and surgery, you will be contacted to see how you feel and if you had any problems. You may receive a telephone call from the surgical facility or a questionnaire to mail back. It is important to use this opportunity to let your caregivers know how you feel so they may provide the best possible care.

### Your Rights as a Patient

Although you will not be spending the night in a hospital, you are still a patient and entitled to the same rights that hospitalized patients receive. You should be given an opportunity to speak to those involved in your anesthesia care. All questions involving how the anesthesia will be administered and the training and qualifications of those providing your anesthesia should be answered fully. Any concerns you have about the facility, billing, pain management, and safety equipment should be addressed to your satisfaction before undergoing anesthesia. The professionals caring for you should treat you ethically and respect your privacy and dignity. If you feel uncomfortable about any aspect of your care, you have the right to refuse the planned treatment.

### Other Questions

Please ask questions! Your experience will be easier if you know what usually happens and what you should expect.

Remember, the focus of ambulatory anesthesia is on you, the patient.

## Sedation Analgesia

Although once referred to as "twilight sleep," over the past few years the term "conscious sedation" has become popular to describe a semi-conscious state that allows patients to be comfortable during certain surgical or medical procedures. There is no universal agreement on the meaning of these terms, however. This chapter will clarify some of the information regarding what is more appropriately called "sedation analgesia" and will describe the different levels of sedation as well as the purposes of sedation analgesia. Analgesia refers to the relief of pain that is often included in sedation techniques.

Sedation analgesia can provide pain relief as well as relief of anxiety that may accompany some treatments or diagnostic tests. It involves using medications for many types of procedures without using general anesthesia, which causes complete unconsciousness.

Sedation analgesia is usually administered through an intravenous catheter, or "I.V.," to relax you and to minimize any discomfort that you might experience. This is often used in combination with an injection of a local anesthetic, or "numbing medicine," at the site of surgery. Oftentimes, sedation analgesia can have fewer side effects than may occur with general anesthesia. Frequently, there is less nausea from sedation techniques, and patients generally recover faster after the procedures.

### Levels of Sedation

Although the effects of sedation are better described in terms of "stages" or being part of a "continuum," sedation is usually divided into three categories:

1. Minimal sedation, or anxiolysis

2. Moderate sedation

3. Deep sedation

During minimal sedation, you will feel relaxed, and you may be awake. You can understand and answer questions and will be able to follow your physician's instructions.

When receiving moderate sedation, you will feel drowsy and may even sleep through much of the procedure, but will be easily awakened when spoken to or touched. You may or may not remember being in the procedure room.

During deep sedation, you will sleep through the procedure with little or no memory of the procedure room. Your breathing can slow, and you might be sleeping until the medications wear off. With deep sedation, supplemental oxygen is often given.

With any of the three levels of sedation, you may receive an injection of local anesthetic to numb the surgical site. You may or may not feel some discomfort as this medication is injected, depending on how sedated you are.

## Monitoring and Safety

As with any type of anesthesia, you will be monitored when receiving sedation analgesia. These monitors are very important to ensure your safety. They are used to monitor your heart rate and rhythm, blood pressure, and the oxygen levels of your blood. During moderate and deep sedation, someone will be solely responsible for monitoring your vital signs and controlling your level of consciousness.

## Your Anesthesia Provider

An anesthesiologist (a physician who has completed a residency in anesthesiology), or a registered nurse or nurse anesthetist working with a qualified physician may administer the sedation. You should know who will be providing your sedation analgesia, what their level of training is, and who will be there to handle any situation during the procedure that might affect you.

## Questions to Ask

Here are a few questions that you may want to ask prior to receiving sedation analgesia:

- Who will be responsible for the administration of sedative medications? What are his or her qualifications?

- How will I be monitored during my procedure?

- Will I have an I.V. (intravenous catheter)?

- Will I be receiving local anesthesia in addition to sedation?

- Will the level of sedation I receive be sufficient to make me comfortable during the procedure as well as the recovery period immediately afterward?

- Who will be monitoring my recovery after the procedure?

- In case of an emergency, what equipment and personnel will be available?

- Who will decide when I am ready to go home?

- Whom can I call if I have any problems or questions once I get home?

### After Sedation Analgesia

If you have received minimal sedation only, you may be able to go home once the procedure is finished. If you have received moderate or deep sedation, you will probably require more time to recover. Often this may be within an hour. In the recovery room, you will be monitored until the effects of the medication wear off.

Any after-effects of the medication must be minimal or gone before you will be discharged from the facility to go home. You will not be allowed to drive yourself, so arrangements should be made for a responsible adult to provide you with transportation. If you think you may need some assistance, you might consider having someone stay with you on the day of surgery.

### Conclusion

When given appropriately, sedation analgesia is safe and effective for many procedures done in hospitals, ambulatory surgical centers, and doctors' or dentists' offices. Ask the physician performing your diagnostic or therapeutic procedure about which level of sedation is appropriate for you, and whether an anesthesiologist will be involved in your care. Remember that anesthesiologists are physicians trained to administer all levels of sedation, including general anesthesia should it be necessary for your comfort or safety.

Chapter 9

# *Information for Patients Considering Laser Therapies*

## *The Laser Revolution*

Lasers were first developed in 1960 for industrial uses like the precise cutting of metals and plastics. During the next 20 years, laser design and engineering were advanced to produce short individual pulses of light energy—necessary for its role in medical care. Today, lasers have revolutionized patient care in dermatology, cosmetic surgery, ophthalmology, oncology, and dentistry, to name just a few. In fact, laser therapy has become the gold standard of care for a wide range of medical therapies and cosmetic conditions.

From wrinkles, acne, sagging skin, and vein disorders to birthmarks, diabetic retinopathy, breast cancer detection, and age-related macular degeneration, lasers, and light and other energy sources offer patients an effective solution that doesn't require incisions, scalpel surgery, and extensive recovery periods. In most cases, laser and related high-tech procedures are performed in a doctor's office using only topical or local anesthesia, providing increased safety, enhanced precision, less bleeding, and faster healing than is generally the case with conventional surgery. The laser revolution has also helped to make certain treatments affordable and accessible to consumers from every walk of life.

---

## Laser Design and Engineering

New advances in photonics and laser design are being developed on an ongoing basis to better serve the needs of medical professionals. Similar to consumer electronics, laser technology is driven by the demand for miniaturization. Diode laser technology is replacing bulky equipment, making utilization by physicians easier and more precise. Advances are also being made in patient safety and comfort. Devices and accessories that cool the skin surface and make skin more transparent allow for superior laser penetration. New designs also lead the way to new applications. For example, lasers for vascular lesions, radiofrequency devices for skin tightening, and light-based acne treatments are now available for patient care, thanks to the scientific developments and technical progress emerging from laser engineering labs.

## Laser Therapy for Acne, Scars, Wrinkles, Unwanted Hair, Birthmarks, and Other Skin Conditions

Lasers, pulsed light treatments, and other high-tech energy sources are being used to combat the most stubborn cases of acne and acne scarring. Some of these systems thermally alter the sebaceous (or oily) glands, which contribute to acne, while others emit wavelengths of light that target the acne bacteria itself. Due to high efficacy, high safety, high compliance, and high patient satisfaction, laser/light therapy is fast becoming a first-line defense against acne and acne scarring. In some cases use of topical agents in combination with laser/light activated therapy is proving beneficial.

The use of ablative, fractional, and nonablative laser/light and radiofrequency technologies have become the established methods for skin resurfacing and photorejuvenation; removal of unwanted hair, red birthmarks, and port wine stains, as well as for the treatment of broken blood vessels, rosacea, and red-nose syndrome.

The $CO_2$ laser beam can also cut the skin, which is useful for removing select skin cancers, treating warts, and for eyelid operations.

## Laser Treatment of Pigmentation Problems

Laser therapy is one of the most exciting treatments for removing unwanted skin pigments, such as brown birthmarks, age spots, freckles, and tattoos. The laser emits a specialized light that passes through the skin and is selectively absorbed by the pigment, causing the targeted pigment or tattoo ink to break up and ultimately disappear. It often takes several treatments to totally eliminate a pigmented lesion or tattoo, depending on the amount of pigment or ink present in the lesion.

### *Guidelines for Laser Safety*

The American Society for Laser Medicine and Surgery (ASLMS) was among the first organizations to develop practice guidelines and safety standards for the use of lasers by physician and health personnel in hospitals and office settings. The Society recommends training devoted to the principles of lasers, their instrumentation and physiological effects and safety requirements. An initial program should include clinical applications of various wavelengths in the particular specialty field and hands-on practical sessions with lasers and their appropriate surgical or therapeutic delivery systems. Further, the ASLMS promotes prudent selection of both procedures and patients appropriate for office-based and institutional laser procedures. To ensure safe and effective selection, ASLMS asserts that a comprehensive knowledge of the disease process and experience in management of patients with the disease is essential. In addition, each patient should have at minimum a brief history and physical examination by the physician. Medical records and the highest level of quality assurance should be maintained.

## *Safety Tips for Patients Considering Cosmetic/ Dermatologic Laser and Light Based Device Procedures*

Laser surgery is a safe and effective therapy for numerous medically necessary and elective cosmetic procedures, offering patients a wide range of non-invasive treatment solutions. Before undergoing a laser procedure, ASLMS recommends that those considering laser surgery keep these safety tips in mind:

**Find out who will be administering the treatment:** If the procedure is not being performed by a physician, make sure that a supervising physician is present on-site and readily available to address any problems that might arise.

**Ask questions:** How many procedures has this person performed? Check the doctor's credentials and ask to see before and after photos of other patients with similar conditions. How long is the recuperation period? What are the risks? What is the cost?

**Discuss your medical history with your physician:** Be sure to mention any pre-existing medical conditions, previous medical, or cosmetic procedures, as well as any current medications you are taking.

**Ask if this laser is right for your skin type:** Has this laser been approved for your skin type, hair color, and complexion and for use on the area of the body where you are seeking treatment?

**Request a patch test:** If you have sensitive skin, ask your physician to perform a patch test. It will be much easier to treat a complication on a small patch of skin than a larger area.

**Manage expectations:** Be sure to discuss with your physician what results can reasonably be expected. Will your condition improve after one treatment or will you require multiple treatments for optimal results?

**Let your physician know in advance if you have a history of scarring or herpes:** Both can affect treatment outcomes.

**Don't delay:** If you experience intense pain or unexpected side effects following a procedure, call your physician immediately. Don't wait to see if it will go away.

# Chapter 10

# *Herbal Supplements Can Cause Dangerous Side Effects during Plastic Surgery*

Natural herbal supplements are supposed to help boost our immune systems, give us more energy and make us generally healthier. However, many of these "harmless" supplements could cause dangerous side effects during plastic surgery, reports a study in the February 2006 *Plastic and Reconstructive Surgery*®, the official medical journal of the American Society of Plastic Surgeons (ASPS). In fact, the study found approximately 55 percent of plastic surgery patients, compared to 24 percent of the general public, take supplements but often do not tell their surgeons.

"When patients are asked about the medications they are taking, many do not mention medicinal herbs because they assume that they are safe," said ASPS member James Bradley, MD, study co-author, University of California, Los Angeles. "What many unsuspecting patients don't know is that the natural herbs they are taking may cause serious complications during and after surgery."

All 55 percent of plastic surgery patients who used herbal supplements took at least two different supplements and at least one on a daily basis. The most popular herbal supplements were chondroitin (18 percent), ephedra (18 percent), echinacea (14 percent) and glucosamine (10 percent).

---

"Herbal Supplements, a Smoking Gun in Plastic Surgery," February 13, 2006. Reprinted with permission from the American Society of Plastic Surgeons, www.plasticsurgery.org.

- Chondroitin is often used to treat osteoarthritis. People using chondroitin may suffer from bleeding complications during surgery, particularly when used in combination with doctor-prescribed blood-thinning medications.

- Ephedra has been known to promote weight loss, increase energy and treat respiratory tract conditions such as asthma and bronchitis. This agent has been banned by the U.S. Food and Drug Administration (FDA) because it can raise blood pressure, heart rate and metabolic rate, ultimately causing heart attacks, heart arrhythmia, stroke, and even death.

- Echinacea is often used for the prevention and treatment of viral, bacterial, and fungal infections, as well as chronic wounds, ulcers, and arthritis. However, it can trigger immunosuppression, causing poor wound healing and infection.

- Glucosamine, often offered in conjunction with chondroitin, contains chemical elements that mimic human insulin and may artificially cause hypoglycemia during surgery.

Other common supplements taken by patients in the study that may cause dangerous side effects included gingko biloba, goldenseal, milk thistle, ginseng, kava, and garlic.

In addition to having a greater tendency toward taking herbal supplements, 35 percent of plastic surgery patients were more likely to engage in homeopathic practices, including acupuncture, hypnosis, chiropractic manipulation, massage, yoga, and Pilates. Only six percent of the general population practiced homeopathics on a weekly basis.

"Patients should tell doctors about all of the medications they are taking—natural or prescribed. Only then can we safely suggest the appropriate discontinuation period, which can range from 24 hours to one month," said Dr. Bradley. "Taking this precaution is essential to a safe surgery and smooth recovery."

The American Society of Plastic Surgeons is the largest organization of board-certified plastic surgeons in the world. With more than 6,000 members, the society is recognized as a leading authority and information source on cosmetic and reconstructive plastic surgery. ASPS comprises 94 percent of all board-certified plastic surgeons in the United States. Founded in 1931, the society represents physicians certified by The American Board of Plastic Surgery or The Royal College of Physicians and Surgeons of Canada.

# Chapter 11

# *What to Expect after Plastic Surgery*

Here are the answers to some questions you may have following your aesthetic surgery procedure.

### *Will there be swelling or bruising?*

Surgical procedures are typically followed by variable amounts of swelling (edema) and bruising (ecchymosis) of the operated area. The extent of swelling and bruising will depend, in part, on the type of surgery performed and the location on the body. Surgery of the face tends to result in more swelling and bruising than surgery of the abdomen or breast because of the relatively greater supply of blood in the face. In most circumstances, obvious swelling usually resolves within five to seven days. In people with thick skin, swelling may take longer to disappear. Bruising may persist for up to two weeks and typically changes from a dark purple color to various shades of brown, red, and yellow during this time. These discolorations are all part of the normal wound healing process and can be camouflaged by special cosmetics as directed by your surgeon.

The extent of swelling and bruising can often be minimized and their resolution hastened by elevation of the operated area above the level of the heart. For example, in surgery of the eyelids, elevation of the head on pillows may greatly reduce the extent of swelling. The application of cold compresses to the operative site during the first 48 hours following surgery may also minimize swelling. Your surgeon will define the techniques most appropriate to your specific circumstances.

Remember that medications containing aspirin (for example, Bufferin, Anacin, and Alka-Seltzer) and other non-steroidal anti-inflammatory agents (Advil, Motrin, ibuprofen) tend to delay blood clotting and increase the risks of bruising and bleeding complications following surgery. These medications should be discontinued at least two weeks prior to your surgery to lessen their undesirable effects on normal blood clotting. You should inform your surgeon about all medications you are taking or have taken within the previous six months so that he/she may evaluate the potential risks these medications may pose for your surgery.

### Will there be pain and discomfort following surgery?

The severity of pain and discomfort following aesthetic surgery procedures is typically low but relates to the type of surgery performed and individual pain tolerances. After 48 hours, most aesthetic surgery patients experience very little pain, with the exception of some abdominal procedures which may result in lingering pain and discomfort for up to one week following surgery. Your surgeon will prescribe pain medications for any postoperative discomfort. Severe or persistent pain or pain unrelieved by analgesics may indicate excessive bleeding or infection complications and should be reported immediately to your surgeon.

### What type of dressing and sutures will be used?

The type of dressing and method of wound closure will depend on the type and location of the surgical procedure performed. Most wounds are protected for at least the first 24 to 48 hours following surgery to reduce bacterial contamination that can lead to infection. Incisions of the head and neck are commonly treated with topical antibacterial ointments preceded by cleansing the incision site with saline or hydrogen peroxide solutions to remove accumulated crusts. Incisions of the breast, trunk, and abdomen are usually protected with skin tapes for one to two weeks following surgery. Specific instructions regarding wound care will be provided by your surgeon.

Every effort is made to make your postoperative dressing as comfortable as possible. For this purpose, custom elastic support dressings are frequently used following surgery on the face, breast, abdomen, or hip regions. These supports are easily applied and removed for wound inspections and showering and they may be washed. For face lift surgery, a bulky compression dressing is applied following surgery to reduce the risks of postoperative bleeding and to minimize swelling. This dressing is usually removed after 24 to 48 hours and replaced with a lighter, custom elastic support dressing. Most support dressings are worn for one to two weeks following surgery. In cases of body contouring (suction lipectomy), support dressings may be worn for up to eight weeks or longer following surgery. These dressing may be removed for showering and can be worn beneath regular clothing.

Skin sutures are removed after the wound has healed sufficiently to withstand local forces, such as motion and stretching. In most cases, the skin sutures are removed within five to seven days to avoid unsightly "stretch marks." Since healing occurs faster in areas having relatively more circulation, facial sutures are removed sooner than sutures of the chest, breast, or abdomen. Following early removal of skin sutures, skin tapes may be applied to help support the wound. In some cases, skin sutures may be placed beneath the surface of the skin to avoid suture marks yet provide greater and more prolonged support of the wound. These "sub-cuticular" sutures may be left in place for up to eight weeks following surgery. Generally, it is safe to shower 48 hours following surgery. Specific instructions regarding the care of your incisions will be provided by your surgeon.

## Are there limitations following aesthetic surgery?

To provide the optimal conditions for normal healing of your surgical incisions and to avoid bleeding complications, it is best to avoid vigorous exertional activities (exercise, bending over, heavy lifting, pushing, pulling) for the first several weeks following surgery. Many people ask when they may return to work. A good rule of thumb is that if you are feeling well and your regular work activities do not require strenuous physical exertion, you may return to work within three to five days following surgery. Similarly, driving may be resumed after one to two weeks providing that you have no visual restrictions or limited use of your arms or legs. In general, allow at least four to six weeks for recuperation before resuming full, unrestricted activity. Your surgeon will instruct you in the gradual increase in your postoperative physical activities.

Also, minimize your exposure to ultraviolet sunlight for the first three to six months following surgery as sun rays can cause permanent pigmentation of your skin and incisions at the operative site. Sun screens with a protection value of SPF 15 or greater will help to reduce the effects of ultraviolet exposure. Use of a hat during this time is also recommended for facial surgery patients.

### *Will I need to make follow-up appointments?*

Follow-up examinations are an important aspect of your aesthetic surgical treatment. The timing and frequency of follow-up examinations will depend on the type of surgery. Initially, patients may be seen 24 to 48 hours after surgery and at the time of suture removal. Weekly or monthly visits are then scheduled as determined by your particular needs. Yearly follow-up appointments are desirable for evaluation of your postoperative result. It is not unusual for the final results of aesthetic surgical procedures to manifest themselves nine to twelve months following surgery with subtle changes occurring even beyond that time. Should you experience any unusual symptoms or are concerned about your condition following surgery, contact your surgeon.

# Chapter 12

# *What Is the Mental Cost of Changing Your Appearance?*

Before the makeover, DeLisa Stiles—a therapist and captain in the Army Reserves—complained of looking too masculine. But on Fox's reality TV makeover show, *The Swan 2*, she morphed into a beauty queen after a slew of plastic surgery procedures—a brow lift, lower eye lift, mid-face lift, fat transfer to her lips and cheek folds, laser treatments for aging skin, tummy tuck, breast lift, liposuction of her inner thighs, and dental procedures. The Fox show gives contestants plastic surgery and then has them compete in a beauty pageant, which last year Stiles won.

*The Swan* and other such plastic-surgery shows, including ABC's *Extreme Makeover* and MTV's *I Want a Famous Face*, are gaining steam, but some psychologists are concerned about the psychological impact on those who undergo such drastic cosmetic surgery—and also on those who don't and may feel inadequate as a result. While such radical transformations are rare, some psychologists plan to investigate the surge in cosmetic procedures and whether these surgeries have any lasting psychological consequences.

The number of cosmetic procedures increased by 44 percent from 2003 to 2004, according to the American Society for Aesthetic Plastic Surgery. Plastic surgeons conducted a record 11.9 million procedures last year, including nonsurgical procedures like Botox and surgical procedures like breast augmentation or liposuction.

Dittman, M. "Plastic Surgery: Beauty or Beast?" *Monitor on Psychology*, September 2005, Volume 36, Number 8. Copyright © 2005 by the American Psychological Association. Reprinted with permission.

How do such procedures affect patients psychologically? A recent analysis of 37 studies on patients' psychological and psychosocial functioning before and after cosmetic surgery by social worker Roberta Honigman and psychiatrists Katharine Phillips, MD, and David Castle, MD, suggests positive outcomes in patients, including improvements in body image and possibly a quality-of-life boost too. But the same research—published in the April 2004 issue of *Plastic and Reconstructive Surgery* (Vol. 113, No. 4, pages 1,229–1,237)—also found several predictors of poor outcomes, especially for those who hold unrealistic expectations or have a history of depression and anxiety. The researchers found that patients who are dissatisfied with surgery may request repeat procedures or experience depression and adjustment problems, social isolation, family problems, self-destructive behaviors, and anger toward the surgeon and his or her staff.

Overall, there are more questions than answers regarding psychological effects of cosmetic surgery: There are few longitudinal studies and many contradictory findings, researchers note. Many studies also contain small sample sizes and short follow-ups with patients, says Castle, a professor and researcher at the Mental Health Research Institute of Victoria in Victoria, Australia.

"We really need good, large prospective studies of representative samples of patients, using well-established research instruments," Castle says. "While most people do well in terms of psychosocial adjustment after such procedures, some do not, and the field needs to be aware of this and to arrange screening for such individuals."

In particular, the extent to which cosmetic surgery affects patients' relationships, self-esteem, and quality of life in the long-term offers many research opportunities for psychologists, says psychologist Diana Zuckerman, PhD, president of the National Research Center for Women and Families, a think tank that focuses on health and safety issues for women, children and families.

"These are fascinating issues for psychologists to look at—from the cultural phenomena to the interpersonal phenomena to the mental health and self-esteem issues," Zuckerman says.

In addition, plastic surgery issues will increasingly affect clinician psychologists, and the area will offer new roles for them—such as conducting pre- and post-surgical patient assessments, says psychologist David Sarwer, PhD, director of the Education, Weight and Eating Disorders Program at the University of Pennsylvania. He has studied appearance-related psychological issues, including cosmetic surgery, for the last 10 years.

"As the popularity of plastic surgery continues to grow, many psychologists likely already have—or will encounter—a patient that has thought about or undergone a cosmetic procedure," he says. Therefore it will be increasingly important for psychologists to be able to talk with patients about their appearance concerns and what may make some one a good or bad candidate for cosmetic surgery, he says.

## Research Directions

Equally pressing, however, is the need for research that sheds light on plastic surgery's psychosocial effects, many psychologists agree. To help fill in the gaps, researchers suggest further studies on the following questions:

### *Does plastic surgery make patients feel better?*

Studies have shown that people report increased satisfaction with the body part they had surgery on, but results are mixed on whether plastic surgery boosts their self-esteem, quality of life, self-confidence, and interpersonal relationships in the long term.

In a recent study, Sarwer—also an associate professor of psychology at the Center for Human Appearance at the University of Pennsylvania School of Medicine—found that a year after receiving cosmetic surgery, 87 percent of patients reported satisfaction following their surgery, including improvements in their overall body image and the body feature altered. They also experienced less negative body image emotions in social situations. The study, which was supported by a grant from the Aesthetic Surgery Education and Research Foundation, appeared in the May/June 2005 issue of the *Aesthetic Surgery Journal* (Vol. 25, No. 3, pages 263–269). Sarwer and his colleagues plan to follow up with the patients next year.

However, Castle's team found in their literature review—besides some positive outcomes—a link between plastic surgery and poor post-surgical outcomes for some patients, particularly for those with a personality disorder, those who thought the surgery would save a relationship, and those who held unrealistic expectations about the procedure.

Some studies have even gone as far as linking dissatisfaction with cosmetic surgery procedures to suicide. For example, in one study, the National Cancer Institute found in 2001 that women with breast implants were four times more likely to commit suicide than other plastic surgery patients of the same age as the women who underwent breast implants, says Zuckerman, who in April 2005 testimony to the Food and Drug Administration (FDA) urged the FDA to deny approval of silicone gel breast implants because of a lack of longitudinal research ensuring their safety.

The other three studies on the topic found the suicide rate to be two to three times greater. Neither of the studies, however, identified a causal relationship between breast implants and suicide. Some researchers speculate that some of the surgery recipients may hold unrealistic expectations of it or have certain personality characteristics that predispose them to suicide.

### How does cosmetic surgery affect those around the recipients?

Physically attractive people often receive preferential treatment and are perceived by others as more sociable, dominant, mentally healthy, and intelligent than less attractive people, according to research by psychologist Alan Feingold, PhD, in the March 1992 issue of the American Psychological Association (APA)'s *Psychological Bulletin* (Vol. 111, No. 2, pages 304–341).

"It's not like looking good doesn't have real advantages—it does," Zuckerman says. "If some people get plastic surgery and other people don't, is that going to put the people who don't at all kinds of disadvantages, such as in finding a job or spouse?"

Nearly 30 years ago, many mental health professionals viewed patients who sought cosmetic surgery as having psychiatric issues, but many studies since then suggest that those who seek cosmetic surgery have few differences pathologically with those who don't have surgery, Sarwer says.

Most people are motivated to undergo cosmetic surgery because of body-image dissatisfaction, says Susan Thorpe, a lecturer in psychology at the University of Surrey in Guildford, Surrey, who conducts cosmetic surgery research.

"They want to look normal—that is, they don't want to stand out in an obvious way or to have features which cause comment or make them feel self-conscious," Thorpe says. "They also want their physical appearance to be more in line with their personalities and feel that they want all the bits of their bodies to match."

### What effect does plastic surgery have on children and teenagers?

In 2004, about 240,682 cosmetic procedures were performed on patients 18 years old or younger, and the top surgical procedures were nose reshaping, breast lifts, breast augmentation, liposuction, and tummy tucks. However, very few studies have been conducted to examine the safety and long-term risks of these procedures on adolescents—an age in which teenagers are still developing mentally and physically, Zuckerman says.

### When does changing your appearance qualify as body dysmorphic disorder (BDD)?

BDD, first introduced in the revised third edition of the *Diagnostic and Statistical Manual of Mental Disorders* in 1987, is characterized by a preoccupation with an aspect of one's appearance. People with BDD repeatedly change or examine the offending body part to the point that the obsession interferes with other aspects of their life. Several studies show that 7 to 12 percent of plastic surgery patients have some form of BDD. Plus, the majority of BDD patients who have cosmetic surgery do not experience improvement in their BDD symptoms, often asking for multiple procedures on the same or other body features.

Sarwer often works with plastic surgeons to help them identify such psychological issues as BDD, so surgeons then can refer patients to mental health professionals. He encourages them to look for the nature of the person's appearance concern, such as whether a patient has an excessive concern with a body feature that appears normal to nearly anyone else. Part of that also includes accounting for patients' internal motivations for surgery—are they doing it for themselves or out of pressure from a romantic partner or friend? And, he encourages surgeons to ensure patients hold realistic expectations about the procedures, rather than expecting the surgery to end long-standing personal issues.

## Psychology's Role

Apart from research, psychologists can find clinical roles in aiding cosmetic surgery patients too, such as helping plastic surgeons conduct such assessments. For example, they can help plastic surgeons identify patients who may not adjust well psychologically or psychosocially after surgery, researchers say.

Castle says that empirically based screening questionnaires will help plastic surgeons select cosmetic surgery patients likely to experience positive psychosocial outcomes.

Sarwer has teamed with other psychologists and plastic surgeons to develop such screening questionnaires, which are included in the book *Psychological Aspects of Reconstructive and Cosmetic Plastic*

*Surgery: Clinical, Empirical and Ethical Perspectives* (Lippincott Williams & Wilkins, 2005). The book, features a chapter on how to help both surgeons and mental health professionals screen for BDD, as well as explore the relationships among physical appearance, body image, and psychosocial functioning.

Sarwer believes more psychologists will begin to examine issues related to cosmetic surgery because of its increasing popularity and the link between appearance, body image, and many psychiatric disorders, such as eating disorders, social phobia, and sexual functioning. "Scientifically, we're just starting to catch up to the popularity of [cosmetic surgery] in the population," Sarwer says.

And, as more studies commence, Castle says they need to characterize the population being studied, clearly identify outcome variables, and use standardized and state-of-the-art measures.

"There may be strong cultural pressures that are so unrealistic in terms of how we're supposed to look," Zuckerman adds. "Psychologists should...figure out why this is happening and what we need to know to make sure that people aren't going to be harmed by this."

## *Further Reading*

Honigman, R., Phillips, K., and Castle, D.J. (2004). A review of psychosocial outcomes for patients seeking cosmetic surgery. *Plastic and Reconstructive Surgery*, 113(4), 1229–1237.

Rankin, M., Borah, G., Perry, A., and Wey, P. (1998). Quality-of-life outcomes after cosmetic surgery. *Plastic and Reconstructive Surgery*, 102(6), 2139–2145.

Sarwer, D.B. (2001). Plastic surgery in children and adolescents. In J. Thompson and L. Smolak (Eds.) *Body image, eating disorders and obesity in youth*. (pp. 341–366). Washington, DC: American Psychological Association.

Thompson, J.K., Heinberg, L.J., Altabe, M.N, and Tantleff-Dunn, S. (2004). *Extracting beauty: Theory, assessment and treatment of body image disturbance*. Washington, DC: American Psychological Association.

# Chapter 13

# *Body Dysmorphic Disorder: When Poor Body Image Is an Illness*

### *What is body dysmorphic disorder (BDD)?*

Body dysmorphic disorder (BDD) is a serious illness when a person is preoccupied with minor or imaginary physical flaws, usually of the skin, hair, and nose. A person with BDD tends to have cosmetic surgery, and even if the surgeries are successful, does not think they are and is unhappy with the outcomes.

### *What are the symptoms of BDD?*

- Being preoccupied with minor or imaginary physical flaws, usually of the skin, hair, and nose, such as acne, scarring, facial lines, marks, pale skin, thinning hair, excessive body hair, large nose, or crooked nose.

- Having a lot of anxiety and stress about the perceived flaw and spending a lot of time focusing on it, such as frequently picking at skin, excessively checking appearance in a mirror, hiding the imperfection, comparing appearance with others, excessively grooming, seeking reassurance from others about how they look, and getting cosmetic surgery.

---

"Body Dysmorphic Disorder (BDD)—When poor body image is an illness," National Women's Health Information Center (www.4woman.gov), U.S. Department of Health and Human Services, August 2004.

Some people with mild symptoms of BDD can function well, despite the stress they feel. For others, the illness can get so serious that they may be unable to work, socialize, or leave their homes. They worry that they look ugly, or that people will laugh at them. Some even commit suicide.

Getting cosmetic surgery can make BDD worse. They are often not happy with the outcome of the surgery. If they are, they may start to focus attention on another body area and become preoccupied trying to fix the new "defect." In this case, some patients with BDD become angry at the surgeon for making their appearance worse and may even become violent towards the surgeon.

### *What is the treatment for BDD?*

**Medications:** Serotonin reuptake inhibitors or SSRIs are antidepressants that decrease the obsessive and compulsive behaviors.

**Cognitive behavioral therapy:** This is a type of therapy with several steps:

- The therapist asks the patient to enter social situations without covering up her "defect."

- The therapist helps the patient stop doing the compulsive behaviors to check the defect or cover it up. This may include removing mirrors, covering skin areas that the patient picks, or not using make-up.

- The therapist helps the patient change false beliefs about appearance.

# Part Two

# Skin and Hair Procedures

# Chapter 14

# *Aging Skin, Wrinkles, and Blemishes: An Overview*

## *Introduction*

As a person ages, the skin undergoes significant changes:

- The cells divide more slowly, and the inner layer of skin (the dermis) starts to thin. Fat cells beneath the dermis begin to atrophy (diminish). In addition, the ability of the skin to repair itself diminishes with age, so wounds are slower to heal. The thinning skin becomes vulnerable to injuries and damage.

- The underlying network of elastin and collagen fibers, which provides scaffolding for the surface skin layers, loosens and unravels. Skin then loses its elasticity. When pressed, it no longer springs back to its initial position but instead sags and forms furrows.

- The sweat- and oil-secreting glands atrophy, depriving the skin of their protective water-lipid emulsions. The skin's ability to retain moisture then diminishes and it becomes dry and scaly.

- Frown lines (those between the eyebrows) and crow's feet (lines that radiate from the corners of the eyes) appear to develop because of permanent small muscle contractions. Habitual facial expressions also form characteristic lines.

- Gravity exacerbates the situation, contributing to the formation of jowls and drooping eyelids. (Eyebrows, surprisingly, move up as a person ages, possibly because of forehead wrinkles.)

- Wrinkles can have a profound impact on self-esteem. Indeed, the stigma attached to looking old is evidenced by the fact that Americans spend more than $12 billion each year on cosmetics to camouflage the signs of aging. Our current society places a premium on youthfulness, and age discrimination in the workplace, although illegal, has stalled many a person's career. Indeed, the emotional ramifications of aging explain in large part why the cosmetics industry and plastic surgeons thrive.

## Ultraviolet Radiation, Sunlight, and Photoaging

The role of the sun cannot be overestimated as the most important cause of prematurely aging skin (called photoaging) and skin cancers. Overall, exposure to ultraviolet (referred to as UVA or UVB) radiation emanating from sunlight accounts for about 90% of the symptoms of premature skin aging, and most of these effects occur by age 20:

- Even small amounts of UV radiation trigger process leading to skin wrinkles.

- Long-term repetitive and cumulative exposure to sunlight appears to be responsible for the vast majority of undesirable consequences of aging skin, including basal cell and squamous cell carcinomas.

- Melanoma is more likely to be caused by intense exposure to sunlight in early life.

**Initial Damaging Effects of Sunlight:** Sunlight consists of ultraviolet (referred to as UVA or UVB) radiation, which penetrates the layers of the skin. Both UVA and UVB rays cause damage leading to wrinkles, lower immunity against infection, aging skin disorders, and cancer. They appear to damage cells in different ways, however.

- UVB is the primary agent in sunburning and primarily affects the outer skin layers. UVB is most intense at midday when sunlight is brightest. Slightly over 70% of the yearly UVB dose is received during the summer and only 28% is received during the remainder of the year.

- UVA penetrates more deeply and efficiently, however. UVA's intensity also tends to be less variable both during the day and throughout the year than UVB's. For example, only about half of the yearly UVA dose is received during the summer months and the balance is spread over the rest of the year. UVA is also not filtered through window glass (as is UVB).

Both UVA and UVB rays cause damage, including genetic injury, wrinkles, lower immunity against infection, aging skin disorders, and cancer, although the mechanisms are not yet fully clear.

**Processes Leading to Wrinkles:** Even small amounts of UV radiation trigger the process that can cause wrinkles:

- Sunlight damages collagen fibers (the major structural protein in the skin) and causes accumulation of abnormal elastin (the protein that causes tissue to stretch).

- In response to this sun-induced elastin accumulation, large amounts of enzymes called metalloproteinases are produced. (One study indicated that when people with light to moderate skin color are exposed to sunlight for just five to 15 minutes, metalloproteinases remain elevated for about a week.)

- The normal function of these metalloproteinases is generally positive, to remodel the sun-injured tissue by manufacturing and reforming collagen. This is an imperfect process, however, and some of metalloproteinases produced by sunlight actually degrade collagen. The result is an uneven formation (matrix) of disorganized collagen fibers called solar scars. Repetition of this imperfect skin rebuilding over and over again causes wrinkles.

- An important event in this process is the over-production of oxidants, also called free radicals. These are unstable molecules that are normally produced by chemical processes in the body, a process called oxidation. With environmental assaults, however, such as from sunlight, they are produced in excessive amounts and damage the body's cells and even alter their genetic material. Oxidation may specifically contribute to wrinkling by activating the specific metalloproteinases that degrade connective tissue.

There is a possible upside to wrinkles and sun exposure. A 2001 study reported that people with more wrinkles were less likely to develop basal cell carcinomas, even among high-risk groups. Some experts

87

suggest that people prone to wrinkles may respond to sun exposure with biologic mechanisms that protect against basal cell carcinoma. More research is needed confirm this.

### Other Factors Responsible for Wrinkles

In addition to sunlight, other factors may hasten the formation of wrinkles:

**Cigarette Smoke:** Smoking produces oxygen-free radicals, which are known to accelerate wrinkles and aging skin disorders and increase the risk for nonmelanoma skin cancers. Studies also suggest that smoking and subsequent oxidation produce higher levels of metalloproteinases, which are enzymes associated with wrinkles.

**Air Pollution:** Ozone, a common air pollutant, may be a particular problem for the skin. One study reported that it might deplete the amount of vitamin E in the skin; this vitamin is an important antioxidant.

**Rapid Weight Loss:** If weight loss occurs too rapidly, the volume of fat cells that cushion the face are also decreased before chemicals in the skin can react. This not only makes a person look gaunt, but can cause the skin to sag.

## Blemishes

Three types of blemishes are covered here: Liver spots, purpura, and seborrheic keratoses, or warts.

### Liver Spots

Liver spots (medically referred to as lentigos or sun-induced or pigmented lesions) are flat brown spots on the skin. They are almost universal signs of aging. Occurring most noticeably on the hands and face, these blemishes tend to enlarge and darken over time. The extent and severity of the spots are determined by a combination of skin type, sun exposure, and age. These spots are harmless, but should be distinguished from lentigo maligna, which is an early sign of melanoma.

Liver spots or age spots are a type of skin change that are associated with aging. The increased pigmentation may be brought on by exposure to sun, or other forms of ultraviolet light, or other unknown causes.

**Treating Liver Spots:** They do not require treatment, although some people are distressed by their appearance. Treatments may include the following:

- Trichloroacetic acid (a chemical peel).

- Tretinoin (Retin-A) alone or in a combination with Mequinol (Solagé). Tretinoin is a vitamin A derivative and is also effective in treating wrinkles.

- Gentle freezing with liquid nitrogen (cryotherapy).

- Laser treatment. Specific lasers, such as the Nd:YAG, are effective in eliminating 80% of liver spots in one treatment. (It may be more effective than cryotherapy and have fewer adverse effects.)

- Bleaching creams. These are commonly available but are not as satisfactory as peels, and high concentrations can sometimes cause permanent loss of color.

## *Purpura*

Purpura occurs when tiny capillaries rupture and leak blood into the skin. In older people, the condition (called senile or actinic purpura) is usually caused by fragile blood vessels. The capillaries appear as flat purplish patches. These patches are called petechiae when they are smaller than 3 mm (about an inch). When they are greater than 3 mm, they are referred to as ecchymoses. Patients typically complain of a rash, which may appear reddish at first but gradually change color, turning brown or purple.

**Treatment:** Although there is no specific treatment for purpura, patients are advised to avoid trauma, including vigorous rubbing of the skin, which may be sufficient to damage the capillaries. Emollients that soften the skin may be helpful. Some doctors also recommend vitamin C, but its effectiveness is unproven.

## *Seborrheic Keratoses*

Seborrheic keratoses, (also called seborrheic warts), are among the most common skin disorders in older adults. Their cause or causes are unknown. They usually appear on the head, neck, or trunk and can range in size from 0.2 cm to 3 cm (a little over an inch). They are well defined and appear to be pasted onto the skin, but their appearance can vary widely:

- They can be smooth with tiny, round, pearl-like formations embedded in them.

- They can be rough and warty.

- They can be brown or black.

Seborrheic keratoses sometimes look like melanoma, since they can have an irregular border, but they are always benign. A dermatologist can tell the difference between them, although experts warn that melanomas may "hide" among these benign lesions and go unnoticed without close inspection. In general, seborrheic keratoses have a uniform appearance while melanomas often have a smooth surface that varies in height, color density, and shading. In some cases, keratoses may cause itching or irritation. They can be easily removed with surgery or freezing. Vitamin D3 ointment is also showing promise in clinical trials.

## Risk Factors

**Exposure to Sun in Childhood:** It is estimated that 50–80% of skin damage occurs in childhood and adolescence from intermittent, intense sun exposure that causes severe sunburns. In spite of this now well-known effect, many people still believe that a tan in children signifies health. And, even many parents who are concerned about sun exposure still rely too much on sunscreen and not enough on protective clothing.

**The Elderly:** Most people over 70 have at least one skin disorder and many have three or four. Everyone experiences skin changes as they age, but a long life is not the sole determinant of aging skin. Family history, genetics, and behavioral choices all have a profound impact on the onset of aging-skin symptoms.

### Activities Leading to Overexposure to Sunlight and Ultraviolet Radiation

Of all the risk factors for aging skin, exposure to UV radiation from sunlight is by far the most serious. Indeed, the vast majority of undesirable consequences of aging skin occur in individuals who are repetitively exposed to the sun, including the following:

- Outdoor workers, such as farmers, fishermen, construction workers, and lifeguards.

- Outdoor enthusiasts.

- Sunbathers.

- People who regularly attend tanning salons or use tanning beds. A 2002 study indicated that regular use significantly increases the risk for nonmelanoma skin cancers. Fair women under age 50 were at particular risk.

### Skin Types

Experts have devised a classification system for skin phototypes (SPTs) based on the sensitivity to sunlight. It ranges from SPT I (lightest skin plus other factors) to IV (darkest skin). People with skin types I and II are at highest risk for photoaging skin diseases, including cancer. It should be noted, however, that premature aging from sunlight can affect people of all skin shades.

**Table 14.1.** Tanning and Sunburn History

| Skin Type | Tanning and Burning History |
|---|---|
| I | Always burns, never tans, sensitive to sun exposure |
| II | Burns easily, tans minimally |
| III | Burns moderately, tans gradually to light brown |
| IV | Burns minimally, always tans well to moderately brown |
| V | Rarely burns, tans profusely to dark |
| VI | Never burns, deeply pigmented, least sensitive |

### Gender

It is commonly believed that women are at greater risk for wrinkles than men. Some evidence suggests, however, that given the same risk factors, men and women in the same age groups have comparable risks for skin photoaging. In fact, in one 1999 study, long-term sun exposure caused a greater number of wrinkles in men than in women. In a French study, the evidence of moderate to severe photoaging was observed in the following:

- In 22% of women and 17% of men between the ages of 45 and 49

- In 36% of women and 38% of men by age 54

- Nearly half of both men and women by age 60

In fact, some studies report that men are more likely to develop nonmelanoma skin cancers.

### Smokers

According to one study, heavy smokers are almost five times as likely to have wrinkled facial skin than nonsmokers. In fact, heavy smokers in their 40s often have facial wrinkles more like those of nonsmokers in their 60s. Studies of identical twins have found smokers to have thinner skin (in some cases by as much as 40%), more severe wrinkles, and more gray hair than their non-smoking twins. And even worse, cigarette smokers are more prone to skin cancers, including squamous cell carcinoma and giant basal cell carcinomas.

## Prevention

The best long-term prevention for overly wrinkled skin is a healthy lifestyle:

**Eat Healthy:** A diet with plenty of whole grains, fresh fruits and vegetables, and the use of healthy oils (such as olive oil) may protect against oxidative stress in the skin. A 2001 study reported that people over 70 years old had fewer wrinkles if they ate such foods. Diet played a role in improving skin regardless of whether the people in the study smoked or lived in sunny countries. Benefits from these foods may be due to high levels of anti-oxidants found in them.

**Exercise:** Daily exercise keeps blood flowing, which brings oxygen to the skin. Oxygen is an important ingredient for healthy skin.

**Reduce Stress:** Reducing stress and tension may have benefits on the skin.

**Quit Smoking:** Smoking not only increases wrinkles, but smokers have a risk for squamous cell cancers that is 50% higher than nonsmokers' risk. Smokers should quit to prevent many health problems, not just unhealthy skin.

### Daily Preventive Skin Care

Some daily measures for skin protection are as follows:

- Don't wash face too often with tap water. (Once a day is enough.) It strips the skin of oil and moisture. In addition, chlorinated water, particularly at high temperatures, poses special risks for wrinkles.

- Wash the face with a mild soap that contains moisturizers. Alkaline soaps, especially with deodorant, should be avoided.

- Pat the skin dry and immediately apply a water-based moisturizer.

- Always apply sunscreen, even if going outdoors for short periods.

- Avoid drinking alcohol within three hours of bedtime. Alcohol increases the risk for leaks in the capillaries, which allows more water in and causes sagging and puffiness. Capillary leakage increases when one is lying down.

- Lie on the back when sleeping. This helps offset the effects of gravity.

### *Avoid Sun Exposure*

One of the most important ways to prevent skin damage is to avoid episodes of excessive sun exposure. The following are some specific guidelines:

- Use sunscreens that block out both UVA and UVB radiation. However, do not rely on them only for sun protection. Also wear protective clothing and sunglasses.

- Avoid exposure particularly during the hours of 10 A.M. to 4 P.M. when sunlight pours down 80% of its daily UV dose.

- Avoid reflective surfaces, such as water, sand, concrete, and white-painted areas. (Clouds and haze are not protective and in some cases may intensify UVB rays.)

- Ultraviolet intensity depends on the angle of the sun, not heat or brightness. So the dangers are greater the closer to the summer-start date. For example, in the Northern Hemisphere, UV intensity in April (two months before summer starts) is equal to that in August (two months after summer begins).

- The higher the altitude the quicker one sunburns. (One study suggested, for example, that an average complexion burns at six minutes at 11,000 feet at noon compared to 25 minutes at sea level in a temperate climate.)

- Avoid sun lamps, and tanning beds or salons. They provide mostly high-output UVA rays. Some experts believe that 15 to 30 minutes at a tanning salon is as dangerous as a day spent in the sun. People should not be misled by advertising claims of "safe" tanning or promotions offering unlimited tanning.

**Sunscreens:** The use of sunscreens is complex and everyone should understand how and when to use them. The bottom line is not that people should avoid sunscreens or sunblocks, but that they should always use them in combination with other sun-protective measures.

**Protective Clothing:** Wearing sun-protective clothing is extremely important and protects even better than sunscreens. Special clothing is now available for blocking UV rays and is rated using SPF ratings or a system called the UPF (ultraviolet protection factor) index, with 50 UPF being the highest. (According to one study, this is a very reliable indicator of protection.) The clothing is expensive, however. The following are some tips for anyone:

- Everyone, including children, should wear hats with wide brims. (Even wearing a hat, however, may not be fully protective against skin cancers on the head and neck.)

- People should look for loosely fitted, unbleached, tightly woven fabrics. The tighter the weave, the more protective the garment.

- Washing clothes over and over improves UPF by drawing fabrics together during shrinkage. An easy way to assess protection is simply to hold the garment up to a window or lamp and see how much light comes through. The less the better.

- Everyone over age one should wear sunglasses that block all UVA and UVB ray.

**Chemical Tanners:** Some research suggests that melanin and dihydroxyacetone (DHA), the active ingredients in many self-tanning lotions, may help filter out UVA and UVB radiation and so be protective against sun damage. More research is underway. A preliminary study funded by the National Cancer Institute found that people who received numerous daily injections of melanotan-1 (MT-1) before going in the sun or a tanning bed tanned more quickly and showed fewer signs of sun-related damage. MT-1 is a synthetic version of the hormone melanin, which helps produce the skin's natural pigment.

## Treatment

An increasing number of dermatology patients are looking for a way to improve the appearance of their skin. As a result, more and more products have become available to treat skin wrinkles and blemishes. From vitamins and supplements to exfoliants and chemical peels—the options can be overwhelming. In some cases, more than one approach may be needed. This section details the risks and benefits of several products.

### *Antioxidant Creams, Lotions, and Ointments*

Antioxidants are substances that hunt oxygen-free radicals, the unstable particles that can damage cells and are believed to cause sun damage and even skin cancers. Antioxidants in the skin are depleted when exposed to sunlight and must be replaced.

Antioxidant ointments, creams, and lotions ("topical products") may help reduce the risk of wrinkles and protect against sun damage. Unlike sunscreens, they build up in the skin and are not washed away, so the protection may last. Selenium, coenzyme Q10 (CoQ10), and alpha-lipoic acid are types of antioxidants that come in topical form. Many are proving to be very beneficial for the skin.

**Vitamin A:** Vitamin A is important for skin health. UV radiation produces deficiencies in the skin. Topical products containing natural forms of vitamin A (retinol, retinaldehyde) or vitamin A derivatives called retinoids (tretinoin, tazarotene) have shown to help repair skin damage due to sunburn and also by natural aging.

- *Tretinoin (Retin-A):* Tretinoin (known commercially as Retin-A) is the only topical agent approved for treating photoaging and is available in prescription form (Avita, Renova, Differin). The June 2004 journal *Dermatology Surgery* reported that tretinoin (0.25% concentration) was an effective and well-tolerated treatment for photodamaged facial skin. This agent produces a rosy glow and reduces fine and large wrinkles, liver spots, and surface roughness. It also may help prevent more serious effects of ultraviolet radiation. Tretinoin may be applied to face, neck, chest, hands, and forearm and should be applied at least twice a week. Noticeable improvement takes from two to six months. Because Retin-A increases a person's sensitivity to the sun, patients should apply just a tiny amount at bedtime. A sunblock should be worn during the day, and overexposure to the sun should be avoided. Almost all patients experience redness, scaling, burning, and itching after two or three days that can last up to three months. In women who experience irritation, a daytime moisturizer or low-dose corticosteroid cream, such as 1% hydrocortisone, may help. There is some concern that overuse of high-dose tretinoin may cause excessive skin thinness over time. Studies now suggest that low concentrations (as low as .02%) of tretinoin can produce significant improvements in wrinkles and skin color, with less irritation than at higher doses.

• *Retinol:* Retinol, a natural form of vitamin A, could not, until recently, be used in skin products because it was unstable and easily broken down by UV radiation. Stable preparations are now sold over the counter. In the right concentrations, retinol may be as effective as tretinoin and studies indicate that it has fewer side effects. An animal study suggests that adding antioxidant creams (such as those containing vitamins C or E) may offer added protection against degradation of retinol, but not tretinoin. The FDA (Food and Drug Administration) warns that over-the-counter retinol skin products are unregulated; the amount of active ingredients is unknown, and some preparations, in fact, may contain almost no retinol.

• *Tazarotene:* Tazarotene (Tazorac, Zorac, Avage) is a retinoid used for acne and psoriasis. It has now been approved for treating wrinkles, skin discoloration, and blemishes due to photoaging. One short-term study suggested that it may be as effective as tretinoin and even slightly better at high doses. At such high doses, however, it can cause very severe irritation. Redness and peeling may be reduced by administering tretinoin first to get the skin acclimated. A randomized study of 562 patients with facial photodamage found that a daily application of tazarotene 0.1% cream resulted in a minimum 1 grade improvement in fine and coarse wrinkling, pigmentation discrepancies, pore size, skin roughness, and overall photodamage. More research is needed to determine if it produces any long-lasting significant benefits.

*Warning:* Any vitamin A derivative, it should be avoided by pregnant women and those who may become pregnant. For example, oral tretinoin causes birth defects, and women should avoid even topical Retin-A when pregnant or trying to conceive.

**Vitamin C:** Vitamin C, or ascorbic acid is a very potent antioxidant and most studies on the effects of antioxidants on the skin have used this vitamin. In laboratory studies, large amounts reduced skin swelling and protected immune factors from sunlight. It may even promote collagen production. Vitamin C by itself is unstable, but products that solve the delivery problem are now available (Cellex-C, Avon's Anew Formula C Treatment Capsules, Physician Elite, and others). Studies using these formations in 2002 (one using Cellex-C) reported reduction in wrinkles and appeared to improve skin thickness. In one of the studies, wrinkle improvement with a time-released vitamin C product was as effective as with topical retinoids and some laser treatments. Of concern, according to one 2002 study, ascorbyl palmitate, a vitamin C derivative found in many skin products, may actually increase skin damage from UV rays. More research is needed, since other studies have found this chemical to be protective.

**Antioxidants Under Investigation for Skin Care:** Other antioxidants are also being investigated for their value in skin protection Even with these antioxidants, however, most available brands contain very low concentrations of them. In addition, they are also not well absorbed and they have a short-term effect. New delivery techniques, however, may prove to offset some of these problems.

- *Vitamin E:* Studies suggest that topical vitamin E, particularly alpha tocopherol (a form of vitamin E) cream decreased skin roughness, length of facial lines, and wrinkle depth. Studies on mice have also reported reductions in UV-induced skin cancer with its use.

- *Both green and black tea* may provide some protection against skin cancers and photoaging. There is also some evidence that pomegranate and soy extracts may help rejuvenate aging skin.

- *Aloe, ginger, grape seed extract, and coral extracts* contain antioxidants and are promoted as being healthy for the skin, although evidence of their effects on wrinkles is weak.

### Vitamins and Supplements

A small study found that taking vitamin C and E supplements by mouth—at the same time—may help reduce sunburn, although it doesn't work as well as sunscreen. Taking the vitamins separately did not have any effect. Vitamin C and E are also antioxidants.

## *Alpha Hydroxy Acid and Home Exfoliation*

One of the basic methods for improving skin and eliminating small wrinkles is exfoliation (also called resurfacing), which is the removal of the top layer of skin to allow regrowth for new skin. Methods for doing this run from simple scrubs to special creams to intensive peeling treatments, including laser resurfacing. People with darker skin are at particularly higher risk for scarring or discoloration with the more powerful exfoliation methods.

**Abrasive Scrubs:** Scrub gently with a mildly abrasive material and a soap that contains salicylic acid to remove old skin so that new skin can grow. The motion should be perpendicular to the wrinkles. Use textured material or cleansing grains with microbeads. Organic materials, such as loofahs or sea sponges may harbor bacteria. Avoid cleansing grains that contain pulverized walnut shells and apricot seeds, which can lacerate skin on a microscopic level. Cleansing grains with microbeads don't have sharp edges and remove skin without cutting it. Exfoliation using scrubs, however, can worsen certain conditions, such as acne, sensitive skin, or broken blood vessels.

**Topical Alpha Hydroxy Acid and Similar Substances:** Alpha hydroxy acids facilitate the shedding of dead skin cells and may even stimulate the production of collagen and elastin. They are found naturally as follows:

- Lactic acid (milk)
- Glycolic acid (sugar cane)
- Malic acid (found in apples and pears)
- Citric acid (oranges and lemons)
- Tartaric acids (grapes)

Most alpha hydroxy acid products contain glycolic acid. Skin care products are also made from polyhydroxy acids (PHAs) and beta hydroxy acids (BHAs). BHAs contain salicylate acid (the primary ingredient in aspirin). PHAs contain gluconolactone. Research suggests that PHA products may cause less skin irritation than AHA or BHA products.

Acid concentrations in over-the-counter AHA preparations are 2% to 10%. One clinical study suggested that 8% concentrations showed modest improvement. Some examples include Avon's Anew Intensive Treatment (8% glycolic), Pond's Age Defying Complex (8%), Elizabeth Arden's

Alpha-Ceramid Intensive Skin Treatment (3% to 7.5%), and BioMedic's home product (10%). Prescription strength creams contain at least 12% glycolic acid, and glycolic acid peels of 30% to 70% concentration may be administered in a doctor's office at weekly or monthly intervals.

Response to AHA varies, and the treatment is not without risk, particularly in high-concentration products. Side effects from over-the-counter creams, prescription products, and professional AHA peels can include burns, itching, pain, and possibly scarring. Studies also suggest that AHA may increase susceptibility to sun damage, even at concentrations as low as 4%. Such effects can persist up to a week after the products have been stopped. Experts advise that people should purchase products with AHA concentrations of 10% or less. (Chemical peels of up to 60% are available without prescription on the internet. Such concentrations are not recommended except in consultation with a doctor.) If any adverse effects occur, the product should be stopped immediately. In all cases, people are advised to avoid sunlight or use proper sun protection when using them.

### Other Skin Treatments

**Copper Peptides:** Certain copper containing compounds may both protect skin and help repair it. Of note, copper itself is a toxic metal and it should only be used in products that contain peptides (small protein fragments) that bind to copper. Most studies have been conducted on a copper peptide glycyl-l-histidyl-l-lysine:copper (II) or GHK-Cu. It is currently used in a number of products (CP Serum, Neutrogena's Visibly Firm, ProCyte's Neova).

**Furfuryladenine:** Furfuryladenine (Kinetin, Kinerase) is a naturally occurring growth hormone found in plant and animal DNA; it has antioxidant and anti-aging properties. Some small laboratory studies suggest that it may both delay the onset and decrease the effects of aging on skin. However, no well-conducted human trials have been performed.

**Vitamin K:** Microsponge-based vitamin K is being promoted to clear bruises, spider veins, and other small blood vessel damage. Vitamin K is important for blood clotting.

### Moisturizers

Moisturizers help prevent dryness, bruising, and tearing but have no effect on wrinkles by themselves. They should be applied while the skin is still damp. These products retain skin moisture in various ways:

- Occlusives, such as petroleum jelly, prevent water from evaporating.

- Humectants, including glycerin, act by pulling water up to the surface of the skin from deep tissues. People with oily skin generally should use the humectant type.

- More powerful compounds, such as one called monolaurin (Glylorin), contain mixtures of fatty molecules called lipids, which may help restore the skin's natural barriers against moisture loss and damage.

Most moisturizers contain combinations of these and usually have other ingredients, such as AHA, sunscreens, collagen, and keratin. (Collagen and keratin leave a protein film and temporarily stretch the skin.) They range widely in price, and a major consumer organization found little difference in general between the more and less expensive products.

### Under-Eye Creams

The skin under the eyes is very thin and does not produce as much of the protective oils that keep skin soft and supple. Under-eye gels are aimed at reducing puffiness and dark circles. They typically work in one of two ways:

- Temporarily constricting blood vessels to prevent the build-up of fluids.

- Firming the skin with an invisible film.

- Never rub under the eyes, as this may cause more wrinkles to form. Instead, apply these products with a light tapping motion to stimulate the skin.

### Cosmetics

Cosmetics, if properly applied, can be surprisingly effective in camouflaging the signs of aging skin, including wrinkles and age spots. Moreover, they offer additional benefits by retarding water loss and providing a physical barrier to UV radiation. However, as women age, less is more. Here are some suggestions for older women:

**Moisturizers:** Moisturizers should be applied before foundation. If reddish discoloration is extensive or the skin is sallow, tinted moisturizers may be helpful and can be worn alone or under foundation.

**Foundations:** Caking on make-up will cause cracks at the wrinkle lines and only increase the appearance of aging. Large areas of the face are best covered with a moderate-coverage foundation with a matte or semi-matte finish. Facial powder reflects light and thus minimizes wrinkles but should be avoided by people with dry skin.

**Correcting Color:** When blemishes are especially prominent, applying color correctors under the foundation can be very effective:

- Green neutralizers mask red lesions.
- Yellow will camouflage dark circles and bruises.
- Mauve (a purplish-pink color) helps neutralize sallow skin or yellowish blemishes.
- A white, pearled base helps to minimize wrinkles.

**Blushes:** Blushes and color washes can help conceal the spidery network of dilated capillaries on the nose and cheeks. Powder blushes are preferred because they blend easily on top of foundation.

**Eyes:** Powder eye shadows applied on top of a moisturizer are preferred to cream-based shadows. The appearance of deep-set eyes is best offset with light-colored shadow, which should be applied along the upper eyelid crease and above the iris. A slightly deeper shade of the same color should then be applied to the lower part of the eyelid and drawn out to the corner.

**Lips:** A lip-setting cream or facial foundation should be applied before lipstick to help prevent it from bleeding into surrounding wrinkles. Try using a stiff bristle brush instead of a lip pencil. The brush will help keep the lipstick on and prevent bleeding. (Some women use the pencil itself for the full lip, which gives color but appears natural.) Some make-up artists recommend cream lipsticks instead of matte.

## Resurfacing Treatments

Those who wear the natural signs of aging with a healthy and happy outlook should be regarded with respect as role models. Before embarking on an expensive and ultimately futile attempt to keep time at bay, consider the real bases for self-esteem and the pursuit of a lifestyle that will bring true health and youthful vigor rather than an imitation of it.

## *Choosing a Resurfacing Approach*

There are many choices for skin resurfacing (also called exfoliation) and the patient must discuss a number of different factors that affect the choice. Resurfacing can achieve the following:

- Removal of abnormal tissue and rough skin
- Stimulation of new skin growth
- Stimulation of collagen and elastin production

In addition to determining the skill of the surgeon and the safety of the procedure, the patient must discuss the desired depth of the resurfacing and the capability of each procedure to reach this safely. All resurfacing procedures require a healing period afterward, during which the skin is red and sensitive. And it should be noted that the deeper the procedure, the higher the risk for complications, including delayed healing, infection, loss of pigment (skin color), and scarring.

For people who make the decision to pursue intensive treatments, individuals should consider the following factors, among others, and discuss them with their dermatologist or plastic surgeon:

- The ability of the procedure to safely reduce wrinkles
- The ease and safety record of the procedure
- The skill of the doctor
- The length of recovery
- Possible complications
- The duration of the benefits

A person's age also helps determine the procedure:

- For people in their thirties, a simple chemical peel is sufficient.
- After age 40, people may benefit from collagen or fat implants.
- At age 50 and over, plastic surgeons recommend laser resurfacing and customized treatments for individual needs.

In older individuals, combination procedures may be beneficial. Some examples include the following:

- Laser surgery may be used for deep lines (such as those around the mouth) and chemical peels used over the rest of the face.

- For enhancing the eye by correcting droopy eyelids and bags and raising the brow, combinations of blepharoplasty (eye lift), Botox, and laser resurfacing may be used.

### *Chemical Peels*

Chemical peels, also known as chemosurgery, help restore wrinkled, lightly scarred, or blemished facial skin. Much like chemical paint strippers, chemical peels strip off the top layers of skin, and new, younger-looking skin grows back. Nearly a million were performed in 2003. The procedure is very effective for the upper lip. It cannot be performed around the eyes. Partial peels are often done in conjunction with a facelift. Combinations of the topical anti-oxidants, such as tretinoin and vitamin C, along with a chemical peel may be particularly effective.

#### The Procedure

- Dermatologist applies chemicals to the skin. They include trichloroacetic acid, high concentrations of alpha hydroxy or beta hydroxy acids, or combinations of them.

- In some cases, tretinoin (vitamin A derivative) or alpha hydroxy is applied four to six weeks before and starting one day after the peel. Such treatments can enhance the effects of a peel and reduce the risk of discoloration in people at risk for this complication. (Tretinoin itself is being tested as a chemical peel. In one small 2001 study, it effectively reduced wrinkles with no side effects.)

- A crust or a scab generally forms within 24 hours after surgery, which can be removed by gentle cleansing with soap and water.

- The skin takes six or seven days to heal.

- After the scab disappears, the visible skin is deep red but gradually lightens as it regenerates.

**Complications:** Complications include white heads, cold sores, infection, scarring, numbness, and permanent discoloration, particularly in people with darker skin. Refinement of chemical peel techniques are now permitting doctors to reach deeper skin, improvements which make it easier to apply peels to non-facial skin and to individuals with darker skin.

## *Dermabrasion*

Dermabrasion affects deeper layers of skin than chemical peels, and may be useful for removing disfiguring marks, such as deep acne scars or deep wrinkles. As with chemical peels, it is effective for wrinkles on the upper lip and chin and cannot be used around the eyes. Some experts prefer dermabrasion to lasers for skin surfacing of people with darker skin colors.

**Standard Dermabrasion:** Standard dermabrasion uses a rotating brush that removes the top layers of a person's skin. As with chemical peels, dermabrasion selectively strips away the upper layers of skin, leaving the underlying dermal layers exposed. As with chemical peels, after the procedure, the treated skin oozes and forms a scab, a reaction that is both unsightly and uncomfortable, but only temporary. Postoperative care is similar for both procedures.

**Microdermabrasion:** A gentler variation called microdermabrasion uses very tiny crystals to polish the skin and a vacuum technique to remove them. It has largely replaced the older dermabrasion, and, in fact, was the third most common cosmetic surgery method performed in 2003 (behind Botox injections and chemical peels) with close to a million procedures. Results are similar to light chemical peels. Patients can have this procedure done on their lunch hour and return to work. Only mild redness occurs after treatment, although for best results five or six repetitive treatments are needed every one or two weeks. To date, overall patient satisfaction has been very high.

## *Laser Resurfacing*

Lasers are currently the most effective exfoliation tools for eliminating wrinkles. Their unique advantages over other resurfacing methods are their ability to tighten the skin. A successful procedure can make patients look 10 to 20 years younger, and the results can last up to 10 years. It should be noted, however, that a 2002 study indicated that this procedure may not protect against skin cancers.

The procedure is most beneficial for the following areas:

- Best around the mouth and eyes. Recent evidence suggests $CO_2$ lasers may be even better than dermabrasion for the upper lip.

- Slightly less beneficial for the area around the nose.

- Used alone, current laser therapy does not eliminate crow's feet, broken blood vessels, or dark circles under the eye.

- Standard laser dermabrasion is too harsh for thinner skin layers, such as on the neck. Newer and gentler laser techniques, however, stimulate collagen without taking off skin layers and may prove to be useful for necklines.

- The evidence of the effects of lasers on acne scars is unknown.

**The Laser Resurfacing Procedure:** In general the procedure works in the following way:

- Laser pulses penetrate the skin quickly, vaporizing water and surface skin without damaging the deeper layers, allowing new top skin to grow.

- In addition, enough heat is applied to shorten collagen fibers, restoring some elasticity to the skin.

**Choice of Lasers:** The lasers used depend on skin type and severity of the condition:

- The carbon dioxide ($CO_2$) laser is the most powerful laser treatment and is used for deep wrinkles and skin imperfections. People who have had silicone injections should not have $CO_2$ procedures, which can burn and scar the skin over the implanted area.

- The erbium: YAG (Er:YAG) laser is gentler than the $CO_2$ and is effective for mild wrinkles and for providing a smooth texture. It has a shorter recovery time. Some experts have even found the YAG laser as effective in removing deep wrinkles as $CO_2$ when used to sufficient depth. A so-called variable pulse YAG laser can shift between pulses that destroy skin to tissue to those that heat the skin; this process effectively resurfaces the skin with fewer side effects than $CO_2$ laser therapy.

- A gentle laser procedure called non-ablative laser resurfacing (NLite), also called photorejuvenation, is now approved for the treatment of all facial wrinkles. The procedure uses light energy to gently stimulate new collagen, and possibly elastin, without removing the skin tissue itself. Its effects are less pronounced than those of other laser procedures. However, because it does not injure the external layers of skin, it can be used on delicate skin areas, such as the neck and around the eyes. It also causes very little irritation afterward.

Some surgeons are using combination techniques that employ more than one laser technology in one session to achieve different effects. For example, one combination technique uses $CO_2$, YAG, pulsed-dye laser, and one other laser technology to both improve wrinkles and clear under-eye dark circles and acne scarring. Pretreatment with botulinum injections before laser resurfacing significantly improved the treatment of crow's feet in one 2001 study.

**Post-Procedure Recovery:** The procedure itself is relatively painless, but the redness and irritation that occur during the healing process can be severe. (Non-ablative laser resurfacing does not have the same severe after effects as other laser treatments.) For eight to nine days, the face looks skinned and swollen and requires continuous moisturizing. (Some experts suggest that people with very sensitive skin who cannot tolerate the medications and lubricants should avoid laser resurfacing.) Redness and sensitivity can persist for one to four months. The patient must stay out of the sun as much as possible during this time and should always avoid sunbathing and damaging their skin again. Early research suggests that silicone dressings may reduce post-procedure pain and crusting.

**Complications:** Scarring and infections can occur in about 1% of procedures, with risk increasing or decreasing depending on the experience of the surgeon. People with a history of herpes simplex may experience flare-ups of fever, facial pain, and flu-like symptoms for five or six days afterward. In addition, people with darker skin may wish to avoid the procedure because it can cause unpredictable and dramatic lightening of the skin.

### Other Exfoliation Procedures

**Cold Ablation:** Cold ablation, called coblation for short, delivers saline (salt water) to the skin through which a cool electric current is passed. A subsequent reaction heats and vaporizes the top shallow layer of skin. The procedure is very specific and appears to minimize any damage to other areas of the skin.

**Radiofrequency Resurfacing:** A promising technique uses low radiofrequency energy to resurface the skin. Preliminary research indicates that this procedure may eventually be as effective as laser surgery in reducing severe wrinkles around the eyes and mouth, with minimal pain and a shorter recovery time. In a 2003 study, one treatment with a topical anesthetic resulted in tighter facial skin for 14 out of 15 patients within 12 weeks. All but one patient returned to normal activity immediately afterward. A small clinical trial published in *Dermatology Surgery* found that a noninvasive radiofrequency technique called NARF safely and effectively improved drooping lower eyelids.

**Intense Pulsed Light:** Intense pulsed light (IPL) uses filters to selectively deliver wavelengths of light. It is being used to treat a number of photoaging skin problems and appears to have long-term effects. Typically, four to six treatments are performed over a four-month period. It takes 15 to 20 minutes. Unlike laser light, which uses one color wave-length (such as green or red), intense pulsed light starts with a full spectrum of light. It then allows the doctor to selectively block off specific wave lengths depending on how shallow or deep the procedure should go. IPL machines are less expensive and safer than lasers.

## Implant Procedures

Implants, also called injectable fillers, are becoming a common means of erasing wrinkles and folds. A number of materials are currently being used for deep wrinkles, depression under the eyes, lip enhancements, and for acne scars. In 2002, more than 1.5 million Americans removed wrinkles with injectables (including Botox).

After being banned from the market in 1992, silicone is making a comeback in research settings as a potential permanent wrinkle eraser. Scientists are looking into a new microdroplet technique combined with purified silicone as a way to eliminate any danger. The past problems with silicone occurred when it was mixed with a foreign substance, like mineral oil, or when it was injected in large doses.

Most implants to date, however, are not completely satisfactory. Collagen implants and biologic fillers from animal, bacterial, or human sources do not provide long-lasting benefits. Synthetic fillers are permanent but may provoke an allergic reaction, which can cause chronic problems. Such reactions are rare, but they can be painful and unattractive.

**Table 14.2.** Implant Procedures (*continued on next page*)

**Implant Procedure and Material Used**
*Procedure; Specific Areas Affected; Benefits; Drawbacks*

**Collagen implants:** Collagen is the protein that forms the structures in the body (e.g., skin, bones, cartilage). The implant procedure has typically used bovine (cow) collagen. A form of human collagen (CosmoDerm, CosmoPlast) has now been approved.

> *Procedure:* Injected into target wrinkles with needle and syringe. Several weeks after injection, cow collagen breaks down and is replaced by newly created human collagen.
>
> *Specific Areas Affected:* Wrinkles around the eyes and mouth; used to give lips greater fullness.
>
> *Benefits:* Very simple with faster recovery than many other implant techniques.
>
> *Drawbacks:* Wrinkles reform and repeat treatments are needed three to 12 months later. Rarely, severe allergic reactions. Should not be used by children, pregnant women, and people with a history of autoimmune disease.

**Microlipoinjection:** Fat tissue from the patients' own thigh or abdomen.

> *Procedure:* Injected into target wrinkles with needle and syringe.
>
> *Specific Areas Affected:* Deep wrinkles around the nose and mouth, folds in the forehead, and wrinkles on the hands.
>
> *Benefits:* No allergic or immune reaction because substance is patient's own fat.
>
> *Drawbacks:* Body eventually absorbs the fat, so multiple injections are needed. Some studies suggest that 70% of the fat may still be viable after at least a year.

**Gore-Tex:** Highly porous and inert (not chemically active) synthetic material.

> *Procedure:* Requires some surgery. Tiny patches are inserted under the skin to fill out wrinkles. Skin cells and blood vessels penetrate the porous material easily, reducing the risk of severe inflammation.
>
> *Specific Areas Affected:* Deep wrinkles.
>
> *Benefits:* Material does not degrade.
>
> *Drawbacks:* Possible scarring from surgical procedure. Allergic reactions are rare but can occur even with chemically inactive materials.

**Artecoll:** Contains PMMA, or polymethylmethacrylate, an inert substance, enclosed in tiny droplets of natural collagen.

> *Procedure:* Material is injected. Body absorbs collagen. PMMA remains and stimulates new collagen growth.
>
> *Specific Areas Affected:* Deep wrinkles.
>
> *Benefits:* Although part of the implant is natural collagen implant, it does not degrade as quickly as a full collagen implant.
>
> *Drawbacks:* Repeat treatments still may be needed. Possible allergic reaction.

**Table 14.2.** (*continued*) Implant Procedures

**Implant Procedure and Material Used**
*Procedure; Specific Areas Affected; Benefits; Drawbacks*

**Hyaluronic acid:** Natural (non-animal) substance acts like a molecular sponge to absorb water. The FDA approved Restylane in 2003, and Captiva, Hylaform-Plus, and Hylaform in 2004.

    *Procedure:* Gel is injected under the skin.

    *Specific Areas Affected:* Moderate-to-severe wrinkles.

    *Benefits:* Low risk for allergic reaction. May last longer than bovine collagen.

    *Drawbacks:* Repeat treatments needed.

**Poly-L-lactic acid:** Synthetic polymer. Approved in U.S. as Sculpta. Approved in other countries as New-Fill.

    *Procedure:* Material is injected under the skin.

    *Specific Areas Affected:* Approved in U.S. only for patients with facial fat loss due to HIV. Approved in other countries for wrinkles.

    *Benefits:* Low risk of allergies. Treatment effects can last 18–24 months.

    *Drawbacks:* Doctors require special training.

## *Botulinum (Botox)*

The popularity of Botox injections has skyrocketed in the United States. Between 2002 and 2003 alone, the number of procedures performed jumped 157 percent. Botox injection was the number one cosmetic plastic surgery technique in 2003, with more than 2.8 million injections. Botulinum, the deadly toxin found in uncooked foods, is also a powerful muscle-relaxant, and tiny amounts of a purified form (Botox) are being injected into wrinkles to relax the surrounding muscles. It may benefit forehead and frown lines, crow's feet, lower eyelids, lines on the side of the nose, and the area between the upper lip and the nose. It is also useful for treating involuntary muscle movements that can occur after a face-lift.

The injections need to be repeated every few months, since the effects wear off. The treatment decreases the ability to frown or squint and may cause the corners of the mouth to turn down. When used for areas around eyes, it produces a rounder appearance afterward, which patients should be aware of before they undertake the procedure.

The drug does not cross the blood-brain barrier, and, to date, the only side effects are temporary muscle weakness near the injection site. Although there have been some reports that Botox can reduce migraine and tension headaches, Botox also causes headaches in about 1% of cases. In some cases, the headaches can be very severe and long lasting (from eight days to a month). Some experts suggest that either a contaminated batch of Botox or a specific injection technique may be the cause, but additional investigation is needed.

## Plastic Surgery

In 2003 there were about 1.7 surgical cosmetic procedures, up 43% from the year before. Most of these surgeries were liposuction and breast surgeries. However, nearly a quarter of a million each of eyelid and nose surgeries were performed. Facial plastic procedures range from being fairly minimal, such as a browlift to a full face-lift.

### Face-Lifts (Rhytidectomy)

A number of face-lift procedures (called rhytidectomies) are available. Face-lifts can provide individuals with a more youthful, if not necessarily younger, look. The degree of improvement, however, depends on a number of factors including age, bone structure, skin type, and personal habits, such as smoking and sunbathing.

**The Procedure:** When a face-lift is a relatively simple procedure, it can take about two hours under local anesthetic in a doctor's office. Complicated face-lifts are done under general anesthesia in a hospital and can take three to six hours. The face-lift procedure may be one of the following:

- SMAS (superficial musculoaponeurotic system) is the most common face-lift procedure. The surgeon makes an incision at the hairline and separates the skin from the underlying tissue and muscles. The muscles are tightened and excess fat and tissue, such as fat under the chin and neck, are removed.

- The endoscopic subperiosteal or subgaleal face-lift is a less invasive surgical technique. The surgeon raises facial structures rather than cutting away flaps of skin. Only a few half-inch incisions are made, and scarring is minimal. Not all individuals are candidates for this procedure, however.

Neither SMAS nor the endoscopic version is effective for the middle part of the face, particularly the deep lines (nasolabial folds) that run down from the nose beside the mouth. Some time after the SMAS face-lift, the upper face begins to age again while the lower area still retains its shape, causing the face to look imbalanced. Other approaches, such as one called composite face-lifts that lift most muscles in the face, are being investigated.

**Recovery Process:** Recovery normally lasts from several weeks to several months. Swelling and discoloration are common. Some patients report tingling or numbing sensations after surgery, which generally subside as damaged nerves regenerate.

**Complications:** Rhytidectomy is not without risks. A postsurgical hematoma is a collection of blood that can occur after a rhytidectomy. In one study, major hematomas occurred in 2.2% and minor hematomas in 6.65% of patients. They generally develop within two weeks of the surgery and require drainage. Even minor hematomas need fast treatment to prevent greater complications, including infection, changes in pigmentation, fluid buildup, and prolonged recovery time.

Other less common complications may include the following:

- Infection
- Excessive bleeding
- Asymmetrical facial muscles
- Delayed healing
- Scarring
- Permanent injury to the nerves that control facial movements

These complications are rare, particularly with a skilled surgeon, but the more complex the face-lifts, the greater the risk.

### _Procedures for the Eyes_

**Blepharoplasty:** Blepharoplasty is the primary surgical procedure for eye lifts. Results usually last between five and ten years. Although simple, it has potential complications, including permanent difficulty in closing the eyes or making a stern expression. Newer techniques, however, are preventing this complication. Assuming the surgeon is experienced, laser surgery is now preferred to the standard surgical scalpel approach; bleeding and bruising are reduced, and both the operation and recovery are faster. Temporary blurred or double vision is common. More serious complications include infection, bleeding, dry eyes, difficulty in closing the eyes, and pulling down of the lower lids. Rare cases of blindness have been reported.

**Transconjunctival Upper Blepharoplasty:** An innovative procedure called transconjunctival upper blepharoplasty removes fat from the membrane that lines the eyelids (the conjunctiva) and is an effective technique for treating both the upper and lower eyelids. Unlike traditional blepharoplasty, this procedure does not cause scarring in the nasal area. In patients who have scars from previous surgeries, transconjunctival removal of fat can also make existing scars less obvious. Long-term side effects and efficacy of this procedure have not been studied.

### *Procedures for the Neck*

**Laser Liposculpture and Platysma Resurfacing:** A procedure called laser neck and jowl liposculpture and platysma resurfacing may prove to be an alternative to face-lifts. The procedure requires only a one-inch incision under the chin and removing excess fat. After the fat is removed, the surgeon tightens the platysma, the thin muscular sheet under the skin of the neck, which improves the shape of the neck. Only local anesthetic is needed and the patient can return to normal activities in two days. The patient's skin should be elastic enough to be able to reform without sagging.

## *References*

Gordon, ML. A conservative approach to the nonsurgical rejuvenation of the face. *Dermatol Clin*. 2005 Apr;23(2):365–71.

Edison BL, Green BA, Wildnauer RH, Sigler ML. A polyhydroxy acid skin care regimen provides antiaging effects comparable to an alpha-hydroxyacid regimen. *Cutis*. 2004;73(2 Suppl):14–17.

Kang S. A multicenter, randomized, double-blind trial of tazarotene 0.1% cream in the treatment of photodamage. *J Am Acad Dermatol*. 2005; 52(2): 268–274.

Mitsuhashi Y, Kawaguchi M, Hozumi Y, Kondo S. Topical vitamin D3 is effective in treating senile warts possibly by inducing apoptosis. *Dermatol*. 2005;32(6):420–423.

Rubino C, Farace F, Dessy LA, Sanna MP, Mazzarello V. A prospective study of anti-aging topical therapies using a quantitative method of assessment. *Plast Reconstr Surg*. 2005;115(4):1156–1162.

Samuel M, Brooke RC, Hollis S, Griffiths CE. Interventions for photodamaged skin. *Cochrane Database Syst Rev*. 2005;(1):CD001782.

Sudel KM, Venzke K, Mielke H, et al. Novel aspects of intrinsic and extrinsic aging of human skin: beneficial effects of soy extract. *Photochem Photobiol*. 2005;81(3):581–587.

Thornfeldt C. Cosmeceuticals containing herbs: fact, fiction, and future. *Dermatol Surg*. 2005;31(7 Pt 2):873–880.

Vochelle D. The use of poly-L-lactic acid in the management of soft-tissue augmentation: a five-year experience. *Semin Cutan Med Surg*. 2004;23(4):223–226.

# Chapter 15

# *Liver Spots and Aging Hands*

As people age, unsightly blemishes, commonly called liver spots, can appear on the face and on the back of the hands. Another upsetting change for many mature adults is the loss of smoothly contoured hands. Dermatologic surgeons can improve both of these distressing conditions safely and effectively with excellent results.

### *What are liver spots?*

Liver spots, also called lentigines or lentigos, are sharply defined, rounded, brown or black, flat patches of skin. The epidermis (top surface layer) is expanding with more pigment, developing what looks like a large freckle. One may appear by itself, or as a few clustered together.

Many people have a hereditary predisposition to them. While liver spots may develop at an early age, even in childhood, they are more common in older people, especially those who have spent too much time in the sun.

### *Are liver spots cancerous?*

The spots are not cancerous, nor do they lead to cancer. However, on skin exposed to the sun, they may be accompanied by precancerous

---

scaly, red elevations of the skin called actinic keratoses. Dark spots, which might be cancerous, may also appear to be lentigines. All of these blemishes should be evaluated by a dermatologic surgeon.

### Can liver spots be prevented?

Although nothing can be done about the role heredity plays, excessive exposure to the sun should be avoided—a precaution that will diminish the threat of skin cancer as well as protect your skin from sun-damage. To moderate exposure, the skin should be protected by a sunscreen having minimum SPF of 15.

### How are liver spots treated?

Treatment of liver spots is usually performed by the dermatologic surgeon in the office or other outpatient facility. Results can be permanent if a sunscreen is used continuously after removal.

Following are common treatment approaches:

**Sunscreens:** The simplest treatment to protect the skin from further damage and worsening of the spots is use of a sunscreen. Sunscreen is also important after other treatment methods so the spots will not recur.

**Bleaching Creams, Tretinoin, and Alpha-hydroxy Acids:** These are topical applications prescribed by the physician to fade small spots. Treatment normally takes anywhere from two months to a year or longer.

**Cryosurgery:** The dermatologic surgeon freezes the skin tissue with liquid nitrogen to remove liver spots and skin growths.

**Peeling:** A chemical solution is applied to peel away the blemished skin. The face and hands usually heal in one to two weeks.

**Dermabrasion:** The skin is sanded lightly with a special instrument to remove the spot. Upon healing, which normally takes a week or so, the liver spot is gone.

**Laser Surgery:** New techniques with various lasers are used to remove the spots. A beam of laser light is directed at the liver spots to selectively eliminate the damaged skin.

### *How are youthful contours restored to the hands?*

The skin of the backs of the hands can be improved by a technique called microlipoinjection, a form of soft tissue filler. The dermatologic surgeon uses a tiny syringe to remove a small amount of a patient's own fat from another part of the body, such as the buttocks or the thigh. The fat is then injected into the back of the hands and molded to restore a youthful contour.

Since one's own fatty tissue is used, there is little risk of the body's rejecting it, as can sometimes occur when a foreign substance is used. Some patients have long-lasting results; others need re-treatment periodically.

# Chapter 16

# *Botulinum Toxin (Botox™)*

## *Botox Cosmetic: A Look at Looking Good*

The promise of a more youthful look was too tempting for 53 year old Mary Schwallenberg to pass up. So, when the Food and Drug Administration (FDA) approved a product that temporarily improves the appearance of frown lines between the eyebrows, the Orlando, Florida, resident took a shot at it. And it wasn't long before she became one of many people clamoring for regular treatments that often include refreshments and friendly conversation, as well as injections.

Botulinum toxin type A (Botox cosmetic) is a protein complex produced by the bacterium *Clostridium botulinum*, which contains the same toxin that causes food poisoning. When used in a medical setting as an injectable form of sterile, purified botulinum toxin, small doses block the release of a chemical called acetylcholine by nerve cells that signal muscle contraction. By selectively interfering with the underlying muscles' ability to contract, existing frown lines are smoothed out and, in most cases, are nearly invisible in a week.

Botox injections are the fastest-growing cosmetic procedure in the industry, according to the American Society for Aesthetic Plastic Surgery (ASAPS). In 2001, more than 1.6 million people received injections, an increase of 46 percent over the previous year. More popular

"Botox Cosmetic: A Look at Looking Good," by Carol Lewis, in *FDA Consumer magazine*, U.S. Food and Drug Administration, July–August 2002. "Questions and Answers about Botox™" is from "Botox™," FDA, August 2005.

than breast enhancement surgery and a potential blockbuster, Botox is regarded by some as the ultimate fountain of youth.

Schwallenberg, a pharmaceutical sales representative who is excited about her next round of injections, says she wants to look her best for her job. "That's corporate America for you," she says. "I have a lot of energy and I just wanted to look good."

Botox was first approved in 1989 to treat two eye muscle disorders—uncontrollable blinking (blepharospasm) and misaligned eyes (strabismus). In 2000, the toxin was approved to treat a neurological movement disorder that causes severe neck and shoulder contractions, known as cervical dystonia. As an unusual side effect of the eye disorder treatment, doctors observed that Botox softened the vertical frown (glabellar) lines between the eyebrows that tend to make people

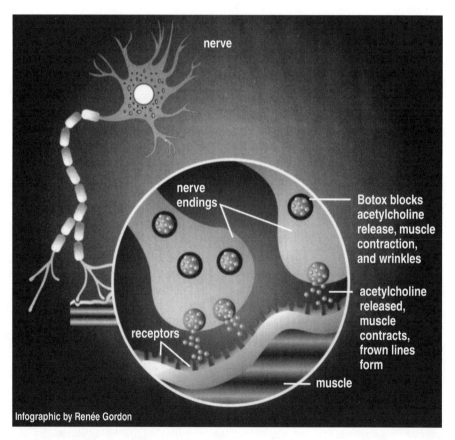

*Figure 16.1.* How Botox Works

look tired, angry or displeased. But until this improvement was actually demonstrated in clinical studies, Allergan Inc., of Irvine, California, was prohibited from making this claim for the product.

By April 2002, the FDA was satisfied by its review of studies indicating that Botox reduced the severity of frown lines for up to 120 days. The agency then granted approval to use the drug for this condition.

The FDA regulates products, but not how they are used. Approved products are sometimes used by a licensed practitioner for uses other than those stated in the product label. Botox Cosmetic, for example, is currently being used by physicians to treat facial wrinkles other than those specified by the FDA. Consumers should be aware, however, that this "off-label" use has not been independently reviewed by the agency, and the safety and effectiveness of Botox injections into other regions of the face and neck, alone or in combination with the frown-lines region, have not been clinically evaluated.

Ella L. Toombs, M.D., a dermatologic medical officer in the FDA's Office of Cosmetics and Colors, says, "Careful deliberation, investigation and evaluation is undertaken by the agency before any prescription product is approved." Drugs such as Botox, which are not indicated for serious or life-threatening conditions, "are subject to a greater level of scrutiny because of the benefit-to-risk ratio." Toombs says this means that the FDA may allow someone to incur a greater risk from products that treat medical conditions, rather than from those that are approved for cosmetic purposes.

### *Botox 'Parties'*

The recent rise in the popularity of Botox has much to do with the manner in which it is frequently marketed. Some practitioners buy the toxin in bulk and arrange get-togethers for people receiving their treatments. As in business, volume discounts can be found in medicine.

Plastic surgery events known as Botox parties—also seminars, evenings and socials—are a key element of Botox marketing in much of the United States. The gatherings are thought to be a convenient means of providing Botox treatments more economically, and may help reduce the anxiety that normally goes along with getting an injection. Doctors are finding that treating people in groups allows them to make the procedure more affordable to their patients.

Here's how a "party" typically works: A group of often nervous, but excited, middle-aged men and women mingle in a common area. Sometimes refreshments are served. One by one, as their name is called, each slips away for about 15 minutes to a private exam room. He or she pays a fee and signs an informed consent agreement. Anesthesia is rarely needed, but sedatives and numbing agents may be available. The practitioner injects about one-tenth of a teaspoon of toxin into specific muscles of the forehead most often targeted for the effect. The person then rejoins the group.

Scott A. Greenberg, M.D., a board-certified plastic surgeon in Winter Park, Florida, has been hosting monthly "Botox Happy Hours" in his medical office since the drug's approval in April 2002. Greenberg feels that these by-invitation-only events to previous patients "are an opportunity to treat a lot of people at one time in a relaxed but professional atmosphere." Greenberg says there is no difference between treating 10 people during individual office visits throughout the day and treating 10 people individually, but in a more socialized setting. "The important thing is that the identical standards of medical care are maintained at these gatherings as in a routine daytime office consultation."

Julianne Clifford, Ph.D., of the FDA's Division of Vaccines and Related Products Applications, explains that "Botox is licensed for marketing and distribution as single-use vials." This means that as packaged, "each vial is intended to be used for a single patient in a single treatment session." Botox does not contain a preservative against potential contamination of the product through repeated use of a single vial. Once opened and diluted, Botox must be used within four hours. Treating multiple people with one vial violates product labeling, which is stated on the package insert, the vial and the carton.

"We lose something when we mass treat," says Franklin L. DiSpaltro, M.D., president of the ASAPS. "One of my concerns is that these parties are a marketing tool—gathering as many patients as possible trivializes a medical treatment, which could deteriorate over time into a nonprofessional environment." DiSpaltro says there's more to medicine "than just dispensing drugs."

Schwallenberg, however, insists that "Dr. Greenberg was very professional. It wasn't a cattle call," she says. "And I don't think I'd go to a doctor I didn't know."

The FDA is concerned that Botox has the potential for being abused. The ASAPS recently reported that unqualified people are dispensing Botox in salons, gyms, hotel rooms, home-based offices, and other retail venues. In such cases, people run the risks of improper technique, inappropriate dosages, and unsanitary conditions. "Botox is a prescription drug that should be administered by a qualified physician in an appropriate medical setting," says Toombs.

Greenberg agrees. "Patient safety has to be of prime concern," he says. "People need to be in the right hands when complications arise." That's why Greenberg does not allow his staff to administer Botox treatments. Even the most skilled health-care providers, he says, can have complications as well as dissatisfied customers.

Although there is no chance of contracting botulism from Botox injections, there are some risks associated with the procedure. If too much toxin is injected, for example, or if it is injected into the wrong facial area, a person can end up with droopy eyelid muscles (ptosis) that could last for weeks. This particular complication was observed in clinical trials.

Other common side effects following injection were headache, respiratory infection, flu syndrome, and nausea. Less frequent adverse reactions included pain in the face, redness at the injection site, and muscle weakness. These reactions were generally temporary, but could last several months.

While the effects of Botox cosmetic don't last, still, people don't seem to mind repeating the procedure every four to six months in order to maintain a wrinkle-free look. Battling the signs of aging in a non-invasive way, after all, is part of the allure of the product—that and the fact that there are no unsightly scars, and that there is very little recovery time with the procedure.

The FDA recommends that Botox cosmetic be injected no more frequently than once every three months, and that the lowest effective dose should be used.

## Question and Answers about Botox

Botox is used to make lines or wrinkles between the eye brows look better. It only lasts for a short time.

### What is Botox?

Botox comes from a kind of bacteria. The bacteria can make you very sick. But doctors have found that a chemical in Botox can also help treat some health problems. They have been using it safely for many years.

### How was this found?

FDA (Food and Drug Administration) approved Botox over 10 years ago to treat certain problems with the eye muscle. Doctors noticed that some wrinkles around the eyes looked better, too. The company that makes Botox tested it. They showed the FDA that Botox worked and was safe for treating some kinds of wrinkles.

### How does Botox work?

Wrinkles may be caused when a muscle tightens. Botox is injected through the skin into the muscle. The Botox keeps the muscle from tightening. When the muscle can't tighten, the wrinkle doesn't show as much.

### You mean you can't move your muscles?

A doctor trained in the use of Botox will inject small amounts of Botox into the muscle. Only the treated muscle can't move.

### What happens over time?

Botox works for about four months. As the muscle returns to normal, you will see the wrinkle again.

### Are there any side effects?

Yes. Side effects may include the following:

- Droopy eyelids, which can last for a few weeks
- Feeling like you have the flu
- Headache and upset stomach
- Risk of botulism (a life or death illness that makes it hard for a person to move the arms and legs or to breathe) is low with Botox, if used the right way

Remember that Botox is a drug, not a cosmetic.

### What should I do if I want to try Botox?

- Ask about how Botox could help or hurt you.
- Make sure your doctor is trained in the use of Botox.
- Make sure you get treatment in a doctor's office or clinic.
- Emergency equipment should be on hand in case of a problem.
- Do not use if you are pregnant or think you might be pregnant.

- Do not use if you are breast feeding.
- Tell your doctor if you are taking antibiotics.
- Tell your doctor if you have any problems with nerves or muscles.

### Are "Botox parties" safe?

No. You should only get Botox in a clinic or doctor's office. You should never share a tube of Botox.

### Can I use Botox on other wrinkles?

Botox is only approved to treat wrinkles between the eyebrows.

### Can I get Botox at any age?

Botox is only approved for people 18–65 years old. It has not been tested on people under 18 or over 65.

# Chapter 17

# *Collagen Replacement and Other Dermal Fillers*

## Collagen Replacement Therapy

Collagen treatment is a safe, non-surgical procedure that softens lines and furrows on the face. Tiny quantities of collagen are injected under the line or scar through very fine needles, boosting the skin's natural collagen. The effects can be maintained by small 'top-up' collagen injections two or three times a year.

### *What is collagen?*

Collagen is a natural substance that is found in skin, muscle, tendons, and bones and provides structural support. In the dermis (the mid-layer of skin), collagen is made by fibroblast cells. It forms a fibrous network on which new cells can grow. Through the natural processes of aging, collagen in the dermis is gradually lost and contributes to the formation facial lines.

---

Text in this chapter begins with information from "Collagen Replacement Therapy," "Hyaluronic Acid Implants," and "Fat Grafting"; this information is reprinted with the permission from DermNet, the website of the New Zealand Dermatological Society. Visit www.dermnet.org.nz for patient information on numerous skin conditions and their treatment. © 2006 New Zealand Dermatological Society. The chapter concludes with "Newly Approved Products," information excerpted from the following U.S. Food and Drug Administration (FDA) announcements: "ArteFill® - P020012," January 10, 2007; "Cosmetic Tissue Augmentation Product - P050033," January 10, 2007; and "Radiesse - P050037," January 23, 2007.

Injectable bovine collagen is made of sterile, purified collagen from cow skin. Human collagen implants are highly purified and isolated from human skin grown in a laboratory. The cells have been grown for the last ten years or so primarily to manufacture living skin-equivalents to treat burns and ulcers.

When injected into the body's skin both forms of collagen are accepted as if they were the body's own collagen, forming a network of collagen fibers.

Zyderm® and Zyplast® are popular brands of injectable bovine collagen. Others include Resoplast®. Human collagen brands include Dermalogen®, Cymetra, CosmoDerm® and CosmoPlast®.

There is also a product derived from porcine collagen, Fibrel®, which is injected with the patient's own serum. The injections are said to be rather painful and may cause allergic reactions.

A person's own skin may be used to produce fibroblast cultures (Isolagen®) or a suspension of collagen (Autologen®). It can also be mixed with synthetic PMMA beads (Artecoll®).

### Where can collagen implants be used?

Collagen injections can be used to improve the skin's contour and fill out depressions in the skin due to scars, injury, or lines. Facial lines and features that can be smoothed out using collagen implants include the following:

- Frown lines that run between the eyebrows (glabellar lines)

- Smoker's lines which are vertical lines on the mouth (perioral lines)

- Marionette lines at the corner of the mouth (oral commissures)

- Worry lines that run across the forehead (forehead lines)

- Crow's feet at the corner of the eyes (periorbital lines)

- Deep smile lines that run from side of the nose to corners of the mouth (nasolabial furrows)

- Cheek depressions

- Redefining lip border

- Acne scars (collagen is not suitable for narrow 'ice-pick' scars)

- Other facial scars, providing they don't have a sharp edge

Collagen treatment can be combined with other cosmetic procedures, including botulinum toxin injections and laser resurfacing.

### Am I suitable for collagen replacement therapy?

Your doctor will take a complete medical history. Medication that reduce blood clotting, such as aspirin, anti-inflammatory agents, warfarin, and some herbal medications, may increase the chance of bleeding. People with severe allergies (anaphylaxis) or allergy to injected local anesthetics should not be treated with bovine or human collagen.

Since injectable bovine collagen is derived from cows it may cause allergic reactions. Approximately 3% of the population is allergic to bovine collagen; these individuals should not receive these implants. Human collagen is a better choice in the following circumstances:

- Allergies to foods, especially meat products

- Family or personal history of severe allergies (including asthma, hay fever and atopic dermatitis)

- Any previous reaction to a test dose of collagen

To see if you are eligible for bovine collagen replacement therapy you will require one or two skin tests. No skin test is necessary for human collagen as allergic reactions are very unlikely.

*Procedure for collagen skin test*

1. Test dose of bovine collagen injected just below the skin's surface on forearm.

2. Observe the site closely for at least four weeks for any of the following signs:
   - redness
   - swelling
   - hardness
   - itching
   - tenderness

3. Most reactions will occur within the first three days, but can happen at anytime within this timeframe.

4. If it appears that you have a very mild reaction, the doctor may need you to have a second skin test on the other arm to confirm sensitivity.

5. Report all reactions to your doctor. After the 4-week observation period (or eight weeks if second test is required) your doctor will advise whether or not you can proceed with bovine collagen replacement therapy.

### How is collagen treatment given?

Collagen treatments are carried out in a medical centre by a specially trained nurse or doctor. The treatment usually take 20 minutes to an hour.

*Procedure for collagen replacement treatments*

1. Wash the face thoroughly.

2. The treatment site is wiped with an antiseptic.

3. Using a very fine needle, the collagen, local anesthetic, and saline are injected just below the skin to fill out the depression.

4. Depending on the area treated, massaging may be used to smooth out the collagen before it firms up.

Immediately after injection the site may be tender, red, and swollen. This will gradually settle over the next few days. It is safe to cover the treated areas with make-up if you wish. Avoid strenuous exercise, sunburn, and alcohol during this time. Your therapist may ask to check the results in two or three weeks and top up with more collagen if necessary.

### How long does the collagen implant last?

Collagen implants are not permanent. Because collagen is a natural protein it slowly breaks down into amino acids that are then absorbed by the body. In most cases, implants last anywhere between one to six months, although in some people one implant may be sufficient for up to two years. Repeat treatments will be necessary to maintain the results.

The longevity of the implant will depend on its location and individual response. Muscular activity such as smiling and frowning will reduce how long it lasts. Conversely, it may last longer than expected in scars because these are not caused by facial muscle movement.

## *Are there any side effects from collagen replacement therapy?*

At the time of treatment most patients report minor discomfort. This is minimized by the addition of lignocaine (lidocaine) to the collagen preparation. This is local anesthetic to numb the treatment area, and is known as 'lidocaine' in America.

Immediately after treatment the area may be red, swollen, and tender; this usually improves over the following days. Temporary bruising and discoloration may also occur. The collagen is sometimes visible for a while in the form of small white bumps at the treatment site. This generally smoothes out within a few weeks.

Very rarely, if a blood vessel is accidentally blocked by the collagen injection, a small area of skin may die resulting in an ulcer that scabs. This reaction may leave a permanent scar. It has most often been reported in the glabellar area.

Injections through the skin carry a risk of bacterial infection (impetigo). This is more likely if inflammation is present in the treated area such as acne or rosacea spots. Injections in and around the lips may also provoke cold sores in those prone to them.

Allergic reaction to bovine collagen is usually recognized after one or two test doses. In rare cases, allergic reactions may occur during the course of treatment even though there was no reaction to the test dose. They may occur rapidly after treatment or arise weeks to months afterwards. The reaction may clear up in a few days or persist for months. See your doctor immediately if you have an allergic reaction. Allergic reactions may include the following:

- Shortness of breath, low blood pressure, and chest pain
- Urticaria (hives)
- Red, itchy, or sore lumps at injection sites
- Scarring when the lumps have resolved
- Shorter lasting effect of collagen injections

People with connective tissue diseases such as rheumatoid arthritis, systemic lupus erythematosus, systemic sclerosis, and dermatomyositis may be more likely to experience an allergic reaction to bovine collagen, and the effect of the treatment might not last as long. There have also been reports of connective tissue disease arising for the first time after bovine collagen injections. However a connection between the injections and the connective tissue disease has not been established.

131

The safety of collagen implants in pregnancy or in children has not been established.

## Hyaluronic Acid Implants

Hyaluronic acid therapy is becoming a popular choice as a temporary filler for facial augmentation. It is a safe, non-surgical procedure that conveniently softens facial lines and furrows. It also has the added benefit of not requiring skin testing before use. Products available include Hylaform®, Restylane®, Perlane® and Esthélis®.

Tiny quantities of hyaluronic acid are injected through very fine needles, boosting the skin's own hyaluronic acid. Depending how many lines are treated, the treatment takes 20 minutes to an hour, with minimal discomfort.

The effects can be maintained by small 'top-up' treatments as required, generally about twice a year.

### *What is hyaluronic acid?*

Hyaluronic acid is a natural substance that is found in all living organisms. High concentrations are found in soft connective tissue and in the fluid surrounding the eye. It is also present in some cartilage and joint fluids, and in skin tissue.

In skin tissue, hyaluronic acid is a jelly-like substance that fills the space between collagen and elastin fibers. The role of hyaluronic acid in skin is to:

- provide a mechanism of transport of essential nutrients from the bloodstream to living skin cells,

- hydrate the skin by holding in water, and

- act as a cushioning and lubricating agent against mechanical and chemical damage.

Over time, either through the natural process of aging or through exposure to environmental factors such as pollutants and sunlight, the body's natural store of hyaluronic acid is degraded and destroyed.

In the last 30 years synthetic forms of hyaluronic acid have been developed and used to correct disorders in the fields of rheumatology, ophthalmology, and wound repair. More recently, synthetic forms of hyaluronic acid are being manufactured for use in facial augmentation. Brand names of manufactured hyaluronic gels for this purpose include Hylaform® (includes Hylaform Fine Line and Hylaform Plus—

Hylan B), Restylane® (non-animal stabilized hyaluronic acid), Perlane®, Juvederm®, Rofilan Hylan® and AcHyal®.

## *Where can hyaluronic acid injections be used?*

Hyaluronic acid injections can be used as a dermal filler to improve the skin's contour and reduce depressions in the skin due to scars, injury, or lines. Facial lines and features that can be corrected using hyaluronic acid implantation include the following:

- Frown lines that run between the eyebrows (glabellar lines)
- Smoker's lines which are vertical lines on the mouth (perioral lines)
- Marionette lines at the corner of the mouth (oral commissures)
- Worry lines that run across the forehead (forehead lines)
- Crow's feet at the corner of the eyes (periorbital lines)
- Deep smile lines that run from side of the nose to corners of the mouth (nasolabial furrows)
- Cheek depressions
- Redefining lip border
- Acne scars
- Some facial scars

## *Am I suitable for hyaluronic acid therapy?*

Almost all people are suitable for hyaluronic acid therapy. Because hyaluronic acid is chemically identical within and between species, allergy to it is very rare. Thus, unlike bovine collagen implants, manufacturers claim there is not the need to perform a skin allergy test and wait up to eight weeks for results before commencing treatments. You should discuss with your doctor about whether or not you require a skin allergy test with hyaluronic acid before commencing therapy.

Hyaluronic acid therapy is suitable for patients allergic to bovine collagen.

## *How is hyaluronic acid treatment given?*

Treatments are carried out at a medical center by a trained doctor or supervised nurse.

*Procedure for hyaluronic acid treatments*

1. Wash your face thoroughly.

2. The treatment area is wiped with an antiseptic.

3. Local anesthetic may be used to numb the treatment area.

4. Injection method used depends on the doctor but will be either the serial intradermal puncture technique (series of small injections with a very fine needle) or tunnel or threading technique (needle is withdrawn as the hyaluronic acid is injected).

5. Depending on the area treated, the skin may be lightly massaged.

6. Immediately or within a few hours after injection the site may be red and swollen. This usually disappears within a week.

7. Another one or two treatments (at least a week apart) may be necessary to achieve the desired correction.

### How long do hyaluronic acid implants last?

Hyaluronic acid implantation is not permanent. Like natural hyaluronic acid, manufactured hyaluronic acid once injected into the skin will gradually break down and be absorbed by the body. In most cases, the augmentation usually lasts anywhere between three and nine months. To maintain the initial results, repeat treatments or top-up treatments will be necessary. Most people have two to three treatments per year.

### Are there any side effects from hyaluronic acid therapy?

Hyaluronic acid therapy is generally very well tolerated. At the time of treatments most patients report minor discomfort. This is minimized by the use of a local anesthetic. Immediately after treatment the area may be red, swollen, and tender, this usually improves within a few days. Rarely, allergic reactions to hyaluronic acid have been reported. These are generally red or thickened nodules arising in the injected sites and may persist for several weeks or months.

## Fat Grafting

Fat grafting is also called free fat transfer, autologous fat transfer/

134

transplantation, liposculpture, lipostructure, volume restoration, microlipoinjection, and fat injections.

This is a procedure which removes surplus fat cells from one area of the body and then re-implants it where needed.

### What is fat grafting?

Fat grafting fills facial features with a patient's own fat. The fat used for fat transfer is extracted from part of your body like the abdomen or thighs and injected into another area that requires plumping.

The advantage of fat grafting is that the fat comes from your own body, so you cannot develop an allergic reaction unlike other external implant substances that are introduced into the body. Your body naturally accepts the injected fat.

### Where can fat grafting be used?

Fat grafting can been used for correcting or improving:

- facial scarring (acne scars);
- facial volume in diseases such as hemifacial atrophy;
- facial aging such as sunken cheeks and facial lines.

Fat grafting lasts longer in larger areas of non-movement, so while it is successful for the correction of grooves under the eyes and sunken cheeks, it may not be as successful for creating fuller lips. Fat grafting can also correct aging of the hands where the natural tissue is lost between the bones.

Fat grafting is not recommended for breast augmentation as the grafted fat can later make it difficult to detect breast cancer.

### How is fat grafting performed?

Fat grafting is performed in your doctor's rooms on an outpatient basis. There are basically three parts to the procedure.

1. Harvest
   - Prepare site for removal of fat by injecting local anesthetic.
   - Insert cannula connected to a syringe through small incision and carefully suck out fat.

2. Purification and transfer

- Fat is purified either by hand or mechanically to get fat cells for grafting.

- Prepare fat cells for transfer.

3. Placement

   - Area for graft is prepared.

   - Needle or cannula is inserted into incision point of the site being augmented. Fat cells carefully injected into area.

   - This is repeated until desired correction has been achieved.

After the procedure, avoid massage and excessive facial movement, as this will stop migration of the fat away from the desired areas of treatment. Ice compresses may be used for 24–48 hours to minimize inflammation.

The doctor will schedule to see you about a week after the procedure to check both the donor and recipient sites. A follow-up appointment six to eight weeks later should see most of the swelling resolved and early results assessed. A repeat procedure may need to be performed if the desired outcome has not been achieved but this should not be within three months of the first graft.

### How long do fat grafts last?

How much of the graft survives and for how long is currently unknown. Over the first few months your body will resorb about 65% of the fat. The remaining 35% will usually stay in place. It appears that the amount resorbed by the body and ultimately the longevity of the graft is highly dependent on the technique used in grafting. Newer techniques are being developed to increase the longevity. For longer lasting results, patients may receive three or four treatments over a period of six months to a year.

### Are there any side effects or complications from fat grafting?

A moderate amount of swelling is expected after the fat graft. This is usually evident for two weeks after the procedure. Some bruising may also be apparent. Some complications of fat grafting include:

- Undercorrection: desired outcome not achieved thus requiring a further graft to complete the correction.

- Overcorrection: too much fat is injected into the area. This prevents new blood vessels growing to supply the graft, leading to cell death and a lumpy consistency.

- Clumping of the graft.

- Accidental damage to underlying structures such as nerves and blood vessels, particularly around the eye.

- Bleeding: usually associated with use of sharp needles for fat injection.

- Infection.

- Scarring of the donor site.

## Newly Approved Products

This is a brief overview of information related to the U.S. Food and Drug Administration (FDA)'s approval to market these product.

### ArteFill® - P020012

**What is it?** ArteFill® is a filler that is injected into the nasolabial folds around the mouth to smooth these wrinkles. The device contains small polymethylmethacrylate beads, collagen, and lidocaine.

**How does it work?** ArteFill® works by adding volume to nasolabial folds and restoring a smoother appearance.

**When is it used?** ArteFill® is injected by a doctor into the facial tissue around the mouth (i.e., nasolabial folds). The device adds volume to the skin and can give the appearance of a smoother surface.

**What will it accomplish?** ArteFill® will help smooth nasolabial folds around the mouth. In a clinical study most patients needed more than one injection to achieve optimal wrinkle smoothing. The average number of treatment sessions was 2.28.

Side effects of ArteFill® include the following:

- Lumpiness at injection area more than one month after injection

- Persistent swelling or redness

- Increased sensitivity

- Rash, itching more than 48 hours after injection

**When should it not be used?** ArteFill® should not be used in patients who have the following characteristics:

- A positive response to the ArteFill Skin Test
- Severe allergies with a history of anaphylaxis or presence of multiple severe allergies
- Allergies to bovine collagen or lidocaine
- Susceptibility to form keloid or hypertrophic scars

ArteFill® should not be used for the following:

- Implantation into blood vessels, because it may obstruct blood flow
- Lip augmentation or injection into the vermilion or the wet mucosa of the lip

**Additional information:** For more complete information on this product, its indications for use, and the basis for FDA's approval, see the Summary of Safety and Effectiveness and product labeling at: http://www.fda.gov/cdrh/pdf2/p020012.html.

### *Cosmetic Tissue Augmentation Product - P050033*

**What is it?** Cosmetic Tissue Augmentation Product (CTA) is a transparent hyaluronic acid gel with 0.3% lidocaine that is injected into facial tissue to smooth wrinkles and folds, especially around the nose and mouth (nasolabial folds). Hyaluronic acid is a protective, lubricating, and binding gel substance that is produced naturally by the body.

**How does it work?** CTA works by temporarily adding volume to facial tissue and restoring a smoother appearance to the face. The effect lasts for about 6 months.

**When is it used?** CTA is injected by a doctor into areas of facial tissue where moderate to severe facial wrinkles and folds occur. The gel temporarily adds volume to the skin and can give the appearance of a smoother surface.

**What will it accomplish?** CTA will help smooth moderate to severe facial wrinkles and folds. In a clinical study most patients needed one injection to achieve optimal wrinkle smoothing; about one-quarter of the patients needed more than one injection to get a satisfactory result. The smoothing effect lasted about six months.

Side effects of CTA include bruising, redness, swelling, pain, tenderness, and itching.

**When should it not be used?** CTA should not be used in patients who have severe allergies marked by a history of anaphylaxis (hypersensitivity to the ingestion or injection of a drug or protein) or severe allergies to gram-positive bacterial proteins or lidocaine. CTA should not be used for the following:

- implantation into bone, tendon, ligament, or muscle
- implantation into blood vessels, because it may obstruct blood flow

**Additional information:** For more complete information on this product, its indications for use, and the basis for FDA's approval, see the Summary of Safety and Effectiveness and product labeling at: http://www.fda.gov/cdrh/pdf5/p050033.html

## *Radiesse - P050037*

**What is it?** Radiesse is an injectable calcium hydroxylapatite implant in the form of a gel.

**How does it work?** Radiesse works by temporarily adding volume to facial tissue and restoring a smoother appearance to the face.

**When is it used?** Radiesse is intended for restoration and/or correction of the signs of facial fat loss (lipoatrophy) in people with human immunodeficiency virus (HIV). It is injected by a doctor into areas of facial tissue where moderate to severe facial wrinkles and folds occur. The gel temporarily adds volume to the skin and can give the appearance of a smoother surface.

**What will it accomplish?** Radiesse will help smooth moderate to severe facial wrinkles and folds. The smoothing effect lasts up to six months.

Side effects of Radiesse include bruising, redness, swelling, pain, tenderness, and itching.

**When should it not be used?** Radiesse should not be used in patients who have a hypersensitivity to any of the components of the product, severe allergies manifested by a history of anaphylaxis, or history or presence of multiple severe allergies.

**Additional information:** For more complete information on this product, its indications for use, and the basis for FDA's approval, see the Summary of Safety and Effectiveness and product labeling at: http://www.fda.gov/cdrh/pdf5/p050037.html.

Chapter 18

# *Dermabrasion*

From the beginning of time, people suffering from the disfigurement of facial scarring have searched for ways to improve these imperfections. Thanks to refinements of a number of dermatologic surgical techniques, there are several safe, effective procedures available today to improve facial scarring, including dermabrasion or scarabrasion.

### *What is dermabrasion?*

While more than 100 years old, dermabrasion has enjoyed a resurgence of popularity since the 1960s. The resurfacing technique has been further perfected over the last few decades.

During dermabrasion, or surgical skin planning, the dermatologic surgeon freezes the patient's skin, scarred from acne, chicken pox, or other causes. The doctor then mechanically removes or "sands" the skin to improve the contour and achieve a rejuvenated appearance as a new layer of remodeled skin replaces the damaged skin. The new skin generally has a smoother and refreshed appearance. Results are generally quite remarkable and long-lasting.

### *When is dermabrasion indicated?*

When dermabrasion was first developed, it was used predominantly to improve acne scars, chicken pox marks, and scars resulting from accidents or disease. Today, it is also used to treat other skin conditions, such as pigmentation, wrinkles, sun damage, tattoos, age (liver) spots, and certain types of skin lesions. The treatment may also be applied to select areas of deformed skin.

The conditions under which dermabrasion would not be effective include the presence of congenital skin defects, certain types of moles or pigmented birthmarks, and scars from burns.

### What happens prior to surgery?

Before surgery, a complete medical history is taken and a careful examination is conducted in order to evaluate the general health of the patient. During the consultation, the dermatologic surgeon describes the types of anesthesia that may be used, the procedure, and what results might realistically be expected. The doctor also explains the possible risks and complications that may occur. Photographs are taken before and after surgery to help evaluate the amount of improvement. Preoperative and postoperative instructions are given to the patient at this time.

### How does the procedure work?

Dermabrasion can be performed in the dermatologic surgeon's office or in an outpatient surgical facility. Medication to relax the patient may be given prior to surgery. The area is thoroughly cleansed with an antiseptic cleansing agent. The area to be "sanded" is treated with a spray that freezes the skin. Sometimes local tumescent anesthesia can be used. A high-speed rotary instrument with an abrasive wheel or brush removes or abrades the upper layers of the skin and improves irregularities in the skin surface.

### What happens after the surgery?

For a few days, the skin feels as though it has been severely "brush-burned." Medications may be prescribed to alleviate any discomfort the patient may have. Healing usually occurs within seven to ten days.

The newly formed skin, which is pink at first, gradually develops a normal appearance. In most cases, the pinkness has largely faded by eight to 12 weeks. Make-up can be used as a cover-up as soon as the crust is off. Generally, most people can resume their normal occupation in seven to 10 days after dermabrasion. Patients are instructed to avoid unnecessary direct and indirect sunlight for three to six months after the procedure and to use a sunscreen on a regular basis when outdoors.

# Chapter 19

# *Chemical Peels*

## *Chemical Skin Peel: Light to Medium*

Skin peeling involves an application of a chemical solution to sun-damaged, unevenly pigmented, and finely wrinkled facial areas. The procedure is meant to diminish imperfections by peeling away the skin's top layers. It has proven to be a very popular non-surgical cosmetic procedure. Chemical peels vary according to their specific ingredients and their strength. Depth of peeling action may also depend on factors such as how long solutions remain on the skin and whether they are lightly applied, or more heavily or vigorously applied.

## *Technique*

The surgeon will select the best chemical or chemical mix for the individual patient. A solution is applied—using a sponge, cotton pad, cotton swab, or brush—to the areas to be treated (or the entire face, avoiding the eyes, brows, and lips). Generally, the most superficial peels are those using alpha hydroxy acids (AHA), such as glycolic, lactic, or fruit acid. Various concentrations of an AHA may be applied

This chapter begins with "Chemical Skin Peel: Deep (Phenol) Peel" and "Chemical Skin Peel: Light to Medium," © 2003 American Society for Aesthetic Plastic Surgery (www.surgery.org). All rights reserved. Reprinted with permission. Additional text is included from "Glycolic Peels" by Sam P. Most, MD, reprinted with permission. Copyright © 2002 Sam P. Most, M.D. For additional information visit http://www.drmost.com.

weekly or at longer intervals to obtain the best result. A trichloroacetic acid (TCA) peel is stronger, and has a greater depth of peel compared to AHA's.

### *Benefits*

#### AHA:

- No anesthesia or sedation is needed, and the patient will feel only a mild tingling or stinging sensation when the solution is applied.
- Sometimes a single treatment will give skin a healthier, radiant look.
- No downtime—patient can immediately resume normal activities.
- Can be mixed with a facial cream or wash in milder concentrations as part of a daily skin-care regimen.

#### TCA:

- TCA is especially effective in treating darker-skinned patients.
- Can possibly be used to achieve some effects of a deep peel, depending on the concentration, and manner of application.
- Generally shorter recovery time than with a deep (phenol) peel.

#### Both:

- Short, safe procedure.
- No covering or after-peel ointment is necessary.

### *Other Considerations*

#### AHA:

- May require multiple treatments.

#### TCA:

- May require pretreatment with AHA or Retin-A creams.
- Repeat treatment may be required.
- Deeper TCA peel may result in 2–3 days of restricted activity.

**Both:**

- Sun block is strongly recommended, especially with TCA treatment. Skin pores may appear larger, and the skin may not tan evenly following a chemical peel.

- Some facial skin disorders do not respond to chemical peeling.

## Chemical Skin Peel: Deep (Phenol) Peel

A deep chemical skin peel, or phenol peel, is the strongest of chemical peels, and is reserved for individuals with deep wrinkles from sun exposure or is used to treat skin wrinkling around the lips and chin area. The procedure diminishes imperfections in sun-damaged, unevenly pigmented, or coarsely wrinkled facial areas by peeling away the skin's top layers.

### *Technique*

A full-face deep chemical peel takes 1 to 2 hours to perform. A more limited procedure (such as treatment of wrinkling above the lip) will generally take less than a half-hour. A solution is applied to the area to be treated (avoiding the eyes, brows, and lips). There is a slight burning sensation, but it is minimal since the solution also acts as an anesthetic. After the peel solution has worked on the skin, it is neutralized with water. Approximately one hour later, a thick coating of petroleum jelly is layered over the patient's face, covering the protective crust which develops rapidly over the area. This stays in place for 1 to 2 days. In an alternative technique, the patient's face is covered by a "mask," composed of strips of adhesive tape, with openings for the eyes and mouth (this is particularly effective in cases of severe wrinkling).

Some patients experience discomfort after a deep chemical peel, but this can be controlled with medication. A few days after the procedure, new skin with a bright pink color akin to sunburn will emerge; the pinkness will fade within a few days. Postoperative puffiness will also subside in a few days, but the skin will remain sensitive. Patients should avoid exposure to sunlight and continue to use sun block.

### *Benefits*

- Effects of a phenol chemical peel are long lasting, and in some cases are still readily apparent up to 20 years following the procedure. Improvements in the patient's skin can be quite dramatic.

- Normal work schedule and other activities can be resumed after 1 to 2 weeks.

- Variants in the phenol peel formula can create a milder solution for broader use.

### Other Considerations

- Possible postoperative complications can include scarring, infection, or abnormal pigmentation. Tends to have a bleaching effect, and patient may need to wear make-up to match treated and untreated areas.

- EKG monitoring is advised.

- Cannot be used on the neck or other parts of the patient's body.

- Not as effective in treating individuals with dark, oily complexions.

- Some facial skin disorders do not respond to chemical peeling.

- Skin pores may appear larger, and the skin may not tan properly.

- Can activate latent cold sore infections.

- All forms of deep skin peels include the risk of delayed healing and scarring.

### ASAPS Position

The effectiveness of phenol chemical peeling has been proven in clinical studies over the last 30 years. Because they are serious procedures, it is the American Society for Aesthetic Plastic Surgery (ASAPS)'s position that phenol chemical peels should only be performed under the direction of a qualified physician.

## Glycolic Peels

### What is a glycolic peel?

A glycolic peel is a technique to gently remove, exfoliate, the uppermost layers of the skin. As the dead outer-most epidermal cells are removed, the skin can regain a more "freshened" look.

### What can a glycolic peel achieve?

Glycolic peels have a "freshening effect" on the skin.

### What are the limitations of a glycolic peel?

It is not a primary treatment for skin discoloration or wrinkles.

### What is the difference between a glycolic and chemical peel?

A chemical peel is also a technique to remove the upper layers of the skin. However, the impact is deeper. As the skin heals, it has a more youthful look. Technically, the application of any chemical that causes skin to peel is a chemical peel. This would include over-the-counter alpha-hydroxy acids, glycolic peels, and the like. However, these are considered "superficial" peels. A chemical peel is a deeper, more intense peel. The results are better, but more "down time" is involved.

### What is the procedure like?

The procedure can be done in the office. Our nurses have extensive experience in application of glycolic peels. Since the effects are mild, we often suggest a series of six peels, with progressively increasing concentrations of glycolic acid with each peel.

### What is the recovery period?

Glycolic peels sometimes result in mild pinkness of the skin for about 24 hours. Often, the peel can be done during the day and you can go back to your activities. Rarely does skin sloughing occur, as is common in traditional "chemical peels."

# Chapter 20

# *Laser Skin Resurfacing*

## *What is a laser?*

Laser stands for "light amplification by the stimulated emission of radiation." Lasers work by producing an intense beam of bright light that travels in one direction. The laser beam can gently vaporize and/or ablate skin tissue to improve wrinkles, scars, and blemishes, seal blood vessels, or cut skin tissue.

The laser has the unique ability to produce one specific color (wavelength) of light, which can be varied in its intensity and pulse duration. The newest laser systems have become remarkably precise and selective, allowing treatment results and safety levels not previously available.

## *What is skin resurfacing?*

Laser resurfacing to improve cosmetic flaws, such as wrinkles, acne scars, and aging and sun-damaged skin, is the latest scientific breakthrough in skin rejuvenation.

Using a wand-like laser handpiece, undesired skin cells and wrinkles literally disappear in a puff of mist and are replaced by fresh skin cells. One of the laser's most significant advantages over traditional

This chapter includes text from "Laser Resurfacing" and additional facts about lasers excerpted from "Laser and Intense Pulsed Light Applications." Reprinted with permission from the American Society for Dermatologic Surgery, http://asds-net.org. © 2005. All rights reserved.

techniques for skin resurfacing is that treatment is relatively blood-less. The procedure also offers more control in the depth of penetration of the skin's surface, allowing an increased degree of precision and safety in treating delicate areas.

### Who is qualified to perform laser surgery?

Dermatologic surgeons have extensive experience with laser surgery and were among the first specialists to use lasers for skin renewal and treating a variety of skin disorders. Since results are technique-sensitive and entail an artistic component, it's important to select a dermatologic surgeon with demonstrated laser expertise

### What conditions can laser resurfacing treat?

Laser resurfacing is performed in the dermatologic surgeon's office to help with the following:

- Erase fine lines and wrinkles of the face
- Smooth and tighten eyelid skin
- Improve crow's feet around the eyes
- Soften pucker marks and frown lines
- Remove brown spots and splotchy, uneven skin color
- Improve and flatten scars
- Repair smoker's lines
- Improve skin tone and texture

### How does the carbon dioxide (CO2) laser work?

The newest generation of the CO2 laser delivers short bursts of extremely high-energy laser light. This revolutionary technology actually vaporizes the undesired skin tissue, one layer at a time, revealing fresh skin underneath. The laser's highly focused aim enables the dermatologic surgeon to gently remove the skin's surface with a low risk of scarring and complications in properly selected patients.

### How does the erbium (Er) laser work?

The high-powered erbium:YAG laser produces energy in a wavelength that gently penetrates the skin, is readily absorbed by water (a major component of tissue cells), and scatters the heat effects of the laser light. These unique properties allow dermatologic surgeons to remove thin layers of skin tissue with exquisite precision while minimizing damage to surrounding skin.

The Er:YAG laser is commonly used for skin resurfacing in patients who have superficial to moderate facial wrinkles, mild surface scars, or splotchy skin discolorations. Skin rejuvenation with the Er:YAG laser offers the advantages of reduced redness, decreased side effects, and rapid healing compared to some other laser systems.

### What other types of lasers are used by dermasurgeons?

**Yellow light lasers:** Through the use of an organic dye, short pulses of yellow-colored light are produced. A popular yellow light laser is the pulsed dye laser. Because yellow light is more precisely absorbed by the hemoglobin than other colors, these lasers are effective in the treatment of blood vessel disorders, such as port wine stains, red birthmarks, enlarged blood vessels, rosacea, hemangiomas, and red-nose syndrome. Certain yellow light lasers may also be used to treat stretch marks and are safe and effective for infants and children. The krypton and Nd:YAG lasers are dual light systems.

The green light, in contrast, is used for the treatment of benign brown pigmented lesions, such as café-au-lait spots, the "old age" spots commonly found on the backs of the hands, and lentigines or freckles. Green light lasers are also used for the treatment of small blood vessels on the face and legs.

**Red light lasers:** The red light spectrum produced by the ruby or alexandrite light laser is emitted in extremely short, high-energy pulses due to a technique known as Q-switching. The Q-switched ruby or alexandrite laser systems were initially used to remove tattoos, but are now commonly used to treat many brown pigmented lesions, such as freckles or café-au-lait spots.

When the pulse duration of the ruby or alexandrite lasers is lengthened, it is effective in removing unwanted hair for long periods of time, sometimes even permanently.

**Q-switched neodymium YAG (ND: YAG):** Delivering infrared light, it is used to remove tattoos and deep dermal pigmented lesions, such as nevus of Ota (oculodermal melanosis). This laser can also be tuned to produce a green light for the treatment of superficial pigmented lesions like brown spots, as well as orange-red tattoos.

151

**KTP:** The KTP emits a green light and is capable of treating certain red and brown pigmented lesions. When the pulse duration is lengthened, the Nd:YAG laser is also effective in removing hair and an inflammatory condition termed pseudofolliculitis barbae for months and sometimes permanently. This is particularly useful in the treatment of dark-skinned patients.

### How do non-ablative lasers work?

Unlike laser resurfacing technologies that heat and remove the top skin tissue, non-ablative or non-wounding lasers actually work beneath the surface skin layer. This novel approach appears to stimulate collagen growth and tighten underlying skin to improve skin tone and remove fine lines and mild to moderate skin damage. It offers the patient the benefits of few side effects and rapid healing with virtually no "downtime."

### What can be expected during and after treatment?

Discomfort is usually minor during the procedure, and your dermatologic surgeon can discuss the administration of any pain medication prior to treatment.

Following skin resurfacing, the treated areas usually are kept moist with ointment or surgical bandages for the first few days. The skin is typically red or pink and may be covered with a fine crust. The treated sites must be protected from sunlight after the procedure. Once healing is completed, sunblock lotion should be applied. In some cases, a pink surface color may remain for several days to several months. Make-up can be worn after about 7–14 days.

### Are there side effects or complications?

Each year thousands of laser resurfacing procedures are performed successfully. Significant complications are rare, and the risk of scarring is low. Some patients may be at risk for varying degrees of pigmentation loss, particularly with the $CO_2$ laser. Common minor side effects may include crusting, mild swelling, redness, or brown discoloration at the treatment sites. These are usually minimized by surgical techniques and pre- and postoperative regimens.

### What are the limitations of laser resurfacing?

Laser resurfacing is not a substitute for a facelift, nor can the procedure eliminate excessive skin or jowls. However, by tightening loose skin, laser resurfacing can improve certain folds and creases. Laser resurfacing offers an alternative to traditional resurfacing methods like dermabrasion, and can also work well in conjunction with or as an additional treatment to other cosmetic skin procedures such as chemical peels, blepharoplasty (eyelid) surgery, and liposuction of the face and neck.

# Chapter 21

# *Permanent Make-Up*

## *What is permanent cosmetics makeup?*

Permanent cosmetic makeup is cosmetic tattooing. The specialized techniques used for permanent cosmetics are often referred to as "micropigmentation," "micropigment implantation," or "dermagraphics". The cosmetic implantation technique deposits colored pigment into the upper reticular layer of the dermis.

## *How are permanent cosmetic procedures cone?*

Permanent cosmetics procedures are performed using various methods, including the traditional tattoo or coil machines, the pen or rotary machine, and the non-machine or hand method. The process includes an initial consultation, then application of pigment, and at least one or more follow up visits for adjusting the shape and color or density of the pigment.

## *Who benefits from permanent cosmetic makeup?*

Everyone, from the young to the elderly, who desires a soft, natural enhancement to their appearance. It is especially beneficial to people who can't wear other cosmetics due to allergies and skin sensitivities;

"Frequently Asked Questions about Permanent Cosmetics," © 2005 Society of Permanent Cosmetic Professionals. Reprinted with permission.

Active people who want to look their best for activities such as swimming, hiking, biking, tennis, aerobics, and those who don't want to worry about "sweating off" or reapplying cosmetics. Also the vision impaired who have difficulty applying their cosmetics, and others with motor impairments such as arthritis, Parkinson's disease, multiple sclerosis, stroke survivors, and those with unsteady hands who cannot apply their own makeup, and busy people who don't have time to spend on their makeup.

### What type of permanent cosmetic procedures can be done?

Permanent cosmetic procedures can be very subtle or dramatic depending on what you are looking for. Options include the following:

- Eyebrows
- Eyeliner, top and bottom
- Full lip color
- Scar camouflage
- Areola repigmentation
- Lash enhancement
- Hair imitation
- Beauty marks
- Lipliner and blend

Note that some of these procedures use more advanced techniques and thus require an experienced technician with advanced training.

### Are permanent cosmetics really permanent?

Technically, permanent cosmetics procedures are considered permanent because the color is implanted into the upper reticular part of the dermal layer of the skin and cannot be washed off. However, as with any tattoo, fading can and often does occur, requiring periodic maintenance, color re-enhancement, or color refreshing. Just like hair color, furniture that may be located near a window, or even house paint, pigment implanted in the skin may fade with time. It is important to consider this and all aspects of the procedure when selecting a potential permanent cosmetic makeup technician.

## How much does permanent makeup cost?

The average cost per procedure varies but usually averages between $400–$800. Advanced work may be charged at $150 to $250 per hour. Many of these procedures are commonly referred to as para-medical procedures. Work performed from physician's offices or specialized clinics may be charged at higher rates. The cost of the procedure should not be the most important issue when consulting a potential technician. Most important is the training and skill of the technician and the confidence of the client in that skill.

## How long does each procedure take?

The initial procedure will generally take approximately one to two and a half hours. Touch up procedures usually do not require as much time.

## Is it painful?

Most people experience some discomfort. This may vary according to each individual's pain threshold and the skills of the technician performing the service. However, there are different methods available to help with pain management, including various topical anesthetic ointments, anesthetic locals, and nerve blocks (administered by a doctor or dentist). Your technician should discuss these methods with you to determine which one suits you best.

## Is it safe?

If proper sterilization and sanitary guidelines are met, permanent cosmetics should be completely safe. These guidelines include the following:

- All needles should be new and sterile for each client. Other machine parts should also be pre-sterilized and disposed of in a sanitary manner. Other equipment and supplies should be kept in a sanitary manner.

- Gloves should be new for each client and changed during the procedure when needed.

- The technician should be clean and neat and knowledgeable of environmental safety requirements.

- Clean sheets should be used for each patient.

- The room or treatment area should be in an area free from other contaminants.

### What if I don't like it?

Although the procedure is considered permanent, these procedures do have flexibility in changing color and shape to some extent, depending on the expertise of your technician. Colors will appear darker immediately following the procedure but will soften and lighten during the healing process. The healing time is different for each individual and procedure.

### Which technician should I choose?

Choose a technician carefully by considering training, experience, and portfolio. It is important to remember that the shape and proper placement of the procedure is as important as the right color. The desired look is obtained during the course of consultation, initial procedure, and follow up procedures. Interaction between the client and the technician should be of utmost importance.

### Are there any after or side effects?

Generally, there is some swelling of the treated area. While eyebrows my show little after effect, eyeliner and lips may show more and the edema may last from two to seventy two hours. During the procedure there may be some bleeding and or bruising. There is usually some tenderness for a few days. The color is much darker than you may expect for the first six to ten days. Sometimes, people have reactions to antibiotics. You may use any type of antibiotic that you prefer for your individual system. There may be other side effects unforeseen due to individuality.

### Do the pigments pose allergy problems?

The application is just deep enough to penetrate the minute capillaries in the dermal layer of skin. There have been so few reactions to the pigments that some doctors are suggesting that the patch test be eliminated. You can develop an allergy to anything, anytime. Some doctors recommend that people with allergies have permanent cosmetic procedures because they can replace cosmetic products that they are sensitive to. There have been very few reactions to pigments and only rarely in the case of blue-based red pigments.

### *Is there any possibility for medical problems?*

The possibility that you would have any problems or reactions from these procedures is almost non-existent with today's health standards. SPCP (Society of Permanent Cosmetics Professionals) member professionals are given continued opportunities for education in practicing precise methods of sanitation and sterilization. Post procedural instructions, if followed carefully, will completely eliminate any risk.

### *What's a touch-up and do I need one?*

A touch-up is a color re-enhancement. Almost always the implanted color is not perfect after the first procedure. These procedures are processes and at least one follow-up to the initial procedure should be scheduled. It is recommended that you do not traumatize the skin again for a minimum of four weeks. Six weeks is better but of course, your individual needs take precedence. Eight weeks is recommended after a lip procedure.

### *Can I still have an MRI scan?*

Numerous studies have shown that even for people who have large body tattoos there is little to no potential for irritation resulting from a magnetic resonance imaging (MRI) scan. In the rare instance where discomfort resulted, it was localized and temporary. Most people have more metal in their fillings than they have in tattoo work. If you need an MRI, however, be sure to tell your healthcare providers that you have cosmetic tattoos so they can evaluate whether any special precautions would be prudent.

159

# Chapter 22

# *Varicose and Spider Veins*

### *What are varicose veins and spider veins?*

Varicose veins are enlarged veins that can be flesh colored, dark purple or blue. They often look like cords and appear twisted and bulging. They are swollen and raised above the surface of the skin. Varicose veins are commonly found on the backs of the calves or on the inside of the leg. During pregnancy, varicose veins called hemorrhoids can form in the vagina or around the anus.

Spider veins are similar to varicose veins, but they are smaller. They are often red or blue and are closer to the surface of the skin than varicose veins. They can look like tree branches or spider webs with their short jagged lines. Spider veins can be found on the legs and face. They can cover either a very small or very large area of skin.

### *What causes varicose veins and spider veins?*

The heart pumps blood filled with oxygen and nutrients to the whole body. Arteries carry blood from the heart towards the body parts. Veins carry oxygen-poor blood from the body back to the heart.

The squeezing of leg muscles pumps blood back to the heart from the lower body. Veins have valves that act as one-way flaps. These valves prevent the blood from flowing backwards as it moves up the

"Varicose Veins and Spider Veins," National Women's Health Information Center (www.4woman.gov), U.S. Department of Health and Human Services, December 2005.

legs. If the one-way valves become weak, blood can leak back into the vein and collect there. This problem is called venous insufficiency. Pooled blood enlarges the vein and it becomes varicose. Spider veins can also be caused by the backup of blood. Hormone changes, inherited factors, and exposure to the sun can also cause spider veins.

### How common are abnormal leg veins?

About 50% to 55% of American women and 40% to 45% of American men suffer from some form of vein problem. Varicose veins affect one out of two people age 50 and older.

### Who usually has varicose veins and spider veins?

Many factors increase a person's chances of developing varicose or spider veins. These include:

- Increasing age.

- Having family members with vein problems or being born with weak vein valves.

- Hormonal changes. These occur during puberty, pregnancy, and menopause. Taking birth control pills and other medicines containing estrogen and progesterone also increase the risk of varicose or spider veins.

- Pregnancy. During pregnancy there is a huge increase in the amount of blood in the body. This can cause veins to enlarge. The expanding uterus also puts pressure on the veins. Varicose veins usually improve within 3 months after delivery. A growing number of abnormal veins usually appear with each additional pregnancy.

- Obesity, leg injury, prolonged standing and other things that weaken vein valves.

- Sun exposure, which can cause spider veins on the cheeks or nose of a fair-skinned person.

### Why do varicose veins and spider veins usually appear in the legs?

The force of gravity, the pressure of body weight, and the task of carrying blood from the bottom of the body up to the heart make legs the primary location for varicose and spider veins. Compared with other veins in the body, leg veins have the toughest job of carrying blood back to the heart. They endure the most pressure. This pressure can be stronger than the veins' one-way valves.

### Are varicose veins and spider veins painful or dangerous?

Spider veins usually do not need medical treatment. But varicose veins usually enlarge and worsen over time. Severe varicose veins can cause health problems. These include:

- Severe venous insufficiency. This severe pooling of blood in the veins slows the return of blood to the heart. This condition can cause blood clots and severe infections. Blood clots can be very dangerous because they can move from leg veins and travel to the lungs. Blood clots in the lungs are life-threatening because they can block the heart and lungs from functioning.

- Sores or skin ulcers can occur on skin tissue around varicose veins.

- Ongoing irritation, swelling and painful rashes of the legs.

### What are the signs of varicose veins?

Some common symptoms of varicose veins include the following:

- Aching pain
- Easily tired legs
- Leg heaviness
- Swelling in the legs
- Darkening of the skin (in severe cases)
- Numbness in the legs
- Itching or irritated rash in the legs

### How can I prevent varicose veins and spider veins?

Not all varicose and spider veins can be prevented. But some things can reduce your chances of getting new varicose and spider veins. These same things can help ease discomfort from the ones you already have:

- Wear sunscreen to protect your skin from the sun and to limit spider veins on the face.

- Exercise regularly to improve your leg strength, circulation, and vein strength. Focus on exercises that work your legs, such as walking or running.

- Control your weight to avoid placing too much pressure on your legs.

- Do not cross your legs when sitting.

- Elevate your legs when resting as much as possible.

- Do not stand or sit for long periods of time. If you must stand for a long time, shift your weight from one leg to the other every few minutes. If you must sit for long periods of time, stand up and move around or take a short walk every 30 minutes.

- Wear elastic support stockings and avoid tight clothing that constricts your waist, groin, or legs.

- Eat a low-salt diet rich in high-fiber foods. Eating fiber reduces the chances of constipation which can contribute to varicose veins. High fiber foods include fresh fruits and vegetables and whole grains, like bran. Eating too much salt can cause you to retain water or swell.

### Should I see a doctor about varicose veins?

Remember these important questions when deciding whether to see your doctor: Has the varicose vein become swollen, red, or very tender or warm to the touch? If yes, see your doctor.

If no, are there sores or a rash on the leg or near the ankle with the varicose vein, or do you think there may be circulation problems in your feet? If yes, see your doctor. If no, continue to follow the self-care tips above.

### How are varicose and spider veins treated?

Besides a physical exam, your doctor can take x-rays or ultrasound pictures of the vein to find the cause and severity of the problem. You may want to speak with a doctor who specializes in vein diseases or phlebology. Talk to your doctor about what treatment options are best for your condition and lifestyle. Not all cases of varicose veins are the same.

Some available treatments include the following:

**Sclerotherapy:** This is the most common treatment for both spider veins and varicose veins. The doctor injects a solution into the vein that causes the vein walls to swell, stick together, and seal shut. This stops the flow of blood and the vein turns into scar tissue. In a few weeks, the vein should fade. The same vein may need to be treated more than once.

This treatment is very effective if done the right way. Most patients can expect a 50% to 90% improvement. Microsclerotherapy uses special solutions and injection techniques that increase the success rate for removal of spider veins. Sclerotherapy does not require anesthesia, and can be done in the doctor's office. Possible side effects include the following:

- Temporary stinging or painful cramps where the injection was made

- Temporary red raised patches of skin where the injection was made

- Temporary small skin sores where the injection was made

- Temporary bruises where the injection was made

- Spots around the treated vein that usually disappear

- Brown lines around the treated vein that usually disappear

- Groups of fine red blood vessels around the treated vein that usually disappear

- The treated vein can also become inflamed or develop lumps of clotted blood. This is not dangerous. Applying heat and taking aspirin or antibiotics can relieve inflammation. Lumps of coagulated blood can be drained.

**Laser surgery:** New technology in laser treatments can effectively treat spider veins in the legs. Laser surgery sends very strong bursts of light onto the vein. This can makes the vein slowly fade and disappear. Lasers are very direct and accurate. So the proper laser controlled by a skilled doctor will usually only damage the area being treated. Most skin types and colors can be safely treated with lasers.

Laser surgery is more appealing to some patients because it does not use needles or incisions. Still, when the laser hits the skin, the patient feels a heat sensation that can be quite painful. Cooling helps reduce the pain. Laser treatments last for 15 to 20 minutes. Depending on the severity of the veins, two to five treatments are generally needed to remove spider veins in the legs. Patients can return to normal activity right after treatment, just as with sclerotherapy. For spider veins larger than 3 mm, laser therapy is not very practical.

Possible side effects of laser surgery include the following:

- Redness or swelling of the skin right after the treatment that disappears within a few days

- Discolored skin that will disappear within one to two months

- Rarely burns and scars result from poorly performed laser surgery

**Endovenous techniques (radiofrequency and laser):** These methods for treating the deeper varicose veins of the legs (the saphenous veins) have been a huge breakthrough. They have replaced surgery for the vast majority of patients with severe varicose veins. This technique is not very invasive and can be done in a doctor's office.

The doctor puts a very small tube called a catheter into the vein. Once inside, the catheter sends out radiofrequency or laser energy that shrinks and seals the vein wall. Healthy veins around the closed vein restore the normal flow of blood. As this happens, symptoms from the varicose vein improve. Veins on the surface of the skin that are connected to the treated varicose vein will also usually shrink after treatment. When needed, these connected varicose veins can be treated with sclerotherapy or other techniques. Possible side effects include slight bruising.

### When is surgery used to treat varicose veins?

Surgery is used mostly to treat very large varicose veins. Types of surgery for varicose veins include the following:

**Surgical ligation and stripping:** With this treatment, problematic veins are tied shut and completely removed from the leg. Removing the veins does not affect the circulation of blood in the leg. Veins deeper in the leg take care of the larger volumes of blood. Most varicose veins removed by surgery are surface veins and collect blood only from the skin. This surgery requires either local or general anesthesia and must be done in an operating room on an outpatient basis.

Serious side effects or problems from this surgery are uncommon, but possible side effects include the following:

- With general anesthesia, a risk of heart and breathing problems.

- Bleeding and congestion of blood can be a problem. But the collected blood usually settles on its own and does not require any further treatment.

- Wound infection, inflammation, swelling and redness.

- Permanent scars.

- Damage of nerve tissue around the treated vein. It is hard to avoid harming small nerve branches when veins are removed. This damage can cause numbness, burning, or a change in sensation around the surgical scar.

- A deep vein blood clot. These clots can travel to the lungs and heart. Injections of heparin, a medicine that reduces blood clotting reduce the chance of these dangerous blood clots. But, heparin also can increase the normal amount of bleeding and bruising after surgery.

- Significant pain in the leg and recovery time of one to four weeks depending on the extent of surgery is typical after surgery.

**Ambulatory phlebectomy:** With this surgery, a special light source marks the location of the vein. Tiny cuts are made in the skin, and surgical hooks pull the vein out of the leg. This surgery requires local or regional anesthesia. The vein usually is removed in one treatment. Very large varicose veins can be removed with this treatment while leaving only very small scars. Patients can return to normal activity the day after treatment. Possible side effects include slight bruising and temporary numbness.

**Endoscopic vein surgery:** With this surgery, a small video camera is used to see inside the veins. Then varicose veins are removed through small cuts. People who have this surgery must have some kind of anesthesia including epidural, spinal, or general anesthesia. Patients can return to normal activity within a few weeks.

### Can varicose and spider veins return even after treatment?

Current treatments for varicose veins and spider veins have very high success rates compared to traditional surgical treatments. Over a period of years, however, more abnormal veins can develop. The major reason for this is that there is no cure for weak vein valves. So with time, pressure gradually builds up in the leg veins. Ultrasound can be used to keep track of how badly the valves are leaking (venous insufficiency). Ongoing treatment can help keep this problem under control.

The single most important thing a person can do to slow down the development of new varicose veins is to wear graduated compression support stockings as much as possible during the day.

# Chapter 23

# *Tattoos and Tattoo Removal*

## *Tattoos, Body Piercings, and Other Skin Adornments*

Tattoos, body piercings, and other skin adornments have become quite popular in modern society. These practices date back almost 5,300 years and may be fascinating as a part of many cultural rituals, or as signs of beauty; however, they may lead to problems such as keloids (thick scars), infections, allergies, growths, or permanent holes when people want them removed.

### *The Five Major Tattoo Types*

Traumatic tattoos are caused by the unwanted imbedding of dirt or debris beneath the skin which leaves an area of pigmentation after healing. This commonly occurs in "road rash" after a bicycle or motorcycle accident, or a puncture injury from a pencil known as a "graphite or pencil-point" tattoo.

Amateur tattoos are placed by the people themselves, or by their friends, and often show very little artistry or detail. The most common method involves placing India ink beneath the skin with a pin. Pen ink, charcoal, or ashes are also used as the pigment.

Professional tattoos take two forms: cultural and modern. Cultural tattoos are placed using the time-honored methods of a certain cultural ethnicity or heritage such as the South Pacific Islands. Modern tattoos are performed using the "tattoo gun" and are placed by "artists" who are paid for their work. A variety of pigments for different colors are used and their artistry varies from poor to fantastic.

Medical tattoos are commonly used to delineate permanent landmarks for radiation therapy and are placed by a physician.

Cosmetic tattoos are used for permanent make-up such as eyeliner, lip liner, lipstick, blush, hair, and eyebrows. Cosmetic tattooing is also used to replace a nipple after breast surgery, to camouflage vitiligo (the absence of pigment color), or to cover an undesired tattoo.

### *Tattoo Complications*

No matter what type of tattoo, there are always risks and possible adverse reactions that may require treatment. Infections may occur directly after tattooing. Impetigo, a staphylococcal (staph) infection, or cellulitis, a deeper skin infection, may develop. There is also a risk of bloodborne diseases such as hepatitis and HIV, although there has been no documented spread of HIV by a professional tattoo artist with experience. Universal precautions should be used by tattoo studios. Look for inspection certificates to be certain.

Hypersensitivity (allergies) may also develop to tattoo pigments. An allergy to mercury in the red color pigment called cinnabar was very common, but is no longer used. A chemical called paraphenylene-diamine, which is applied to the skin in temporary henna tattoos, frequently causes contact dermatitis.

Tattoos may interfere with proper medical tests like an MRI; misdiagnoses could be made due to the iron oxide and heavy metal pigments in the tattoos.

Scarring and keloid formation may also develop.

### *Tattoo Removal*

With time, many patients decide they no longer want to have a tattoo. Although there are many improved methods for the removal of tattoos like laser surgery, excision, dermabrasion, salabrasion, and cosmetic over-tattoo, it is still time-consuming, expensive, and may leave scars or discolorations. The treatment of tattoos with laser may entirely remove the pigment or only bring fair results. The skin is rarely as perfect as it once was prior to getting the tattoo.

## Body Piercing

Body piercing is another form of skin adornment. Jewelry is worn through the skin. Female ear piercing has long been accepted in Western culture, but in the last 25 years, male ear piercing and the piercing of other body areas has become widespread. Navel piercing has become fashionable. More extreme piercings of the eyebrows, nipples, lips, tongue, and genitals have also become common. Oral and genital piercing is often associated with reported sexual enhancement. Originating in Asia, artificial penile nodules (penis marbles) are made by placing plastic beads or pearls, beneath the skin of the penis.

## Body Piercing Complications

The most common complication of piercing is the development of keloids. This is seen frequently in African Americans. Treatment of keloids can be difficult requiring surgery, injections of steroids, or interferon. Topical creams, cryosurgery (liquid nitrogen), and a combination therapy can be used.

Vascular growths called pyogenic granulomas. These may bleed and must be removed.

Infection may be a problem. Cartilage piercing at the edge of the ear (pinna) increases the chance of a bacterial infection called pseudomonas. Abscess formations, chondritis (inflammation of cartilage) of the ears, Candida (yeast) infections, toxic shock syndrome, and sepsis (severe total body infections) may occur. There is risk of bloodborne diseases such as hepatitis and HIV especially among amateur piercers who do not clean equipment properly.

Embedding of jewelry (where the skin grows over the jewelry) may occur, and is often the result of studs that are too tight.

Hypersensitivity (allergies) to the nickel in some jewelry develops as an itchy, red skin reaction (dermatitis), and is chronic. People who are allergic to nickel should only wear stainless steel, platinum, or gold jewelry.

## Piercing Removal

The forcible removal of the jewelry by accidental trauma may cause a permanent deformity which can be repaired with surgery. Trauma to the teeth from oral jewelry may require restorative (crowns or bonding) dentistry.

Since piercing is not "accepted" by many employers, removal of the jewelry may leave unsightly "holes," which also requires surgery to correct.

### Other Skin Adornments

Some individuals want to form a keloid.

The more permanent the scar, the better. Scarification is a skin adornment that takes two forms—branding and cutting. Branding is the use of a hot metal design, which burns the design into the skin. This is a recognized ritual behavior in some college fraternities. Cuttings are also done in the skin using a sharp knife or scalpel to leave permanent scarifications.

A newer body modification procedure includes tongue splitting which gives a person a forked split tongue. Besides the complications of infection and bloodborne disease, this may lead to a permanent lisp.

Think before attempting any of the procedures. Only use a trained professional with experience and proper hygienic technique. Be sure of what you want and discuss it. If there is a problem, see a dermatologist quickly.

## Tips to Consider when Obtaining a Tattoo or Piercing

Without giving it much thought, many choose to brand themselves with a tattoo or body piercing to express their personality, but today's trend may be tomorrow's regret. As a result, many of yesterday's trendsetters choose to remove piercings and undergo laser tattoo removal. According to the American Society for Dermatologic Surgery (ASDS), there are several dos and don'ts people should consider before getting a tattoo or piercing that would help if and when the removal process comes along.

### Dos

- Do choose a facility carefully: Make sure the establishment is reputable and licensed to perform these procedures.

- Do keep things simple: A small tattoo or one with two or three colors is the easiest to remove, as well as conceal; and simple piercings in the ear are classic symbols of style that never get out of style.

- Do choose an appropriate location: Because outlandish piercings or tattoos in unusual and sensitive areas can lead to scarring and holes that never heal, you may want to think twice about where to place these items on your body. Also, think carefully about where you want it and how big it should be. A good tip is to place it in an area that can be covered by clothing traditionally worn in the work place. For example, a belly button piercing can easily be covered but shown off if you wish, whereas an eye brow piercing can not.

- Do remember what's "hot" today may not be tomorrow: Today, the latest fad may be tribal or flower tattoos, but tomorrow's trends may be different. That lip ring may not be so popular when you are a soccer mom driving the car pool. So, think about down the road and what you'll be happy with in the years ahead.

*Don'ts*

- Don't administer self-piercings or tattoos: Attempting to pierce yourself or give yourself a tattoo is extremely dangerous and can lead to infections, serious health complications, and even death.

- Don't have a procedure in unsanitary conditions: Sterile equipment and supplies should always be used for tattoos and piercings. Look out for unacceptable conditions, such as the use of needles on more than one patient and technicians who don't wear gloves.

- Don't let an infection go: If you suspect any problems, or experience considerable redness or soreness, see your dermasurgeon immediately—it may signal an infection.

## Tattoo Removal

### Tattoos

A tattoo used to be a permanent and irreversible adornment to one's skin. However, in recent years dermatologic surgeons have developed safe and effective techniques to successfully remove unwanted tattoos.

Patients request removal of a tattoo for a variety of reasons—social, cultural, or physical. Some patients develop an allergic reaction to a tattoo several years after the initial application. Because each tattoo is unique, removal techniques must be tailored to suit each individual case. For instance, professionally applied tattoos tend to penetrate the deeper layers of the skin at uniform levels. This uniformity allows dermatologic surgeons to use techniques that remove broader areas of inked skin at the same depth.

Homemade tattoos are often applied with an uneven hand and their removal may be more difficult. Deeper blue and black ink colors are particularly difficult to remove. Professional tattoos made with some of the newer inks and pastel colors may also be difficult to remove entirely.

### Removing Tattoos

Tattoos can be removed by a dermatologic surgeon on an outpatient basis with local anesthesia. The most common techniques used are:

**Laser Surgery:** The surgeon removes the tattoo by selectively treating the pigment colors with a high-intensity laser beam. Lasers have become the standard treatment because they offer a "bloodless," low risk, highly effective approach with minimal side effects. The type of laser used generally depends upon the pigment colors. In many cases, multiple treatments may be required.

**Dermabrasion:** The surgeon "sands" the skin, removing the surface and middle layers of the tattoo. The combination of surgical and dressing techniques helps to raise and absorb the tattoo inks.

**Surgical Excision:** The surgeon removes the tattoo with a scalpel and closes the wound with stitches. This technique proves highly effective in removing some tattoos and allows the surgeon to excise inked areas with great control.

### Are There Side Effects or Complications?

Side effects are generally minor, but may include skin discoloration at the treatment site, infection of the tattoo site, lack of complete pigment removal, or some scarring. A raised or thickened scar may appear three to six months after the tattoo is removed.

# Chapter 24

# *Hair Removal*

As you browse the aisles of your local drugstore, you may feel a little dizzy. There are hundreds of products devoted to making the hair on your head more lustrous, clean, fragrant, and full—and just steps away, dozens more promise to get rid of your unwanted hair just as easily. Which ones work best? How do they work? And do you need any of them?

## *Different Types of Hair*

Before removing hair, it helps to know about the different types of hair on our bodies. All hair is made of keratin, a hard protein that's also found in your fingernails and toenails. Hair growth begins beneath the surface of your skin at a hair root inside a hair follicle, a small tube in the skin.

You have two types of hair on your body. Vellus hair is soft, fine, and short. Most women have vellus hair on the chest, back, and face. It can be darker and more noticeable in some women than others—especially women with darker complexions. Vellus hair helps the body maintain a steady temperature by providing some insulation.

Terminal hair is coarser, darker, and longer than vellus hair and is the type of hair that grows on your head. When a teen reaches puberty,

This information was provided by TeensHealth, one of the largest resources online for medically reviewed health information written for parents, kids, and teens. For more articles like this one, visit www.TeensHealth.org, or www.KidsHealth.org. © 2004 The Nemours Foundation.

terminal hair starts to grow in the armpits and pubic region. On guys, terminal hair begins to grow on the face and other parts of the body such as the chest, legs, and back. Terminal hair provides cushioning and protection.

In some cases, excess hair growth, called hirsutism, may be the result of certain medical conditions. In girls, polycystic ovary syndrome and other hormonal disorders can cause dark, coarse hair to grow on the face, especially the upper lip, and on the arms, chest, and legs. Some medications, like anabolic steroids, can also cause hirsutism.

## Getting Rid of Hair

### Shaving

**How It Works:** Using a razor, a person removes the tip of the hair shaft that has grown out through the skin. Some razors are completely disposable, some have a disposable blade, and some are electric. Guys often shave their faces, and women often shave their underarms, legs, and bikini areas.

**How Long It Lasts:** 1 to 3 days

**Pros:** Shaving is fairly inexpensive. All you need is some warm water, a razor, and if you choose, shaving gel or cream. You don't need an appointment—shaving is a do-it-yourself endeavor, resulting in smooth, hairless skin.

**Cons:** Razor burn, bumps, nicks, cuts, and ingrown hairs are side effects of shaving. Ingrown hairs occur when hairs are cut below the level of the skin. When the hair begins to grow, it grows within the surrounding tissue rather than growing out of the follicle. The hair curls around and starts growing into the skin, and irritation, redness, and swelling can occur at the hair follicle.

**Tips:** Look for blades that have safety guard wires—they minimize nicks and cuts. Also, you'll get a closer shave if you shave in the shower after your skin has been softened by warm water. Go slowly, change your blades often to avoid nicks, and use a moisturizing cream to soften the hair. Although most people shave in the opposite direction from the hair growth, if you want to avoid ingrown hairs it can help to shave in the direction the hair grows. If you have an ingrown hair, try exfoliating (removing dead skin cells with a loofah), sterilizing a pointed pair of tweezers with rubbing alcohol, and attempting to pluck out the ingrown hair.

## *Plucking*

**How It Works:** Using tweezers, a person stretches the skin tightly, grips the hair close to the root, and pulls it out.

**How Long It Lasts:** 3 to 8 weeks

**Pros:** Plucking is time-consuming because you can only remove one hair at a time. However, it's inexpensive because all you need are tweezers.

**Cons:** Plucking can be painful, so it's best to do it only on small areas, such as the eyebrows, upper lip, and chin. If the hair breaks off below the skin, a person may get an ingrown hair. After plucking, you may notice temporary red bumps because the hair follicle is swollen and irritated.

**Tips:** Make sure you sterilize your tweezers with rubbing alcohol before and after use to reduce the chance of infection.

## *Depilatories*

**How They Work:** A depilatory is a cream or liquid that removes hair from the skin's surface. They work by reacting with the protein structure of the hair, so the hair dissolves and can be washed or wiped away.

**How Long They Last:** Several days to 2 weeks

**Pros:** Depilatories work quickly, are readily available at drugstores and grocery stores, and are inexpensive. They're best on the leg, underarm, and bikini areas; special formulations may be used on the face and chin.

**Cons:** Applying depilatories can be messy and many people dislike the odor. If you have sensitive skin, you might have an allergic reaction to the chemicals in the depilatory, which may cause a rash or inflammation. Depilatories may not be as effective on people with coarse hair.

**Tips:** Read product directions carefully and be sure to apply the product only for the recommended amount of time for best results.

## Waxing

**How It Works:** A sticky wax is spread on the area of skin where the unwanted hair is growing. A cloth strip is then applied over the wax and quickly pulled off, taking the hair root and dead skin cells with it. The wax can be warmed or may be applied cold. Waxing can be done at a salon or at home.

**How Long It Lasts:** 3 to 6 weeks

**Pros:** Waxing leaves the area smooth and is long lasting. Waxing kits are readily available in drugstores and grocery stores. Hair regrowth looks lighter and less noticeable than it is after other methods of hair removal, such as shaving.

**Cons:** Many people mention that the biggest drawback to waxing is the pain when the hair is ripped out by the root. A person may notice temporary redness, inflammation, and bumps after waxing. Professional waxing is also expensive compared to other hair removal methods.

People with diabetes should avoid waxing because they are more susceptible to infection. Also, teens who use acne medications such as tretinoin and isotretinoin may want to skip the wax because those medicines make the skin more sensitive. Teens with moles or skin irritation from sunburn should also avoid waxing.

**Tips:** For waxing to work, hair should be at least 1/4 inch (about 6 millimeters) long, so skip shaving for a few weeks before waxing. Waxing works best on legs, bikini areas, and eyebrows.

## Electrolysis

**How It Works:** Over a series of several appointments, a professional electrologist inserts a needle into the follicle and sends an electric current through the hair root, killing it. A small area such as the upper lip may take a total of 4 to 10 hours and a larger area such as the bikini line may take 8 to 16 hours.

**How Long It Lasts:** Permanently

**Pros:** Electrolysis is the only type of hair removal that is permanent.

**Cons:** Electrolysis takes big bucks and lots of time, so it's usually only used on smaller areas such as the upper lip, eyebrows, and underarms. Many people describe the process as painful, and dry skin, scabs, scarring, and inflammation may result after treatment. Infection may be a risk if the needles and other instruments aren't properly sterilized.

**Tips:** Talk to your doctor if you're interested in this method. He or she may be able to recommend an electrologist with the proper credentials.

### Laser Hair Removal

**How It Works:** A laser is directed through the skin to the hair follicle, where it stops growth. It works best on light-skinned people with dark hair because the melanin (colored pigment) in the hair absorbs more of the light, making treatment more effective.

**How Long It Lasts:** 6 months

**Pros:** This type of hair removal is long lasting and large areas of skin can be treated at the same time.

**Cons:** A treatment session may cost $500 or more. Side effects of the treatment may include inflammation and redness.

**Tips:** Using cold packs may help diminish any inflammation after treatment. Avoiding the sun before a treatment may make results more effective.

### Prescription Treatments

A cream called eflornithine is available by prescription to treat facial hair growth (generally in women). The cream is applied twice a day until the hair becomes softer and lighter—more like vellus hair. Side effects may include skin irritation and acne. Talk to your doctor or dermatologist if you are concerned about hair growth and removal.

Antiandrogen medications are another method that doctors prescribe to reduce the appearance of unwanted hair. Because the hormone androgen can be responsible for hair growth in unwanted areas, anti-androgens can block androgen production. Oral contraceptives are frequently used in conjunction with these medications to enhance their effect and to help regularize the menstrual cycle in girls who need it.

Deciding to remove body hair is a personal choice—getting rid of body hair doesn't make a person healthier, and you shouldn't feel pressured to do so if you don't want to. Some cultures view body hair as beautiful and natural, so do what feels right to you!

# Chapter 25

# *Hair Restoration*

## *Medical Hair Restoration for Hair Loss*

When you consult family, friends, library, and the internet about hair loss treatments, you will find a host of "do-it-yourself" hair loss products such as creams, ointments, lotions, nutrition supplements, scalp stimulants, and other "miracle cures", all promising to stop hair loss and regrow hair.

Among all the options for nonsurgical treatment of androgenetic alopecia (pattern baldness), you will find only two that have been approved by the U.S. Food and Drug Administration (FDA), and are recommended by physician hair restoration specialists. Hair restoration products not approved by the FDA are often a waste of money and can be harmful.

---

This chapter includes "Medical Hair Restoration for Hair Loss," © 2005 International Society of Hair Restoration Surgery; "Hair Transplant Surgery for Hair Restoration," © 2005 International Society of Hair Restoration Surgery; "Scalp Reduction Surgery for Hair Restoration," © 2005 International Society of Hair Restoration Surgery. "Scalp Expansion Surgery and Bald Scalp Excision," © 2005 International  Society of Hair Restoration Surgery; "Scalp Flap Surgery for Hair Restoration," © 2005 International Society of Hair Restoration Surgery; and "Hair Loss and Restoration in Women," © 2004 International Society of Hair Restoration Surgery. All six documents are reprinted with permission. For additional information, visit www.ishrs.org, or call toll free 800-444-2737.

## Using Rogaine for Hair Loss

Minoxidil (Rogaine®) is applied topically to the scalp in 2% or 5% solution. Minoxidil is available over-the-counter in 2% solution, but is best and most effectively used in a treatment program planned and supervised by a physician hair restoration specialist. Rogaine tends to be more effective in women than in men.

## Using Propecia for Hair Loss

Finasteride (Propecia®) is an orally-administered medication that influences the response of scalp hair follicles to androgenic hormones. Finasteride is available only by prescription to men.

Determining which medicine or combination of medicines is right for you will depend on your age, degree of hair loss, and budget. For many people, the best results will be achieved by combining Rogaine or Propecia treatments with hair restoration surgery.

## About Hairpieces and Extensions

When custom-made under the supervision of a hair specialist, hairpieces and hair additions can meet the needs of selected patients who may not be suitable candidates for hair restoration surgery.

# Hair Transplant Surgery for Hair Restoration

Hair transplantation is an operation that takes hair from the back of the head and moves it to the area of hair loss. The fringe (back and sides) of hair on a balding scalp is known as donor dominant hair which is the hair that will continue to grow throughout the life of most men. The transplantation of this hair to a bald area does not change its ability to grow. Donor dominance is the scientific basis for the success of hair transplantation. Dr. Okuda of Japan first described the use of transplanted hair to repair scarred eyelashes and eyebrows. Unfortunately, the outbreak of World War II prevented his valuable discovery from reaching the rest of the world for two decades. Dr. Norman Orentreich published the first widely read report on hair transplantation surgery in 1959 and the field of hair transplant surgery was born.

Candidates for hair transplant surgery are those individuals with hair loss that have sufficient donor hair from the fringe of the scalp to transplant to the balding area. In the past, many bald patients were not suitable candidates for hair transplant surgery but modern techniques have advanced the art of hair transplant surgery so that many more men are candidates.

Hair transplantation surgery has improved in leaps and bounds over the past decade. The days of the "plugs and corn rows" are gone and the age of single hair-, micro-, and mini- grafting has arrived. Through the use of the these variable sized hair grafts along with new and improved instrumentation, the accomplished hair transplantation surgeons can create a natural hair appearance that is appropriate for each individual patient. Single hair-grafts have the finest and softest appearance. Although they do not provide much density, they do provide the critical soft hairline that is the transition to thicker hair. Reconstructing a new hairline is a skill requiring surgical as well as artistic skill. It is critically important to get it right the first time and thus requires considerable forethought and planning. Examining the hairline of a non-balding person will show the presence of numerous single hairs in the very frontal hairline. Micrografts are small grafts containing two to three hairs that are placed behind the hairline to provide a gradually increasing hair density. Lastly, minigrafts contain four or more hairs are placed well behind the hairline so that the single hair and micrografts can blend naturally into the density provided by these larger grafts.

There is different terminology and techniques used by many ISHRS (International Society of Hair Restoration Surgery) surgeons. This is because ISHRS surgeons are innovators and are on the cutting edge of hair transplant surgery. New techniques naturally give rise to new terms. Although there are variations in the techniques of individual surgeons, the combination use of these grafting techniques provide the most natural and pleasing results.

The side-effects of hair transplantation surgery are relatively minor consisting of mild pain and discomfort after the operation, swelling which may move down to the eyes, and the formation of scabs over the grafts which take approximately one week to resolve. Serious problems of bleeding, scarring, and infection are rare. Modern hair transplantation surgery is comfortable, predictable, and the results are pleasing to most patients.

Hair loss, however, is a life long process, most men will develop male pattern baldness (due to male hormones) until approximately 40–45 years of age. After that, the aging process thins the entire head of hair. Progressive hair loss or the desire for more density, will require more transplant procedures. Modern techniques, however, allow hair transplant surgery specialists of transplant larger number of grafts, greatly reducing the number of procedures needed to complete the result.

## Scalp Reduction Surgery for Hair Restoration

Alopecia reduction—also called scalp reduction—is a surgical hair restoration procedure that surgically removes bald scalp, and stretches hair-bearing scalp upward to replace bald scalp that has been removed. In selected patients alopecia reduction is a very effective method of hair restoration when performed by a skilled and experienced physician hair restoration specialist. Depending on individual patient characteristics, alopecia reduction may be performed as the only hair restoration procedure desired by the patient, in combination with hair transplantation to achieve a desired aesthetic effect, or occasionally in combination with the aesthetic surgical procedure called brow lifting to remove frown lines from the forehead and crow's feet from around the eyes.

Good candidates for alopecia reduction are patients with excellent donor hair on the sides and back of the scalp that can be stretched upward to cover areas of excised bald scalp. A good supply of donor hair is also needed to provide donor grafts for any supplementary hair transplantation. Alopecia reduction may, in selected patients, be carried out by using a scalp extension or scalp expansion device—a technique that stretches hair-bearing scalp skin to provide greater coverage in bald areas.

### *Indications and Patient Selection: Is Alopecia Reduction Right for You?*

Any non-emergency surgical procedure must be justified by its applicability and ultimate value to the patient. This is especially true for elective cosmetic procedures such as hair restoration. Full and frank discussion between patient and physician hair restoration specialist is essential to determining whether an elective procedure is right for you, the patient.

Alopecia reduction can be a very successful approach to hair restoration. Is it right for you? A number of factors can bear upon that decision:

- **Physical condition:** The patient should be in good general health and have no medical conditions that would rule out a surgical procedure.

- **Degree and pattern of hair loss:** The patient and the physician hair restoration specialist should together make the final decision as to whether alopecia reduction is a good choice for hair restoration. In general, alopecia reduction is likely to be most useful in a patient who has a large area of scalp baldness and an adequate supply of good-quality donor hair on the sides and back of the scalp. Another consideration is the rapidity of alopecia progression and the likelihood that alopecia will significantly progress in the future. These factors will influence the need to consider future hair transplantation to keep pace with an ever-expanding zone of baldness. The patient who undergoes alopecia reduction should be willing and able to have future alopecia reduction and/or hair transplantation and/or correction of surgical complications as the need arises.

- **Tightness or laxity of scalp skin:** Scalp skin that has very little laxity (the ability to stretch) may not be a good foundation for alopecia reduction. The rationale for alopecia reduction is that bald scalp can be surgically removed and hair-bearing scalp skin stretched up to cover the excised area. A substantial degree of scalp skin laxity is required to make the procedure work well.

- **The patient's objectives:** What do you, the patient, want hair restoration to accomplish? Your objectives, discussed thoroughly with the physician hair restoration specialist, will be a major factor in determining if alopecia reduction is a good option for you. For example, alopecia reduction may be a good option for a patient who wants to "pull up" all available donor hair to provide dense coverage of the scalp—given that other factors such as scalp laxity are favorable to that decision.

## *Alopecia Reduction and Hair Transplantation*

Alopecia reduction is often combined with hair transplantation. Hair transplantation may be combined with alopecia reduction to "fine tune" hair restoration in aesthetically sensitive areas, such as the frontal hairline that is not treated with alopecia reduction. Hair transplantation may be necessary in future years to keep pace with continued loss of hair. In younger patients, hair transplantation may be done first to restore the frontal one-third of the scalp, with alopecia reduction reserved for later years if hair loss progresses.

Alopecia reduction surgery can be done before, during or after hair transplantation, as indicated by the needs and wishes of the patient and the assessment of the physician hair restoration specialist. The timing of combined alopecia reduction and hair transplantation can be a critical decision that requires full discussion and understanding

185

between patient and physician hair restoration specialist. The decision must be individualized to the patient, based upon considerations that include the patient's objectives for hair restoration, cost of multiple procedures, degree of likely progression of hair loss, and the patient's age as a factor in likely progression of hair loss over a longer or shorter period of time.

### Alopecia Reduction Techniques

A number of alopecia reduction techniques have been developed. No one technique is adaptable to all patients. Choice of technique is based upon considerations that may include degree of hair loss, scalp laxity, amount and quality of donor hair, and whether hair transplantation is to be a complementary procedure. Alopecia reduction technique is largely a matter of the pattern of scalp incision—for example, "Y" pattern, "star" pattern, or "lateral crescent" pattern. The choice of technique and rationale for the choice should be discussed by patient and physician.

### Potential Complications and Side Effects

Careful planning and expert surgical skills are required to achieve good results in alopecia reduction. Complications are uncommon but there can be postoperative complications such as scarring at the suture lines, "stretch back" of scalp skin at the excised bald area, and a central midline scar called a slot deformity.

Side effects of alopecia reduction surgery are temporary discomfort, swelling, and numbness in the operated area.

## Scalp Expansion Surgery and Bald Scalp Excision

As a method of alopecia reduction for surgical hair restoration, scalp expansion surgery using a balloon-type device implanted under the scalp is called volumetric expansion. Scalp expansion using implanted physical instrumentation is called nonvolumetric expansion or scalp extension. The expansion and excision of bald scalp creates the conditions for subsequent approximation of hair-bearing scalp to cover the area of bald scalp excision. The man most likely to benefit from bald scalp excision and hair-bearing scalp advancement is a man who has enough hair at the sides and back of the head to provide adequate coverage after bald scalp excision, and does not have rapidly progressive male-pattern hair loss.

Although hair transplantation is by far the most commonly performed type of surgical hair restoration procedure some patients may be candidates for scalp reduction or scalp flaps. Some surgeons advocate the use of these procedures in some patients, and the procedures may be choices recommended by a surgeon in selected patients. The scalp reduction of scalp flap procedures can be performed with or without scalp expansion.

Skin has an enormous capacity to expand in response to under-the-skin pressure. The degree to which scalp tissue can expand in response to under-the-scalp pressure is seen naturally in people who have untreated hydrocephalus or large epithelial tumors of the scalp. A more common example of skin expansion in response to under-the-skin pressure is the remarkable ability of skin to "stretch" during pregnancy.

### *Volumetric Scalp Expansion*

The basic principles of volumetric scalp expansion are to expand the bald scalp over a period of time with a balloon-type device implanted under the scalp, collapse and withdraw the device when scalp expansion reaches a predetermined extent, excise the excess scalp skin, advance hair-bearing scalp to cover the area of bald scalp excision, and suture the hair-bearing scalp to complete the correction of male-pattern hair loss.

An implantable balloon-type scalp skin expander was first used for medical purposes about 25 years ago to facilitate surgical removal of a tattoo. By the early 1980s the technique of tissue expansion and bald scalp excision was being pioneered at Hershey (Pennsylvania) Medical Center for treatment of massive scalp defects in children. By the mid-1980s the technique was being used by physician hair restoration specialists to treat selected patients with male-pattern hair loss.

Volumetric scalp expansion begins with the insertion of a Silastic (non tissue reactive) envelope beneath the scalp. The envelope is inserted into the subgaleal plane, a space of loose tissue between the overlying scalp and the blood vessel-rich tissue underneath. The subgaleal space is nearly devoid of blood vessels, so insertion of the envelope causes little bleeding and does not compromise blood or nerve supply to the scalp. As a rule, envelopes are inserted on right and left sides of the head to fit the distribution of bald scalp.

About two weeks after insertion of the device, a small amount of saline fluid is injected into the envelope through self-sealing ports to begin inflation of the devices and to begin the process of scalp expansion.

Injections of saline are repeated at intervals over succeeding weeks and the scalp responds by expanding. If there are scalp expanders on opposite sides of the head they may be injected in alternate weeks.

Volumetric scalp expansion causes a visible change in head shape as the device inflate. Friends and relatives can be prepared for this temporary change. Strangers may be less prepared. Hats or other head covering can be worn to make the change in head shape less apparent. A good relationship between patient and physician hair restoration specialist can prepare the patient for managing any psychological, emotional, or social problems that may arise during the temporary period of scalp expansion.

When scalp expansion is judged to be satisfactory the devices are drained and removed. The patient is taken to an operating room for gathering expanded bald scalp into a "pleat" for excision, excising the pleated bald scalp, advancing hair-bearing scalp to cover the areas of excised bald scalp, and suturing the hair-bearing scalp to create a total or near-total correction of hair loss.

Individual patients may require follow-up treatment such as "fill-in" hair transplantation and use of hair restoration pharmaceuticals (minoxidil or finasteride) to achieve the maximum cosmetic improvement. "Fill-in" hair transplantation may be made more difficult and costly by scalp expansion and excision, however; bald scalp excision and hair-bearing scalp approximation may reduce the number of donor follicles that can be harvested in a single transplantation session, thus increasing the time and dollar investment of "fill-in" hair transplantation.

Patients can usually shower and shampoo the day after surgery, not waiting until sutures are removed. Healing takes place over the following two to six weeks. Postoperative bleeding and infection are potential complications of volumetric scalp expansion and bald scalp excision. Sometimes a postoperative scar forms at the site of hairline suturing. A scar can be revised later to make it unapparent, but revision is more technically difficult when the scar is a so-called "slot defect" that forms where two previously non-adjacent areas of scalp are sutured together.

### Nonvolumetric Scalp Expansion

Nonvolumetric scalp expansion is accomplished with a physical device. Expansion may be over a period to time (one to three months) using a stretchable band implanted in the subgaleal space under constant tension. Scalp expansion may also be accomplished during a scalp reduction procedure using a skin-stretching device.

Advantages cited for the implanted nonvolumetric scalp expander include:

- 50% increase in the amount of bald scalp removed in scalp reduction.

- fewer procedures are needed to accomplish a final result.

- reduced "stretchback" of scalp skin and subsequent scarring.

- reduced postoperative hair loss.

- early development of postoperative scalp laxity.

Potential complications and side effects of nonvolumetric scalp expansion include:

- mild to severe pain during the first 24 hours after the scalp-expanding device is implanted.

- occasional bruising or edema in scalp over the implanted device.

- reduction in the number of donor grafts that can be harvested per session later for "fill-in".

- hair transplantation should this be needed to achieve the desired hair restoration goal.

- postoperative scarring at the site where hair-bearing scalp is sutured together—most difficult to revise when the scar is a so-called "slot defect" the forms at the site where two previously non-adjacent scalp areas are now joined by suturing.

- postoperative drainage and delayed wound healing for up to several weeks rarely, infection in the tissue around the implanted device.

## Scalp Flap Surgery for Hair Restoration

Skin flap surgery is a method of moving a "flap" of skin and underlying tissue from one area of the body to another. It is surgery performed to repair a non-traumatic cosmetic defect such as male pattern hair loss, repair a site of traumatic injury to restore its functionality and cosmetic appearance, or repair a skin defect caused by a congenital malformation.

The flaps used in both cosmetic and reconstructive surgery are either "pedicle" flaps or "free" flaps:

- Pedicle flaps are flaps that are surgically removed from a donor site and transferred to a recipient site with an attached pedicle of tissue that contains the flap's artery-vein blood supply along with the flap tissue. Transfer of artery-vein blood supply along with the flap improves the survival and health of the transferred tissue. Pedicle flaps are the type most often used for cosmetic hair restoration.

- The free flap is called "free" because it is transferred from donor site to recipient site without any attached pedicle. However, it must contain arteries and veins that are reattached to blood vessels at the recipient site by microvascular surgery. Free flaps are often used in reconstructive surgery when local skin is not sufficient to raise a pedicle flap to cover a defect—for example, to cover a substantial area of scarred scalp tissue. In recent years, free flaps have been used for cosmetic hair restoration by skilled and highly trained physician hair restoration specialists.

Scalp flap surgery has an important but limited role in hair restoration. The surgeon who performs the procedure must be a skilled physician hair restoration specialist with specific training and experience in use of skin flaps for hair restoration. In the hands of an appropriately trained and experienced surgeon, scalp flap surgery can be a highly successful approach to hair restoration in carefully selected patients.

### Patient Selection

Patients with frontal baldness exclusively are good candidates for scalp flap hair restoration, but many physician hair restoration specialists do not regard scalp flap surgery as first-choice treatment for frontal baldness. The choice of scalp flap surgery, hair transplantation, scalp extension, or scalp expansion as first-choice treatment for frontal baldness should be weighed carefully in discussions between patient and physician hair restoration specialist.

Frontal baldness may be in any degree from "frontal only" to "frontal to mid-scalp". When scalp flap surgery is the treatment selected, the rotation of one flap or multiple flaps from the hair-bearing donor area of the scalp to the bald area provides instantaneous full hair coverage; narrow gaps between transferred flaps may require some subsequent "touch-up" by hair transplantation or alopecia reduction procedures.

More extensively bald men with vertex (crown of the head) balding may benefit substantially from scalp flap hair restoration with proper preoperative planning, and when the procedure is performed by a skilled, experienced physician hair restoration specialist.

## *Evolution of Scalp Flap Surgery for Hair Restoration*

Scalp flap surgery for hair restoration was performed as early as the 1930s but did not become an established technique at that time. In 1969, plastic surgeon Dr. José Juri, Buenos Aires, Argentina, reported development of the scalp flap techniques that are the basis for practically all scalp flap techniques for hair restoration in use today. A master of flap surgery, Dr. Juri uses both pedicle and free flaps as a method of choice for treating baldness of various types and degrees as well as baldness due to various causes.

However, since the 1980s, the majority of physician hair restoration specialists prefer hair transplantation and alopecia reduction as first-line treatments for cosmetic hair restoration because of the success of these methods. Scalp flaps now tend to be reserved to correct traumatic and congenital defects in reconstructive hair restoration.

## *Facts about Scalp Flaps*

**Pedicle flaps:** The transfer of tissue from one site to another on the scalp is usually done in a series of procedures a week or more apart. These procedures include planning and marking the flaps and recipient sites, incising the flap, raising and transferring the flap with its attached pedicle of blood vessels, and closing the wound at the donor site. The same series of procedures are carried out for any subsequent flap procedures.

Planning for flap transfer to a bald area must include a consideration of hair direction in the transferred flap. Hair does not grow in a uniform direction on all areas of the scalp-it grows in several different directions on various scalp areas. Planning of flap transfer from donor to recipient area should aim to avoid the potential problem of distorted hair pattern that can be a complication of scalp flap surgery.

Although scalp flap surgery produces immediate heavy growth of hair over bald areas, there may be narrow gaps of thin or no hair between multiple flaps. Subsequent hair transplantation or alopecia reduction may be necessary to close these gaps. Adjustments in hair styling may be all that is needed to disguise small differences in hair growth direction and narrow bands of thin hair growth between flaps.

Some potentially serious complications of scalp flap surgery are:

- Failure of blood supply to the flap due to "kinking" or pressure on the flap's blood supply, resulting in partial or total loss of the flap;

- Transection of nerves during surgery with resulting loss of feeling over all or part of the scalp;

- Scarring at donor or recipient sites; and, Permanent loss of hair at donor sites that could be necessary for future hair transplantation.

**Microsurgical free flaps:** The "free" flap is surgically removed from the donor site and transferred to the recipient site without any attached blood supply. The free flap must, however, have a well defined arteriovenous system that can be reattached to the recipient site's circulation by microsurgery.

Surgeon innovators of microsurgical free flaps for cosmetic hair restoration have presented results showing that use of microsurgical flaps can eliminate the complications of distorted hair pattern and inconsistent hair density. They recommend microsurgical free flaps as a treatment of choice of various types and degrees of baldness. It is important to note that microsurgery is an advanced technique in cosmetic and reconstructive surgery that requires great skill, training and experience. Most physician hair restoration specialists have not sought such training and would not recommend use of microsurgical flaps for cosmetic hair restoration.

**Scalp expansion:** Expansion of hair-bearing scalp by the technique of scalp expansion can also be characterized as a scalp flap technique. The expanded hair-bearing scalp created by scalp expansion makes more hair-bearing scalp available for a variety of flaps useful in the treatment of alopecia. Several procedures are necessary to achieve a final result: placement of the expander under the scalp, inflation of the expander over a period of weeks, removal of the expander, creation and transfer of flaps from donor to recipient area, and closure of the wound at the donor site. Patients with an extensive area of baldness may require a second expansion series to achieve complete coverage.

Skilled and experienced physician hair restoration specialists who use this technique cite its advantages as:

- Excellent frontal coverage,

- Natural horizontal frontal hairline,

- Excellent design of hair placement in temporal areas, and

- Good hair direction and avoidance of distorted hair pattern.

Scarring at the temple regions is a potential complication of the expansion/flap technique.

As for other flap procedures, the expansion/flap procedure should be performed only by skilled and experienced physician hair restoration specialists who have training in dermatologic or plastic surgery.

## Hair Loss and Restoration in Women

A man may expect to lose hair as he gets older, especially if his father, uncles, or other near relatives had male-pattern baldness. A woman does not generally expect to lose hair even if there is a history of hair loss in male or female relatives. In the United States, at least, there has been a general belief that thinning hair and baldness is a "male thing."

A woman also usually feels she must have a full head of hair to meet societal expectations. Thinning hair is acceptable only when a woman is very old.

Societal expectation run counter to reality, however. The fact is, many women do experience hair loss at young to middle age and the incidence of the most common type of female hair loss (female androgenetic alopecia) seems to be increasing [Norwood OT. Incidence of female androgenetic alopecia (female pattern baldness). *Dermatol Surg* 2001; 27:53-54.].

Many women today recognize the reality of hair loss and choose to do something about it by seeking hair restoration treatment or procedures. In the hands of a physician specialist in hair transplantation, most hair loss in women can be successfully treated.

### What Causes Hair Loss in Women?

The most common type of hair loss in women is female androgenetic alopecia (female pattern baldness). It occurs in about 20% of American women overall. In one study of 1,008 Caucasian women, female androgenetic alopecia was found in 3% of women aged 20–29 years, 16–17% of women aged 30–49 years, 23–25% of women aged 50–69 years, 28% of women aged 70–79 years, and 32% of women aged 80–89 years. [Norwood OT. Incidence of female androgenetic alopecia (female pattern baldness). *Dermatol Surg* 2001; 27:53–54.]. The statistics reflect the increased incidence of female androgenetic alopecia during and after menopause.

The underlying cause of female androgenetic alopecia is believed to be related to production of androgenetic (male) hormones and the effect of androgenetic hormones on the hair follicle—the same underlying cause responsible for male androgenetic alopecia (male pattern baldness). The pattern of hair loss in female androgenetic alopecia has some distinctive features that differentiate it from male-pattern hair loss. In general, there are three patterns of hair loss in female androgenetic alopecia:

**Grade I:** Thinning hair on the central scalp (top of the head).

**Grade II:** Thinning hair and patches of greater scalp hair loss.

**Grade III:** Male-pattern alopecia with hair loss at the front of the scalp to mid-scalp. However, it is very rare to see complete male-pattern "cue-ball" baldness in a woman.

Other causes of hair loss in women include scalp scarring from injury or an underlying disease, traction alopecia due to injury from tight braiding or corn-rowing of hair, and trichotillomania (compulsive hair plucking).

## Consultation with a Hair Restoration Doctor

A woman who is experiencing hair loss should consider consulting a hair restoration doctor. The consultation has both medical and esthetic aspects.

### Medical

The focus of the medical examination is the reason for hair loss. In a healthy woman the most common reason for hair loss is female androgenetic alopecia in a Grade I, II or III pattern as described earlier. If the patient's medical history and physical examination indicate no underlying medical conditions, and the hair-loss pattern is clearly that of female androgenetic alopecia, no further tests may be necessary. However, if the hair-loss pattern is not clearly that of female androgenetic alopecia, or suggests the possibility of an underlying medical condition, further medical tests, and inquiry into personal and family medical history may be indicated. A scalp biopsy can be helpful in establishing a reason for hair loss when the reason is not immediately apparent.

While the primary reason for the medical examination is to determine the reason for hair loss, the examination may occasionally result in diagnosis of a previously unsuspected underlying disease. Hair loss can be a symptom of certain autoimmune diseases and diseases that cause overproduction of androgenic (male) hormones. An underlying disease does not necessarily preclude hair restoration. However, it may be necessary to treat the underlying condition before hair restoration can proceed.

## *Esthetic*

The rationale for hair restoration is primarily esthetic—how a woman feels about her appearance and how she wants others to perceive her. The esthetic consultation with the physician hair restoration specialist is every bit as important as determining the reason for hair loss. The patient has esthetic goals that she hopes hair restoration can achieve. The physician helps the patient refine her goals within the context of what surgical and/or nonsurgical hair restoration can accomplish. Many questions can be raised and discussed in the esthetic consultation:

- What hair styles has the patient been using to minimize the appearance of thinning hair?

- What hair styles would the patient hope to use after hair restoration?

- Would the patient change her hair style, curl, color, etc., to get the most out of hair restoration?

- Does the patient want a "luxurious head of hair" that might require procedures such as hair weaving or hair extenders? Does the patient want to be able to swim and/or exercise heavily without worrying about her hair?

- What can hair transplantation accomplish and is transplantation an option for the patient?

- If transplantation is not an option because of scalp scarring or underlying disease, what options for hair restoration can be considered?

195

Results of the medical and esthetic consultation are the primary considerations that guide the selection of a surgical or non-surgical hair restoration treatment appropriate to the patient's needs.

## Treatment of Female Hair Loss

Hair restoration treatments for women are primarily surgical, or treatments such as hair weaving or extending. Medical treatments for hair loss are largely directed at male androgenetic alopecia. A surgical treatment for female androgenetic alopecia may occasionally be combined with finasteride or minoxidil, the two products approved by the Food and Drug Administration (FDA) for non-surgical treatment of androgenetic alopecia. The physician hair restoration specialist may be able to determine whether the patient's alopecia would be responsive to one of the FDA-approved drugs.

## Hair Transplantation in Women

Hair loss occurs in women as well as in men, and increasing numbers of women seek medical or surgical treatment for thinning hair. The time is long past when women were unwilling to recognize their hair loss, or accept it as an inevitable consequence of aging.

Hair transplantation is a hair-loss treatment option chosen by many women whose loss of hair has a hereditary basis—the type known as female pattern hair loss. Like male pattern hair loss, female pattern hair loss is genetic in origin and "runs in the family". It is the most common form of permanent hair loss in women.

## Be Certain about the Cause of Hair Loss

No treatment for a woman's hair loss should be undertaken until the cause and permanence of her hair loss is diagnosed with certainty. While hereditary female pattern hair loss is the most common cause of permanent loss of hair in women, there are other causes of both permanent and temporary hair loss that should be ruled out before hair transplantation is undertaken.

Hair transplantation is not an option for treatment of temporary hair loss. Temporary hair loss should never be treated by hair transplantation or other surgical intervention.

Hair transplantation may be a treatment option for some non-pattern causes of permanent hair loss such as physical trauma to the scalp, but female pattern hair loss is the most frequent indication for hair transplantation in women. No treatment should be undertaken until the patient thoroughly understands the rationale for treatment.

## *What Causes Hair Loss in Women?*

Androgenetic alopecia—inherited pattern hair loss—is the most common cause of permanent hair loss in women as it is in men. Female pattern androgenetic alopecia usually occurs as diffuse thinning of hair rather than the frank baldness often seen in men. However, patterns in hair loss vary greatly in women and every case of hair loss in women should be considered for individual diagnosis. Correctly diagnosed hair loss can usually be treated medically or surgically.

Other common causes of hair loss in women include:

- **Alopecia areata:** Patchy loss of hair from the scalp and sometimes eyebrows or other hair-bearing areas of the body; thought to be due to an autoimmune disorder. Hair loss can be episodic and recurrent.

- **Traction alopecia:** Hair loss associated with consistent traction pressure on hair follicles, as may occur with tight braiding or corn-rowing of hair.

- **Trichotillomania:** Compulsive hair plucking, believed sometimes associated with emotional stress or a psychological disorder.

- **Telogen effluvium:** Unusually accelerated hair loss that may have hormonal, nutritional, drug-associated or stress-associated causes.

- **Loose-anagen syndrome:** A condition in which scalp hair is easily pulled out by normal combing or brushing; more common in fair-haired individuals.

- **Triangular alopecia:** Due to unknown cause, hair is lost from areas around the temples.

- **Scarring alopecia:** Caused when physical trauma or burns damage scalp hair follicles. Traction alopecia can lead to scarring alopecia.

Remember that most female hair loss can be treated medically or surgically, but successful treatment requires correct diagnosis by a physician hair restoration specialist.

As noted in the discussion in female hair loss, hair loss in women can sometimes have an underlying hormonal or dermatologic cause,

197

or be associated with severe emotional or physical stress. When such an underlying cause is suspected, a physician hair restoration specialist will refer the woman to an appropriate medical specialist for further examination and diagnosis. Hair loss can be a first sign or symptom of an underlying medical condition.

Appropriate treatment of an underlying medical condition may resolve the problem of hair loss, and no treatment for hair loss will be indicated. Some causes of temporary hair loss—such as hormonal changes during pregnancy—will resolve spontaneously. When a prolonged period of temporary hair loss seems likely—for example, while a woman undergoes prolonged treatment for a medical condition such as cancer—the patient may consult a physician hair restoration specialist regarding a full or partial temporary hair prosthesis.

### When Is a Woman with Female Pattern Hair Loss a Good Candidate for Hair Transplantation?

After it is determined that a woman's thinning hair is due to female pattern hair loss and no other cause, hair transplantation can be considered as a treatment.

When is a woman a good candidate for hair transplantation? The criteria for candidacy are largely the same for both women and men, with some specific considerations that apply more often to women than to men. The best approach to the question is open and honest discussion between the woman and the physician hair restoration specialist.

A woman should not be "sold" hair transplantation as a hair-loss treatment; she should choose it as a treatment only if she fully understands the reasons for the physician's recommendation. Neither should a woman "push" for hair transplantation that the physician is unwilling to recommend. The decision to undergo hair transplantation should be made on the basis of the physician's professional judgment after complete examination of the patient, and full and honest discussion between patient and physician regarding cost, time, details of the procedure, potential side effects and complications, and anticipated result.

Hereditary hair loss patterns differ in women as compared to patterns in men. Hereditary hair loss in women tends to be more diffuse than in men, presenting as areas of patchy thinning rather than the areas of total hair loss more common in men.

The extent and rapidity of patchy hair loss are considerations in determining whether a woman is a good candidate for hair transplantation.

The physician hair restoration specialist will use scalp examination as well as the patient's personal and family history to determine whether there will be enough donor hair currently and in the future to make transplantation a viable treatment option, and if hair transplantation is undertaken, will the result meet the patient's expectations for cosmetic improvement? Inadequate donor hair could rule out hair transplantation as a viable option for hair loss treatment. In some women, for example, the diffuse pattern of hair loss is widespread and rapidly advancing, and this may make it difficult for the physician hair restoration specialist to find scalp hair that is dense enough to provide adequate donor hair (the hair that is taken from one site on the scalp and transplanted to a balding recipient site).

Other scalp and hair characteristics that the physician may consider include hair color, hair texture, degree of hair curl, and skin-to-scalp hair color contrast—all characteristics that the physician hair restoration specialist may be able to use to achieve maximum cosmetic improvement. For example, the physician hair restoration specialist may creatively use color, texture and curl of transplanted hair to complement existing hair and recreate an appearance of density in an area of diffuse hair loss.

If donor hair is limited by overall hair thinning, hair transplantation may be able to offer an improvement in recipient areas by creative use of hair characteristics, but may not be able to offer full density that returns the patient to complete pre-hair loss appearance. Another consideration—applicable to both women and men—is the rapidity and extent of hair thinning. Rapid and extensive hair loss may deplete the amount of donor hair available for future use in keeping pace with continued loss of hair. If this appears to be a possibility, the patient and physician hair restoration specialist should discuss realistic expectations for hair transplantation over a period of years. The patient must determine whether the anticipated result justifies the time, cost and discomfort of hair transplantation.

Women more than men are bombarded with advertising images of models with luxuriously dense hair—images that establish a standard which women are challenged to emulate. These unrealistic images may be in the background when a woman discusses realistic expectations for hair transplantation with her physician hair restoration specialist. Unrealistic images promoted by hair-product advertising should not cloud judgments regarding realistic expectations for cosmetic improvement from hair transplantation.

In the great majority of cases, women who have hair transplantation performed by a skilled, experienced physician hair restoration specialist are highly satisfied with the result. While satisfaction is due in large part to the physician's technical skill and expertise, it also reflects the feeling of patients who find that their realistic expectations were achieved.

## Hair Transplantation Technique

Hair transplantation techniques are adapted to the necessity for placing grafts in multiple areas of patchy hair loss. The types of grafts used and the number of transplantation sessions scheduled for the patient are decisions influenced by the patient's objectives for hair density in the final result.

## Combination Treatments

The topically-applied hair loss remedy minoxidil (Rogaine®) is sometimes used in selected female patients to complement hair transplantation by stimulating new hair growth, or to prevent the temporary postoperative loss of transplanted hair that occurs in a percentage of transplant patients.

When donor hair is limited and hair loss areas are relatively extensive, the patient and physician hair restoration specialist may agree on a treatment plan that combines hair transplantation and hair styling. If all hair loss areas cannot be effectively treated by transplantation, the transplanted areas may be configured to maximize the future use of hair styling to achieve maximum cosmetic improvement.

## Scalp Reductions and Scalp Flaps

A scalp problem such as traumatic scarring may make a patient unsuitable for hair transplantation. A reconstructive procedure such as scalp reduction or a scalp flap may be necessary to restore a suitable hair pattern.

Advances in hair transplantation have made transplants in a scarred scalp possible in some patients. The possibility of hair transplantation should be discussed with the hair restoration doctor.

Perhaps because "baldness" was long believed to be a male characteristic, hair loss in women was often ignored or dismissed as a socially unacceptable topic. Hair loss in women is now fully recognized as a medical problem and esthetic concern that can be treated by a physician hair restoration specialist.

# Part Three

# Facial and Neck Surgical Procedures

# Chapter 26

# *Eyelid Surgery (Blepharoplasty)*

Eyelid skin is the thinnest skin on your face and is likely to be the first facial feature to reveal signs of aging. Wrinkled folds of skin on the upper eyelids, bags under the eyes, and sagging eyebrows can make a person look older, tired, or sad. Plastic surgery can reshape the eyelid area and improve appearance.

### *What is a blepharoplasty?*

A blepharoplasty is a surgery that removes excess skin and fat on upper and/or lower eyelids. It is commonly done for cosmetic reasons. It may also be done to improve vision if the skin folds interfere with normal vision.

Blepharoplasty is a common form of cosmetic surgery. Thousands of these procedures are performed successfully each year.

### *Who performs a blepharoplasty?*

Most blepharoplasties are performed by oculoplastic surgeons (physicians who specialize in plastic and reconstructive surgery of the eye), by plastic surgeons or by ear-nose-throat surgeons. Dermatologists (skin doctors), general ophthalmologists, and oral-maxillofacial surgeons are also performing more of this surgery currently.

"Cosmetic Eyelid Surgery (Blepharoplasty)," University of Illinois Eye Center (www.uic.edu/com/eye), © July 2003. Reprinted with permission.

## What types of cosmetic eyelid surgeries are done?

The most common type of oculoplastic surgery is removal of excess skin and fat on the upper eyelids.

Often, the surgeon simultaneously reconstructs the eyelid creases to create a more pleasing appearance. This method may also be used to make oriental eyes look more western.

Excess skin and fat can also be removed from the lower eyelids (bags under the eyes). Additionally, drooping eyebrows may be lifted. This is done by one of several different methods. The most common techniques involve lifting the brow through the same incision made for the blepharoplasty or by endoscopically elevating the brow. The brow can also be lifted by removing excess skin above the brow or on the scalp. Droopy eyelids also may be corrected by tightening eye muscles. If required, all these changes may be made during a single surgery.

## What results can the patient expect?

During the first visit to the surgeon, the patient and doctor discuss the surgery and the expected results of the surgery. The patient looks in a mirror and points out what he or she would like to improve in appearance. The surgeon then evaluates the patient's facial features to determine if surgery can help the problems the patient wants corrected. The amount and type of surgery done depends on the patient's goals, medical history, general health, age, and skin texture.

The surgeon and patient discuss the patient's motives for and expectations of the surgery as well. It is important to have realistic expectations. Cosmetic eyelid surgery can improve appearance, not make it perfect. Moreover, eyelid surgery cannot correct some blemishes, such as skin discoloration, fullness of cheeks, and deep eyelid creases. The surgery improves this condition, but does not remove wrinkles on the outer edges of the eyelids.

What blepharoplasty does is to create a smoother area around the eyes, giving a more youthful look. A brow lift results in a more alert appearance.

Most of the cosmetic changes occur in the first few weeks after surgery. However, the entire effect of the surgery may not be apparent for a year.

Depending on the patient's physical traits and the type of procedure applied on the patient, one may decide to repeat the surgery in five to 20 years.

## *How and where is blepharoplasty performed?*

Most patients are operated on in an out patient surgical facility or may have surgery as an outpatient at a hospital. The choice depends on the patient's preference and health. Generally, sedating as well as anesthetic agents are used during the procedure to keep the patient comfortable.

## *How safe is cosmetic eyelid surgery?*

Modern cosmetic surgical procedures are very safe. Complications such as infection or blood clots are rare. However, aspirin, aspirin products, non-steroidal anti-inflammatory drugs (NSAIDs) such as ibuprofen (Motrin, Advil), naproxen (Naprosyn), and others can cause excessive bleeding during and after the surgery. The patient should therefore not take aspirin or NSAIDs for two weeks before the surgery. In addition, "blood thinners" such as warfarin (Coumadin) must be managed by the appropriate attending physicians before the time of surgery.

It is normal to have some bruising and swelling for a week or so after surgery. Cold compresses applied to the eyes can help reduce these problems. If there are obvious bruises even after a week of healing, they can be covered with makeup.

The stitches will be removed several days after surgery, leaving very fine scars. These scars will be barely visible within two months. Sometimes, however, a noticeable scar remains after a brow lift as excess skin is removed directly above the brow. A scar can be avoided by lifting the brow through the upper eyelid incision.

Noticeable scars or more severe problems result from poor healing after eyelid surgery. Such problems may require a second, touch-up operation. The likelihood of complications is reduced by adhering to the doctor's instructions on follow-up care.

One lower lid blepharoplasty method avoids even the smallest scars. This technique involves making a cut on the inside, rather than the outside, of the lower eyelid. A dissolving suture is used, so there is no need for suture removal and consequently there are no visible scars. There also is less bruising and swelling. The "internal" approach is best for persons younger than 50 or others who need only fat removed (rather than fat and skin).

## *Can laser be used for blepharoplasty?*

A new way to perform eyelid surgery is with a contact laser that has a probe like a scalpel. This scalpel uses heat energy to cut through skin, muscle, and fat.

The advantages are a faster operating time and less bleeding and pain. When done by an expert, this procedure appears to be as safe as traditional blepharoplasty. However, very little is known about the risks of laser.

### How much does a blepharoplasty cost?

Surgical fees vary widely depending on the length and complexity of the operation. They range from $1,000 to $4,000 or more, according to the American Society of Plastic and Reconstructive Surgeons. Most insurance plans do not cover the cost of blepharoplasty unless the surgery is needed to improve vision.

# Chapter 27

# *Nose Reshaping (Rhinoplasty and Septorhinoplasty)*

### *What is rhinoplasty or septorhinoplasty?*

Rhinoplasty refers to surgery performed on the nose to remodel or reconstruct the external nose. Septorhinoplasty refers to rhinoplasty in addition to reconstruction and remodeling of the nasal septum, the internal wall which separates the two sides of the nose. The two terms are often used interchangeably because reconstructive and aesthetic nasal surgery almost invariably includes the nasal septum.

### *When should septorhinoplasty be performed?*

Septorhinoplasty is performed for reconstructive or aesthetic purposes. Following trauma, the nose may be severely fractured which may lead to blockage of nasal breathing or a severely deformed external nasal appearance. In this instance, septorhinoplasty is performed for reconstructive purposes and to improve function (breathing). However, the majority of septorhinoplasties are performed for cosmetic reasons to enhance the aesthetic appearance of the nose. This is performed for both men and women.

"Rhinoplasty and Septoplasty," © 2006 Canadian Society of Otolaryngology–Head and Neck Surgery. All rights reserved. Reprinted with permission.

### *Who is qualified to perform this type of surgery?*

As with any surgical procedure, septorhinoplasty should be performed by a well-trained surgeon. Specialists who perform "plastic" surgery of the face include ENT (ears, nose, and throat) specialists, plastic surgeons, and others. Facial plastic surgery is one of the areas of expertise of ENT surgeons. It is an integral part of specialty training in ENT and a requirement to obtaining a specialist's license in ENT in Canada and the U.S.

### *What can be achieved in terms of improving the appearance of the nose?*

Much can be achieved in terms of enhancing the appearance of the nose. However, what can be achieved is not necessarily what should be performed. The nose sits amidst the framework of the face and as such needs to fit within this framework. Therefore, the proportions of the nose must be in harmony with the existing facial proportions. For example, shortening the nose excessively in a tall person with long and narrow facial dimensions leads to an undesirable overall result. In addition, while most requests for modifying nasal features are realistic, certain requests such as "I would like to make my whole nose smaller" may or may not be feasible or desirable. These considerations need to be discussed openly with your surgeon to insure a positive outcome.

### *Should I ask to see a digital image of the possible modifications which will be made?*

This may give you an idea of the possible outcome of your nasal surgery, but can occasionally lead to disappointment. It is important to remember that every person's anatomy is different and everyone does not heal in the same fashion. This is where the surgeon's advice enters. He or she is able to assess how the nose will be shaped and heal after surgery based on assessing multiple factors, including the anatomy, skin type, and tissues of a particular patient's nose.

### *What questions should I ask my surgeon?*

It is a good idea to ask the surgeon about his or her training, including additional training or courses particular to septorhinoplasty, level of comfort performing such a procedure, and the number of septorhinoplasties he or she has performed. In addition, there should be a frank and open discussion about the realistic expectations of surgery as well as what can or cannot be achieved.

### *What are the risks involved with septorhinoplasty surgery?*

The risks of bleeding and infection are common to any surgical procedure. These risks are small in the case of nasal surgery. The use of foreign materials such as implants or grafts in nasal surgery slightly increases the risk of infection. Other risks and complications specific to the procedure depend on what procedures are performed by the surgeon for a particular desired result. It is important to discus these risks and possible complications with your surgeon.

### *Should septorhinoplasty be performed under local or general anesthesia?*

The type of anesthesia administered—general or local—does not significantly affect the level of discomfort or the final outcome of the nasal appearance, but may influence the overall experience of the patient. Frequently, patients who undergo surgery under local anesthesia report a very positive experience. However, this choice remains between surgeon and patient and is determined by multiple factors such as the patient's preference, the planned procedure, the surgeon's preference, and the institution where surgery is to take place.

### *Is it painful?*

Overall, this is not a very painful or uncomfortable procedure, with relatively little discomfort. The level of discomfort is dependent on multiple factors, mainly the patient and the extent of surgery. Everyone has a different pain threshold and tolerance level. Other factors which influence the level of discomfort include whether a packing is left in the nose for a prolonged period after surgery and whether the procedure includes breaking the bones of the nose (whether or not this is performed depends on the surgical plan and the modifications to be performed).

### *How much does it cost?*

This is highly variable according to local norms and rates, surgeon's reputation (name recognition and brand name), surgeon's experience, operating room fees, and the planned procedure. The latter depends on the complexity of the nose to be operated on, and the planned maneuvers. These factors may not seem obvious to the untrained eye, but often, what may might appear to be a minor deformity requiring a minor alteration, is, in fact, a highly delicate task that requires skill, experience, and finesse. In addition, whether the planned procedure is a primary (first time) or revision (previously operated) surgery impacts on the skill, experience, and time required in the operating room.

### *How long do I need to book off work or school?*

Patients are usually mobile and able to carry on normal activities very quickly after surgery. By two or three days after surgery, healthy patients are usually recovered to 90%. If the procedure was done under general anesthesia, it may take four to five days to regain one's energy level. Usually, it is safe to take seven or eight days after surgery to completely recover. Another factor which may preclude work is the bandage/splint placed on the bridge of the nose in the vast majority of patients. Depending on the nature of the patient's work, he/she may chose not to return to work until the splint is removed approximately one week following surgery.

# Chapter 28

# *Ear Reshaping (Otoplasty)*

Otoplasty is one of the most common plastic surgery procedures for children. The majority of patients who undergo otoplasty are between four and 14 years old, according to the American Society of Plastic Surgeons, although many adults also elect to have the procedure.

Children's ears are most often fully developed by the age four. There are no additional risks associated with age. Typically, the procedure is performed to improve the appearance of the ears so that the child would not have to endure ridicule from peers throughout their childhood.

Though ridicule from the appearance of ears is not a part of adult life, adults who elect this procedure often feel better with their improved appearance. Individuals may seek ear surgery to correct protruding ears (excessive ear cartilage), large or otherwise deformed earlobes, the "lop ear" (where the ear tip bends down and forward), and a "cupped" or "shell ear" (which could be a very tiny ear or an ear without natural creases). Today a select number of surgeons have developed techniques to create ears for patients who do not have a portion or any ears as a result of a birth defect or traumatic injury.

## *Malformed Ears*

Malformed ears are a broad definition for cupped or shelled ears or ears that are otherwise not visible due to a birth defect. In such cases, the ears are assessed for excessive cartilage, malformed carti-lage, mal-positioned cartilage, and soft tissue (skin and fat) deformity. By conducting a formal physical assessment, each case is then ap-proached diagnostically and the surgery is individualized. For total ear reconstruction, otherwise known as congenital microtia (ear ab-sence), a common approach begins with developing a framework from the ribs, then elevating the back, and placing a skin graft. Next, the ear canal is carved out and often it is necessary to rotate the lobule. Ears that are malformed due to trauma (including burns) may un-dergo a variation of the above description but could require more ex-tensive skin grafting, depending upon the extent of the tissue damage.

## Making the Decision about Otoplasty

Your choice of a qualified facial plastic surgeon is important. Dur-ing the consultation, your surgeon will examine the structure of the ears and discuss possibilities for correcting the problems. Even if only one ear needs "pinning back," surgery will probably be recommended on both ears to achieve the most natural, symmetrical appearance.

After the surgeon and patient decide that otoplasty is needed, your surgeon will discuss the procedure. Following a thorough medical his-tory, your surgeon will explain the kind of anesthesia required, sur-gical facility, and costs. Typically, your surgeon will suggest a general anesthesia for young patients and a local anesthetic combined with a mild sedative for older children and adults. Under normal condi-tions, otoplasty requires approximately two hours.

## About the Otoplasty Procedure

It is important to understand that otoplasty will not alter hearing ability. What is important for successful otoplasty is that the ears be in proportion to the size and shape of the face and head.

Adult candidates for otoplasty should understand that the firmer cartilage of fully developed ears does not provide the same molding capacity as in children. A consultation with a facial plastic surgeon can help parents decide what is best for their child, not only aestheti-cally, but also psychologically and physically. Timing is always an important consideration. Having the procedure at a young age is highly desirable in two respects: the cartilage is extremely pliable, thereby permitting greater ease of shaping; and secondly, the child will expe-rience psychological benefits from the cosmetic improvement.

The otoplasty procedure is performed in an outpatient medical surgery center, physician's office or hospital. The procedure may be performed under local anesthesia—while you are sedated, numbed and awake. Less often, general anesthesia is the appropriate choice—whereby you are asleep throughout the procedure. In the case of a child, the surgeon may recommend general anesthesia so that the child can sleep through the procedure. For certain general anesthesia cases, an overnight hospital stay may be appropriate. Otherwise, patients return home within hours of the procedure on the same day.

## How Otoplasty Is Performed

The otoplasty procedure may be performed through a variety of techniques. Techniques vary among surgeons and patients. Factors that may impact the choice of technique include the general anatomy of the ears, the extent of the ear cartilage, excessive skin in the surrounding area or level of deformity in other areas of the ears. Most often, surgery is performed on both ears to create the best balance between the ears.

During the procedure, the surgeon first determines the incision location in order to identify the most inconspicuous site on the back of the ear. Once the incision is made, the surgeon will sculpt the exposed ear cartilage and re-position it closer to the head for a more natural looking appearance. The surgeon may use non-removable stitches to help the cartilage maintain its position. In some cases, the surgeon will remove more excessive cartilage in order to enhance the ultimate appearance of the ear.

In the second common technique, skin is removed and the ear cartilage is folded back. There is no cartilage removed in this technique. Non-removable stitches are used to help the cartilage maintain its position. Dissolvable or removable stitches are used for the incision location (which are removed or dissolve within seven days).

## After Otoplasty Surgery

After the procedure, the head is wrapped in a thick bandage. The fitting of the bandage helps to maintain the new position of the ears and also enhances the healing process. Patients usually return to the surgeon's office within the first few days to exchange the bandage for a lighter one. Your surgeon will provide specific instructions regarding the use of lighter bandage. Your surgeon will provide a complete post surgery instruction list that must be followed in order to reduce the risk of complications.

Young patients are often required to refrain from normal activity for at least seven days after the procedure. In fact, special care must be given to children throughout the first three weeks of recovery as to avoid playful activities that may disrupt the ears. Adult patients usually return to normal activity within three days of the procedure. More complicated procedures may require a longer recovery time. In all cases, the ears should not be bent for at least a month or more.

During recovery, otoplasty patients may experience the following:

- **Temporary discomfort and numbness:** Managed with oral medications

- **Headaches:** Relieved through use of long acting local anesthetic

- **Swelling:** Managed with head elevation, decreased within a week

- **Unusual sensations:** May include itching or the lack of sensation at the incision line which can disappear over the course of six months

Complications are typically rare. However, there are risks associated with all medical procedures. Although rare, a small number of patients may have a blood clot form on the ear. Other patients may develop an infection in the cartilage area. The surgeon will treat infections with medications. In the case of blood clot or infection, the surgeon may recommend a waiting period to see if the clot or infection (with antibiotic treatment) resolves itself. Should the clot not dissolve, it can be removed with a needle. Rarely, an infection may require surgical drainage. Scar tissue formation is a possibility. However, all complications are infrequent and there are options available to treat complications. Many patients may have a slight visible scar on the back of the ear. However, surgeons take special care to place the incision in an inconspicuous location.

## Average Otoplasty Costs

Average fees for the otoplasty procedure can range from $4,800 to over $7,000. These estimated costs vary based on the extent of the procedure, expertise of the surgeon, and the length of recovery. It is best to ask your surgeon and insurance plan administrator about what is covered and the amount you are responsible for.

As with most medical procedures, many surgeons offer payment plans. If the out-of pocket cost is too large for you ask your surgeon about payment plan options. Many payment plans allow monthly installments over an extended period. Also, ask about medical financing companies. Many practices are familiar with these companies and can provide information.

# Chapter 29

# *Facelift (Rhytidectomy)*

## Commonly Asked Questions about Facelifts

Aging of the face is inevitable. As the years go by, the skin begins to loosen on the face and neck. Crow's feet appear at the corners of the eyes.

Fine forehead lines become creases and then, gradually, deeper folds. The jaw line softens into jowls, and beneath the chin, another chin or vertical folds appear at the front of the neck.

Heredity, personal habits, the pull of gravity, and sun exposure contribute to the aging of the face. As the aging population grows, it is obvious why the face lift has become the third most desired facial plastic surgical procedure in the United States.

If you ever wondered how a facelift could improve your looks or self-confidence, you need to know how a facelift is performed and what you can expect from this procedure.

### *What are the factors for success?*

- Good rapport, communication, and trust between you and your surgeon are critical for success. A thorough consultation

This chapter begins with "Commonly Asked Questions about Facelifts" from "Cosmetic Enhancements - Facelifts (Rhytidectomy)," © 2007 Washington University School of Medicine in St. Louis (http://wuphysicians.wustl.edu). Reprinted with permission. It continues with "Mini Facelift/S-Lift" and "Midface Lift/Cheek Lift" by Sam P. Most, M.D., Reprinted with permission. Copyright © 2002 Sam P. Most, M.D. For additional information visit http://www.drmost.com.

is crucial to both parties understanding of the procedure and outcomes.

- Surgical skill of the surgeon.

- Realistic expectations of the patient.

- Good general health of the patient.

Understanding the limitations of the face lift is crucial and psychological stability is vital. There is no ideal in a facelift. Rather, the goal is to improve the overall facial appearance. Skin type, ethnic background, degree of skin elasticity, individual healing, basic bone structure, as well as a realistic attitude are factors that should be discussed prior to surgery.

This procedure is sometimes performed on patients in their thirties, and successful surgery has been performed on patients in their eighties. A facelift cannot stop aging, nor can it turn back the clock. What it can do is help your face look its best and give you a look of health and a more youthful appearance. A side benefit is that many patients experience increased self-confidence.

Before deciding on a facelift, you should discuss with your facial plastic surgeon whether the overall effect will be more successful if additional changes are made in the chin and neck areas through other facial surgery. Many patients decide to have facial liposuction to remove excess fatty deposits in conjunction with a facelift. If several flaws need correction, more than one procedure may be necessary for the best overall result.

### What is the procedure for evaluation?

During the preliminary consultation, the surgeon will examine the structure of your face, skin texture, color, and elasticity. Photographs will be taken so the surgeon can study your face. Individual risks will also be examined, especially those related to medical situations such as high blood pressure, a tendency to scar, smoking, and any deficiency in blood clotting. The surgeon will take a thorough medical history, as well as assess the patient's mental and emotional attitudes toward the surgery. Because a realistic attitude is crucial to the success of the surgery, the surgical procedure and realistic expectations will be discussed.

After the decision to proceed with a face lift is made jointly by you and your surgeon, the surgeon will describe the technique indicated, the type of anesthesia, the surgical facility, any additional surgery, the pros and cons to include possible complications, and costs of the procedure.

## *What is the surgical procedure?*

The surgeon begins the incision in the area of the temple hair, just above and in from of the ear, and then continues around the lobe, circling the ear before returning to the point of origin in the scalp. The skin is raised outward before the surgeon repositions and tightens the underlying muscle and connective tissue. Some fat may be removed, as well as excess skin. For men, the incision is aligned to accommodate the natural beard lines.

In all cases, the incision is placed where it will fall in a natural crease of the skin for camouflage. After trimming the excess skin, the surgeon closes the incisions with fine sutures or metal clips, which permit surgery without shaving hair from the incision site.

Depending on the extent of the surgery, the process can take from three to four hours. Most often a full facelift is performed under general anesthesia to maximize patient comfort. Following the surgery, the surgeon will apply a dressing to protect the entire area where the incisions have been made.

## *What can I expect after surgery?*

Even though most patients experience very little pain after surgery, the surgeon will still prescribe medication. Some degree of swelling and bruising is unavoidable, and your surgeon may instruct you to use cold compresses to keep swelling to a minimum. If a dressing has been applied, it will be removed within one to two days.

The surgeon will also instruct you to keep your head elevated when lying down, to avoid as much activity as possible, and to report any undue discomfort. Though there are few risks in facelift surgery and thousands are performed every year, some risk exists in any surgery.

In some cases, a drainage tube may have been inserted during surgery. This will be removed on the first or second day after surgery. All sutures and staples are usually removed within 5 to 10 days following surgery. Surgeons generally recommend that patients avoid vigorous activity. Patients should prearrange for post-surgery support from family and friends.

Recovery usually takes two to three weeks, though many patients go back to work in two weeks. Scars are usually not noticeable after enough time has passed for them to mature. In any case, they are easily disguised in natural skin creases, by the hair, or, in persistent cases, by makeup until total healing has occurred.

Bear in mind that the aging process continues after surgery and that some relaxation of tissues will occur over the first few weeks. Facial plastic surgery makes it possible to correct many facial flaws and signs of premature aging that can undermine self-confidence. By changing how you look, cosmetic surgery can help change how you feel about yourself.

### *Is this covered under my insurance?*

Insurance does not generally cover surgery that is done purely for cosmetic reasons.

## *Mini Facelift/S-Lift*

### *What is a mini facelift/S-lift?*

A number of different names are used to describe what is essentially a "mini facelift." These procedures use slightly smaller incisions and have quicker recovery than standard facelift surgery. As in a standard facelift, the goal of the surgery is to enhance the appearance of the aging face and neck by tightening the sagging tissues of the face and neck and by removal of excessive skin and fatty tissue.

### *What can a mini facelift/S-lift achieve?*

The goal of mini facelift is to rejuvenate the lower ½ of the face and the neck. Generally speaking, the results are less dramatic than in facelift surgery. The results with this procedure should last a few years (not as long as with standard facelift surgery).

### *What type of anesthesia is used?*

The procedure can be done awake or asleep. For patient comfort and safety, this procedure may be done asleep.

### *What is the procedure like?*

Incisions are placed in front of and behind the ear.

### *What is the recovery like?*

Patients may expect 1–2 weeks of swelling in the cheeks and neck. Some patients recover more rapidly, some may take a few days longer.

## Midface Lift/Cheek Lift

### What is a midface lift/cheek lift?

A midface lift refers to "lifting" of the tissue in the triangle formed by the two corners of each eye and the corner of the mouth. This area, known as the midface, can begin to descend in one's 30s or early 40s.

### What can a midface lift/cheek lift achieve?

A midface lift can reverse the subtle changes that occur with age. The restoration of a youthful, "mounded" cheek is the goal.

### What type of anesthesia is used?

The procedure can be done under "twilight" anesthesia or completely asleep. Your physician can help you decide which type of anesthesia will work best for you.

### What is the procedure like?

Physicians use advanced endoscopic techniques to perform this surgery. A small incision is made in the hairline above the ear, and another above the gum line in the mouth.

### What is the recovery like?

Patients may expect 7–10 days of swelling in the cheeks and some mild bruising.

## Additional Information

### Department of Otolaryngology
Washington University Physicians
605 Old Ballas Road
Creve Coeur, MO 63131
Phone: 314-432-7760 or 314-632-7509
Website: http://wuphysicians.wustl.edu/dept.asp?pageID=43&ID=8

### Sam P. Most, M.D
Stanford Facial Plastic Surgery
Phone: 650-736-3223
Website: http://www.drmost.com
E-mail: info@drmost.com

# Chapter 30

# *Facial Implants*

Many patients who are seeking a younger looking appearance and refinement of their profile are happy with the results of facial implants. Facial plastic surgeons are able to replace bony deficiency, to improve balance of facial features, or to reposition the sagging skin upward and outward to fill hollows and depressions.

## *Mid-Face Implants*

One of the strongest characteristics of youth is fullness of the cheeks, indicating an abundance of healthy soft tissues and fat that is present under the skin. Also a sign of vitality, the cheekbones are responsible for defining the face, highlighting the eyes, and adding overall balance to your features. Not everyone can retain contour and fullness with age. Not everyone has prominent cheekbones.

When there is depletion of tissue and fat and minimal cheekbones, the skin sags, appears flattened or sunken, and may cause folds and wrinkles around the mouth. The mid-face implant can hold up the collapsed tissue and restore the youthful appearance of adequately padded skin at healthy levels of distention and elasticity. This improves the contour, creates balance, and bolsters self-esteem.

Mid-face implants are performed under local anesthesia with sedation. It may be combined with other cosmetic procedures such as

"Achieving a Younger, More Striking Appearance with Implants," *Facial Plastic Surgery Today*, Volume 18, Number 4, 2004. Reprinted with permission from the American Academy of Facial Plastic and Reconstructive Surgery, www.aafprs.org. © 2004.

rhinoplasty or facelift or chin augmentation. After the face is thoroughly cleansed with an antiseptic cleansing agent, a small incision is made inside of the mouth in the crease above the upper lip. A pocket is created over the bone.

The implants come in a variety of sizes and shapes ranging from three to six millimeters. Each patient is evaluated for proper sizing and shape of the implant that will provide the desired effect.

The sterile implant is placed into the pocket. The implant is secured and the incision is sutured closed. Supportive tissue forms around the implant after a few weeks; and once healed, it will feel like your normal underlying bone structure.

## Chin Implants

Many people have a chin that is too small for their face. Flat, under-projected chins are usually genetic, although traumatic injury or previous jaw surgery can also result in deformity. Chin augmentation can help restore balance to the lower face and jawline.

Take a look at your profile. A weak or receding chin can sometimes make your nose seem larger or more projected. During consultation, you can discuss if a chin implant will bring your profile back into balance or if a combination of rhinoplasty (nose surgery) and chin augmentation is the solution.

Some patients seek to reduce the appearance of deep grooves from each corner of the lip down to the chin. These "marionette lines" can be improved by placing small implants along each side of the jaw, just in front of the jowl.

Implants for the chin area come in a wide variety of sizes and shapes. Your implant will be custom fit to the configurations of your face for optimal results.

Chin augmentation is performed under local anesthesia with sedation. The face is cleansed and a small incision is made underneath the chin or inside the mouth, where gum and lower lip meet. A pocket is created by gently stretching the tissue. The sterile implant is then inserted in front of the bone. The implant is secured and the incision is sutured. When the incision is inside the mouth, no scarring is visible. If the incision is under the chin, the scar is usually imperceptible.

## After Implant Surgery

Immediately after surgery, you will probably have a dressing that will remain in place for two to three days. There will be some tenderness;

however, any postoperative discomfort can be controlled with prescribed medications. Most patients feel a stretched, tight sensation after the surgery, but this usually subsides in a week.

Normal activity can be resumed after approximately 10 days. After two weeks there are very little activity restrictions. And, after six weeks, most swelling will be gone and you can enjoy the results of your procedure.

## Making the Decision

Facial plastic surgery makes it possible to enhance your appearance, reduce signs of aging and deformities that undermine self-confidence. Facial plastic surgery can improve your looks and your self-image, as well.

If you are considering implants to sculpt and restore the youthful contour of your face, answer these questions:

- Are you in good health?

- Do you have realistic expectations?

- Why do you want to change your appearance?

- Do you understand how the procedure(s) is performed?

- How do you feel this will change your life?

Implants for the mid-face and chin area provide a safe, effective, and long-lasting way to a more youthful appearance. After careful deliberation, make an appointment and discuss any questions, concerns, or ideas about your treatment plan.

# Chapter 31

# *Forehead Lift Surgery*

The effects of aging are inevitable, and, often, the brow and forehead area show the first signs. The skin begins to lose its elasticity. Sun, wind, and the pull of gravity all affect the face, resulting in frown lines, wrinkling across the forehead, and an increasing heaviness of the eyebrows. Even people in their thirties may have faces that look older than their years. Your tired, angry, or sad expression may not reflect how you actually feel. As a result, many people have opted for a procedure known as the forehead lift. Based on variations in how men and women age and on new advances in medical technology, different methods are used to perform this procedure.

If you are wondering how a forehead lift could improve your appearance, you need to know how these procedures are performed and what you can expect. This text can address many of your concerns and provide you the information you need to begin considering forehead surgery.

Successful facial plastic surgery is a result of good rapport between patient and surgeon. Trust, based on realistic expectations and exacting medical expertise, develops in the consulting stages before surgery. Your surgeon can answer specific questions about your specific needs.

## *Is a Forehead Lift for You?*

As with all elective surgery, good health and realistic expectations are prerequisites. When a surgeon tightens loose skin and removes

"Forehead Lift Surgery," reprinted with permission from the American Academy of Facial Plastic and Reconstructive Surgery, www.aafprs.org. © 2002.

the excess, forehead wrinkling and drooping brows are modified. The procedure is called a forehead lift or brow lift. If necessary, the surgeon removes part of the muscle that causes vertical frown lines between the brows. The result can be a smoother brow and a more youthful expression. To see what a forehead lift can do for your face, put your hands above your brows and outside the edges of your eyes and gently raise the skin upwards. Forehead lifts are an option if you have a sagging brow or deep furrows between the eyes. This procedure is usually done between age forty and sixty-five, although it may be necessary at an earlier age.

Incisions can be placed at the hairline, behind the hairline, or in some cases, above the brow or in the mid-forehead. Your surgeon can help you select the best technique suited to your particular situation.

## Making the Decision for a Forehead Lift

Whether you are having surgery for functional or cosmetic reasons, your choice of a qualified facial plastic surgeon is of paramount importance. During the consultation, the surgeon will examine your facial structure, the condition of your skin, and your hairline in order to decide where incisions should be made. A thorough medical history will be obtained so that your surgeon can consider any medical conditions that may heighten surgical risks. A detailed description of the procedure will also include a discussion of risk involved.

After the decision to proceed with surgery is made, the surgeon will describe the technique indicated, the type of anesthesia, the surgical facility, any additional surgery, and the risks and costs.

The main difference among the various options for forehead lifting consists of the placement of the incision.

## Understanding the Surgery

The original technique is the coronal incision, which is made slightly behind the natural hairline. An alternative is the pre-trichial incision. This is similar to the coronal incision except that the mid-portion of the incision is made directly at the hairline. This incision generally heals favorably and has the advantage of lowering the hairline. The disadvantage could be noticeable scarring. An option is to place the incision within the midforehead creases. This is primarily used in men with deep pre-existing forehead lines.

The newest approach is endoscopic surgery. Several small one-half-inch to one-inch incisions are placed just behind the hairline. Although this technique may require more surgery time, it is less invasive and results in a smaller chance of temporary scalp numbness.

This procedure takes between one to two hours to perform. It is most commonly performed under IV sedation or twilight anesthesia.

## What to Expect after the Surgery

You will experience a certain amount of swelling and bruising in the 10-day period following surgery. In some patients, this condition may include the cheek and eye area as well as the forehead. You will be advised to keep your head elevated in order to reduce swelling. Cold compresses may further reduce swelling. As the incisions heal, you may experience some numbness as well as itching, both of which will diminish with time. The sutures are usually removed within seven to 10 days following surgery. If bandages have been used, they are removed in one to three days. It is important to follow the advice of your surgeon on resuming normal activities. For most patients, the recovery time will not exceed two weeks, but patients may still be advised to avoid strenuous activities for longer periods. Any prolonged bruising can be camouflaged with standard make-up techniques.

Not infrequently, a brow lift is combined with blepharoplasty (an eyelid tuck) or face lift to provide a harmonious rejuvenation.

Facial plastic surgery makes it possible to correct many facial flaws and signs of premature aging that can undermine self-confidence. By changing how you look, cosmetic surgery can help change how you feel about yourself.

Insurance does not generally cover surgery that is purely for cosmetic reasons. Surgery to correct or improve sagging foreheads and brows which interfere with vision may be reimbursable in whole or in part. It is the patient's responsibility to check with the insurance carrier for information on the degree of coverage.

# Chapter 32

# *Lip Augmentation*

There are many options to improve the appearance of your lips. The methods used may also reduce fine lines and wrinkles around your lips.

## *Who Are the Best Candidates for Lip Augmentation?*

You must be in good general health. You might not a good candidate for lip augmentation if you have oral herpes, scarring, or certain diseases such as diabetes, lupus, connective tissues disorders, or blood clotting problems.

Like any other cosmetic surgery, lip augmentation requires a lot of responsibility. You can only determine for yourself if you're ready. We've included the most popular injections and implants here; this information should serve as a general overview only and should not replace your doctor's advice. Once you've selected a doctor, you will communicate with him or her and decide together which option best suits your needs.

Good candidates for lip augmentation are those who have realistic expectations of the outcome. Injections or implants can enhance and improve your natural look, but they're not designed to create a radical change in your appearance.

As with any medical procedure, you should tell your doctor of any allergies or any medications that you are taking, and you will be required to discuss your medical history. Certain conditions or diseases can increase your chances of complications, such as blood clots, diabetes, or poor circulation. If you are a smoker, this may also be a complicating factor.

## Injectable Fillers

These are performed on an outpatient basis in your doctor's office or an outpatient center and you will be sent home the same day. Your surgeon may use local anesthesia to make you more comfortable during the injection of the filler. The local anesthetic (pain killer) may be topical (applied to the skin) or injected prior to the procedure.

### Artecoll

- **What it is:** Synthetic microbeads of polymethylmethacrylate (PMMA) suspended in partially denatured bovine (cow) collagen.

- **Benefits:** More staying power than standard collagen or fat injections.

- **Drawbacks:** Some risk of allergic reaction, due to the use of partially denatured cow collagen.

### Autologen

- **What it is:** This is your own collagen, extracted from your body and sent to a lab outside the hospital where it is processed into an injectable form.

- **Benefits:** Because your own body made the collagen, there's no risk of an allergic reaction to it. However, the effects are temporary, as your body will slowly reabsorb the collagen.

- **Drawbacks:** It requires a surgical procedure to extract the tissue to be sent for processing and a second appointment at a later date for the injection.

### Bovine Collagen

- **What it is:** This version of collagen is extracted from cows.

- **Drawbacks:** It's a temporary fix, and can last from as little as four weeks to three months. Use of this product is good if you just want to get an idea of what lip augmentation might be like without having to make a more permanent decision. There is also a risk of allergic reaction. Your surgeon will give you a test dose to check for allergies before treatment can begin.

### Dermalogen

- **What it is:** This material is extracted from deceased human donors. It's also called injectable Human Tissue Matrix.

- **Drawbacks:** This is also a temporary fix, but your body should not reject it.

### Hylaform

- **What it is:** This is tissue that is created from a molecular component of the human body.

- **Drawbacks:** Hylaform is only a temporary fix and repeat treatments are needed.

### Restylane

- **What it is:** This is a clear gel used to increase volume in the lips. It contains hyaluronic acid (a complex sugar naturally found in the body), so there's little chance for an allergic reaction.

- **Drawbacks:** It's biodegradable, so your body will absorb it within about six months of the injection.

### Juvederm

- **What it is**: Smooth long lasting dermal gel filler. Like Restylane, Juvederm is also made of hyaluronic acid.

- **Benefits:** Biosynthetic with little chance of allergic reaction.

- **Drawbacks:** Temporary: Lasts six months to one year.

## Implants and Surgeries

You will most likely receive local anesthesia. A procedure can take up to two hours at your doctor's office or outpatient center, depending on the complexity, and you will be sent home the same day.

## *Alloderm*

- **What it is:** This material is a collagen sheet created from deceased humans. Your surgeon will insert these through tiny incisions made on the inside part of the lip. This material offers a temporary fix, lasting up to 12 months.

## *Fascia*

- **What it is:** Fascia (also known as white connective tissue) may be obtained from deceased humans or from your own body and implanted surgically.
- **Benefits:** Your own tissue. Can be relatively long lasting.
- **Drawbacks:** Within about one year of the procedure, your body will reabsorb the fascia.

## *Fat Injection*

- **What it is:** This comes from you, too. Your surgeon will usually obtain this from your thighs or abdomen.
- **Benefits:** Again, like Autologen, there is no risk of allergic reaction because it's from you.
- **Drawback:** Requires a surgical procedure to obtain the fat for injection.

## *Fat Grafting*

- **What it is:** This is the surgical method of inserting your own fat into your lips to achieve the desired fullness.
- **Benefits:** Because it's your own fat, there is into chance of a reaction.
- **Drawback:** Although there is a chance that some of the fat will stay permanently that amount of survival is very unpredictable and the procedure may need to be repeated more than once for the desired effect.

## *Gore-Tex, SoftForm and Soft ePTFE*

- **What it is:** These are white, microporous implants made from the same type of material as Gore-Tex boots and raincoats, but of course a sterile medical grade. ePTFE is a non-reactive, non-toxic polymer that has been used in medical implants throughout the body without ill effects for many, many years.

- **Benefits:** Results are permanent unless the graft is removed.

### *Local Flap Grafts*

- **What it is:** This takes a flap of tissue from the inside of your mouth. It requires a longer incision and sutures inside the mouth.

## How Long Will My Recovery Take?

Your recovery will depend on your lifestyle and which procedure you undergo. Most people having injections are fine within a day or two. There might be bruising or swelling however that can last as long as two weeks depending on the type of injection. If you are having surgical implants or grafts, you should plan on it taking two weeks before you will feel comfortable in public. As with any procedure it is recommended that you stop aspirin or any type of blood thinner two weeks prior to treatment to help minimize bruising and swelling.

It's important that you know yourself. Discuss how much time you think you'll need for recovery with your doctor. It may be necessary to take some time off work. You also may not be able to exercise for a few days to a few weeks depending on the type of procedure.

## How to Prepare

It's important that you have someone with you who can drive you home from the operation. If you are a smoker, you may be required to stop smoking for a period of time before and after the procedure. You should follow your doctor's instructions carefully on this. Make sure you wear loose, comfortable clothing. Be especially mindful of the shirt or blouse you choose to wear that day—it should be a button down, if possible, so you do not have to pull it over your face.

Before your procedure, establish a home recovery area with the following:

- ice
- comfortable pillows on which you can prop yourself
- ointment or cream if recommended by your doctor

- plenty of soft foods, such as Jell-O, pudding, oatmeal and yogurt that do not require chewing

- telephone within reaching distance of your recovery area

## Risks and Complications

As with any surgery, there are risks and complications. You can experience bleeding that might require going back to surgery to stop the bleeding. There is also a risk of infection that may require antibiotics or implant removal. It's very important that you discuss any concerns with your doctor prior to surgery and that you make your doctor aware of any existing medical conditions that may cause further complications. Call your doctor immediately if you:

- Experience extreme swelling associated with pain and pressure; or

- Develop a fever.

## Does Insurance Cover Lip Augmentation?

Insurance may cover lip augmentation if the procedure is being completed for reconstructive purposes, such as a congenital defect or as reconstruction after an injury or accident. If you are undergoing this procedure purely for cosmetic purposes, you will be responsible for the cost. Make sure you understand all of your doctor's charges, including anesthesia, follow-up care, etc. Make sure to obtain an estimate of the charges beforehand and work out a payment plan if necessary.

It's also very important that you realize elective cosmetic surgery may impact your current insurance. Your carrier can increase your premiums and it can affect future coverage. Make sure you ask your insurance carrier about its policy on elective, cosmetic surgery so you're not surprised in the future.

# Chapter 33

# *Chin Surgery (Mentoplasty)*

## *Surgery of the Chin*

A well defined chin helps give balance to the face and creates a major part of one's profile. When people look in the mirror, most focus on the size and shape of their noses, their ears, sagging jowls, or fine wrinkling of the skin. But even though few examine their chins with the same discerning eye, having a "weak chin" is certainly not an asset. Surgeons who specialize in rhinoplasty, or surgery of the nose, are often the first to suggest that changes in chin size or shape may enhance a profile as much as rhinoplasty. It is common for the facial plastic surgeon to recommend chin surgery in addition to nose surgery when the surgeon sees that chin augmentation is necessary to achieve facial balance and harmony. Fortunately, this is a relatively straightforward procedure that can make a major difference.

If you are wondering how chin surgery could improve your appearance, you need to know how the surgery is performed and what you can expect from this procedure. This text can address many of your concerns and provide you the information to begin considering chin surgery.

Successful facial plastic surgery is a result of good rapport between patient and surgeon. Trust, based on realistic expectations and exacting medical expertise, develops in the consulting stages before

"Understanding Mentoplasty Surgery," reprinted with permission from the American Academy of Facial Plastic and Reconstructive Surgery, www.aafprs .org. © 2000.

surgery. Your surgeon can answer specific questions about your specific needs.

## Is Chin Surgery for You?

As with all elective surgery, good health and realistic expectations are prerequisites. It is also key to understand all aspects of the surgery. A pleasing, balanced profile can be achieved by inserting an implant or moving the bone forward to build up a receding chin, or by reducing a jutting or too prominent chin. The result can be greater facial harmony and an increase in self-confidence.

Another possibility for improvement through chin surgery is submental liposuction in which excess fatty tissue is removed to redefine the chin or neckline. When there is a contributing problem of dental malocclusions or birth defects in the structure of the jaw itself, surgery of the jaw can improve the form and function of the lower face and greatly enhance appearance.

Your consultation can help you decide on the type of surgery that addresses your concerns. Your surgeon can also provide information on new medical techniques for chin surgery and offer recommendations for supplementary surgery that can ensure the greatest improvement.

## Making the Decision for Chin Surgery

Whether you are interested in chin surgery for functional or cosmetic reasons, your choice of a qualified facial plastic surgeon is extremely important. During the consultation, your surgeon will thoroughly examine your chin and jaw to pinpoint problems. In some instances, the surgeon will suggest chin surgery as a supplement to rhinoplasty because a small chin can make the nose appear larger. Your surgeon will weigh other factors that could influence the outcome of surgery such as age, skin type, and attitudes toward surgery. The surgical procedure will be described in detail along with reasonable projections. If you opt for surgery, your surgeon will describe the technique indicated, the type of anesthesia to be used, the surgical facility, any additional surgery, and risks and costs.

## Understanding the Surgery

To augment the chin, the surgeon begins by making an incision either in the natural crease line just under the chin or inside the mouth, where gum and lower lip meet. By gently stretching this tissue, the surgeon creates a space where an implant can be inserted. This implant, made of synthetic material that feels much like natural tissue normally found in the chin, is available in a wide variety of sizes and shapes. This allows custom fitting of the implant to the configurations of the patient's face. After implantation, the surgeon uses fine sutures to close the incision. When the incision is inside the mouth, no scarring is visible. If the incision is under the chin, the scar is usually imperceptible.

In chin reduction surgery, incisions are made either in the mouth or under the chin. The surgeon sculpts the bone to a more pleasing size. For orthognathic surgery, the surgeon will make an incision inside the mouth and reposition the facial bones. The procedure, depending on the extent of the work, takes from less than an hour to approximately three hours.

## What to Expect after the Surgery

Immediately after surgery, the surgeon usually applies a dressing that will remain in place for two to three days. You will experience some tenderness. Postoperative discomfort can be controlled with prescribed medications. Chewing will probably be limited immediately after chin surgery, and a liquid and soft food diet may be required for a few days after surgery. Most patients feel a stretched, tight sensation after the surgery, but this usually subsides in a week.

After approximately six weeks, most swelling will be gone, and you can enjoy the results of your procedure. Rigorous activity may be prohibited for the first few weeks after surgery. Normal activity can be resumed after approximately ten days.

Facial plastic surgery makes it possible to enhance your appearance and eliminate signs of premature aging that undermine self-confidence. By changing how you look, facial plastic surgery can improve your self-image.

Insurance does not generally cover surgery that is purely for cosmetic reasons. Surgery to correct or improve genetic deformity or traumatic injury may be reimbursable in whole or in part. It is the patient's responsibility to check with the insurance carrier for information on the degree of coverage.

Chapter 34

# Neck Lift (Platysmaplasty)

For some individuals, the neck begins to show age faster than whole face and many times patients only need a neck lift, rather than a full face lift. However, when a face lift is chosen and a neck lift is included—these two together can complete the rejuvenation package. Sometimes, it isn't age that determines the need for a neck lift, but rather having lost considerable weight or it may even be hereditary feature you'd like to remedy. In fact, many younger people undergo platysmaplasty. Many men and women who have undergone neck lift are often thought to have lost a lot of weight or toned up rather than having had surgery.

Jowls can form from fatty deposits at the jaw line and laxity in the muscles, the neck muscles may begin to separate and hang, creating bands and the skin may hang more that we'd like creating the "turkey waddle" look. If this is the case perhaps you'd like to further research the platysmaplasty procedure.

## What Is a Neck Lift?

A neck lift, or platysmaplasty and even submental platysmaplasty, is a surgery designed to reduce the loose look of sagging skin in the neck area and under the jaw line. Some patients who complain of having a fleshy neck, jowls, plastysma or neck banding, or a turkey waddle can benefit from this procedure. Many times patients choose to have

From "Neck Lift (Platysmaplasty)," reprinted with permission from www .facialplasticsurgery.com. © 2005 Enhancement Media.

a neck lift with their face lift procedure. You must realize that the neck lift or face lift procedure is not designed to rejuvenate the area above the brow or around the eyes. If this is what you seek a brow (forehead) lift or blepharoplasty may benefit you. These four procedures can be performed in conjunction with one another for a complete transformation. You may even wish to have laser resurfacing, if you are a candidate, for increased wrinkle ablation and facial rejuvenation.

## Are You a Candidate for a Neck Lift?

First and foremost, an individual must be in good health, not have any active diseases or pre-existing medical conditions, and must have realistic expectations of the outcome of their surgery. Communication is crucial in reaching one's goals. You must be able to voice your desires to your surgeon if he/she is to understand what your desired results are. Discuss you goals with your surgeon so that you may reach an understanding with what can realistically be achieved.

You must be mentally and emotionally stable to undergo an cosmetic procedure. This is an operation which requires patience and stability in dealing with the healing period. There is sometimes a lull or depression after surgery and if there is already a pre-existing emotional problem, this low period can develop into a more serious issue. Please consider this before committing to a procedure. If the above describes you and you have the desire to rid yourself of loose, sagging skin around the neck, you may be a good candidate for platysmaplasty (neck lift).

## What to Expect at Your Consultation

After checking a few surgeons' backgrounds and credentials, you will make an appointment for a consultation. You will meet with these surgeons and discuss your goals and you will disclose all information regarding your health: if you smoke, what medications or vitamins you presently take, etc.—this is very important. You really should consider smoking cessation as smoking can significantly decrease healing.

You will discuss your complaints and concerns and discuss the various looks one can achieve, the amount that can be removed and tightened, etc. Your surgeon will explain the technique (corset platysmaplasty, hammock platysmaplasty, mini-platysmaplasty, etc.) and incision placements that may be most appropriate for you. He or she should discuss the risks associated with neck lift with you, as well.

You will also discuss the available anesthesia that will be used for your procedure. Most neck lift procedures are performed under general anesthesia, light sleep sedation, twilight, regional, or even an oral sedative (Valium) and local anesthetic for less extensive plastysma work. Either way, discuss this beforehand as many people are not aware of the risks of anesthesia. If you do go under deep general anesthesia, ascertain that the anesthesiologist is certified. The risks regarding anesthesia should be considered for a fully informed choice.

If you should choose to book or reserve a surgery date you will usually give a deposit to hold your surgery date. Most times if you cancel a few days beforehand, this amount is non-refundable. After paying your deposit and scheduling a surgery date, you will also schedule a preoperative appointment.

## Your Preoperative Appointment

This appointment addresses more questions you may not have thought to ask at the initial consultation, such as more surgical details, concerns, and even ascertaining that your surgeon is aware of what you desire from your procedure. Your surgeon will make certain that you know what is realistically possible from this procedure.

You will also discuss your preoperative instructions and speak about the recovery period instructions and what to expect in the months ahead. You will be given prescriptions for antibiotics, pain relievers, perhaps blood pressure medicines, prescription anti-inflammatory drugs, and perhaps a box or directions for gaining a box of SinEcch—a pharmaceutical grade form of *Arnica Montana* (a homeopathic preparation used for the reduction of swelling and bruising). Perhaps you will be instructed to obtain Bromelain (a homeopathic preparation used for anti-inflammatory purposes) or other types of remedies, although many surgeons would rather have you not take anything other than your prescription medications. Please do not go against your surgeon's wishes. Remember, always ask your doctor before taking any of these products.

Please do not hesitate to address any concerns that you may have during this time and even after your preoperative appointment. If you remember something when you get home or the next day or even the day of surgery—don't be afraid to ask.

## Preparing for Your Surgery

You should be given a preoperative information packet that explains everything you should do and know before your surgery date. The packet should include a list of all the medications you should not take starting usually at two weeks before your surgery. These medications will include—but are not limited to—aspirin containing products, stimulants, serotonin supplements, etc. If your surgeon advised that you may take *Arnica montana*, Bromelain, Vitamin K, etc. for swelling and bruising, you should either have this in your packet or begin shopping for your necessities.

It is quite possible that you will have blood work performed. This is normally an extra out-of-pocket expense that the patient must participate in to check your white and red blood cell count and check for disease or disorders beforehand. If you are a female they may take an extra vial for a pregnancy test. Some surgeons ask that you have physical. This can be yet another out of pocket expense so ask at your consultation what will be needed when you are quoted a price.

## How a Neck Lift Is Performed

A neck lift procedure normally takes two to three hours to perform. However, if you will be having other procedures performed with your neck lift—this time will be increased and you will more than likely have general anesthesia.

First, you will have monitoring pads attached to you so that the surgical team can properly monitor your vital statistics before, during, and after your operation. When you are brought to the operating room, electrodes will be plugged into these pads which are connected to the monitoring equipment.

Once you are on the operating room table, you will then be given your choice or your surgeon's preference in anesthesia as discussed prior to your surgery date. If you had been given an oral sedative or Valium prior you will have less anxiety. Technicians will likely insert an IV for a saline drip to keep you hydrated and have a vascular doorway for anesthesia, antibiotics, and other medications. If you haven't been given a sedative, it is more stressful for some patients. If you feel that you may experience anxiety inquire beforehand regarding an oral sedative. Having an IV inserted feels sort of like blood being drawn, but for a shorter period of time. The initial placement of the IV that may sting a bit. Some people get their IV placed in the crook of the elbow, some the hand—it all depends upon your veins though; so if your veins are not very prominent this can be a problem. You are then brought to the operating room (OR) if you aren't on the table yet. After the needle is injected into the vein, it is pulled out and a little plastic tube is left in your vein. This is called a catheter. The catheter is taped to your skin so it is not accidentally knocked or pulled out and is ready to be used as a sort of entryway for anything the surgical team deems necessary for your body. This is usually done before you get into the actual OR—by a nurse—and you have a saline bag hooked up to you. The medications will usually be given with a drip system with this saline. As said before, the saline will keep you hydrated both during and post-operatively.

If you have chosen an IV liquid sedative, they will insert a hypodermic into the tube you are attached to or they will attach the bag of sedative with a drip system to add a few drops every few seconds. When they spring open the stopper the sedative starts heading towards your body. The effects of the anesthesia are felt soon whether after injection or opening of the stopper—a few seconds in fact. It may feel similar to a sensation of heat entering your arm or hand at the catheter site. It then feels as though it is creeping up your arm. Then it jumps from your shoulder to produce a metallic-like taste under your tongue. Then you are anesthetized. The anesthesiologist or surgeon will then determine if you are sedated properly, your stats are stable, and if you are ready for the surgery to begin.

You will then be marked with a magic marker type pen for the placement areas if your placement is to be performed intradermally. You will then be scrubbed with Betadine, the surgical marker markings will remain—although not as dark. You will be injected with a solution of lidocaine, epinephrine, and saline. The epinephrine is a vasoconstrictor. This will impede your skin's ability to bleed excessively. Lidocaine is an anesthetic.

## *For a Neck Lift Only*

The skin only lift can be done with two incisions under or behind the ear, the platysmaplasty with the additional skin lift can be accomplished with a small incision under the chin and the behind or under the ear. With the skin only procedure, sections of skin are trimmed and lifted into place and sutured or fixed with tissue glue. With the platysmaplasty, a section fat muscle is removed if need be and the ends are sutured to bring them together at the mid-anterior (front) section of the neck. The skin can be brought together under or behind the ear to further firm up appearance of the neck.

Some surgeons may use suture, mesh, or even AlloDerm suspension as a sort of hammock to keep the neck tight and waddle-free. Whatever the case, please know that surgeons may have different techniques so please discuss this at your consultation.

The surgical team then performs a sponge and instrument count and your surgeon then closes your incision, likely with a non-dissolvable type suture or tissue glue. You will have a pressure dressing placed around your head. If you are not familiar with this look, it involves wrapping a dressing around the top of your head to underneath your chin, and covering your ears. Of course there may be differences in surgical technique depending upon the preference of your surgeon.

You are then gently awakened and brought into the recovery room where the recovery nurse will monitor your vital stats until you are ready to be released. This is dependent upon the individual but may take up to two hours. Your neck may feel tight and quite tender as the anesthesia wears off. You may even feel emotional or upset—this will depend upon your body's reaction to anesthesia. You may also experience rigors or shivering. This may feel uncontrollable and is usually from the medications—likely the epinephrine, which is used as a vasoconstrictor. The recovery nurse usually has wrapped you in a warm blanket but if not, request one. It certainly makes things more tolerable.

Some patients feel nothing different, although if you have had general anesthetic you may feel a little sick—hopefully your surgeon gave you something to lessen this. Your prescribed medication should alleviate pain and discomfort. However, if you believe your pain to be out of the ordinary once you get home, call your surgeon or the on call staff immediately. You should be driven home by your spouse, significant other, or friend as you will not be able to see, much less drive yourself home

## The Road to Recovery

You may get sick on the ride home from the surgical center or hospital so have a bucket or can with a lid as well as water and some Ritz or Goldfish crackers. Bring pillows and a blanket if need be. If you hurt, take your pain relievers. There is simply no reason to suffer; besides, studies have shown that patients with increased pain heal slower than patients who are not in pain.

You may be groggy from the anesthetic and or oral medications and probably won't remember much of the first day or two. You will have to take it easy and sleep on two pillows to keep your head elevated for about 14 days, or however long your surgeon suggests. A recliner is the best for this. Please keep your head and neck still. Do not turn your head from side to side. Move your whole body if you must move. When you wake up you will notice that your lower face and neck will look even more swollen in the first three days. You won't usually be extremely swollen until late that night or the next day, and then the third is by far usually the worst. But, as the days go on the swelling will dissipate. There may be a lot of bruising, but this will go away, as well. So make a mental note of this or you may be shocked into a depression. Bruising and swelling are a normal occurrence in most surgeries. Don't worry, it is all a part of the natural healing process. You shouldn't really look at yourself in the mirror, but rather have your partner or nurse care for you instead (even take photos if you wish it).

Although any discomfort should be alleviated by your prescribed pain medication if you have excessive pain, redness, pus, or other symptoms that do not appear normal, contact your surgeon immediately. Take your temperature regularly. An elevated temperature could mean an infection. Take those antibiotics on time. Also, if you are a female taking birth control pills don't forget that some antibiotics can interfere with the effectiveness of oral contraceptives, so in the event that you do have relations, use another form of protection as well.

Your back will likely cramp up from not being able to lie completely stretched out and flat, so some patients prefer heating pads or hot water bottles. Remember not to sleep while using any of these devices. This can result in severe burns—especially if you are heavily medicated and don't feel the heat or pain.

You will likely go to your first postoperative visit in the next few days. The surgeon may change your bandages or may wait until the end of the week—depending upon the seepage or the extent of work. Your sutures won't be removed until the seventh to tenth day and staples in your scalp (if applicable) not until around day ten. Your scalp takes longer to heal.

Your skin will be numb. Don't be afraid or worried, this is quiet normal. Remember your nerves and all have been partially separated from their source. Give them time to recuperate—just as you, yourself, need time to heal. Please take it easy and try not to do too much, too soon. You should be up and about in the first few days but don't feel guilty if you don't. Listen to your body.

Even though you may feel better, you must take it easy for the first three weeks. Be careful not to bend over or lift heavy objects. And be careful not to raise the blood pressure for at least three weeks as this could cause internal bleeding at your treatment area. Your blood vessels dilate to allow increased blood flow when you raise your heart rate. This may cause problems at internal wound sites. Do not participate in contact sports for at least six to eight weeks—although ask your surgeon what he recommends specifically. Usually, you are instructed not to go into any steam rooms or use steam devices, saunas, face and neck masks, or products containing niacin, niacinamide, or niacinate (these products cause flushing and make your face and neck red); use no products of any kind to promote major flushing of the skin.

Please continue to avoid alcohol and aspirin containing products for a few days to weeks (or until your surgeon tells you) as these have anti-platelet properties and could cause bleeding. Also, you are going to be bruised and swollen for quite some time. If you quit smoking before the procedure you really should not start back up. Smoking greatly increases lack of vascularity, promoting necrosis (death) of skin, improper healing, and excessive scarring. Quit beforehand and stay such.

You may notice a change in your smile, odd sensations of tightness, tingling, the sporadic sharp pain, or pulling, burning, and cold sensations. These usually subside within the first few weeks. Your swelling will subside, revealing a more defined, youthful version of your former self. This may take some time, so please prepare yourself emotionally. Some patients experience a lull or down period where they become depressed or feel unattractive. This is very normal.

## Risks and Complications of a Neck Lift

Unfortunately, all surgery has risks and potential complications. With platysmaplasty, these include an allergic reaction to the anesthetic used and infection. There could be asymmetry, general dissatisfaction, hematoma or seroma, lumpiness, and/or mottling of the skin. Other risks include cording and laxity relapse of the platysma and skin of the neck.

Numbness is possible. It usually subsides within the first few weeks but it may become a permanent issue. Puckering of the skin may occur and deeper than desired depressions may result. Excess scar tissue and lumps are possible as well. Please go over all risks with your surgeon at your consultation and your preoperative appointment.

## The Average Prices of a Neck Lift

The approximate costs of a platysmaplasty, or neck lift, can vary greatly due to region and the surgeon chosen. However, the average prices may be anywhere from $3,000. to $6,500. (U.S.) in itself—and does not include other procedures such as face lift. Some surgeons include submental lipectomy (fat removal under the chin) along with this procedure so determine this beforehand.

# Part Four


# Body Shaping Procedures

# Chapter 35

# *Liposuction (Lipoplasty)*

### *What is liposuction?*

Liposuction is a surgical procedure intended to remove fat deposits and shape the body. Fat is removed from under the skin with the use of a vacuum-suction cannula (a hollow pen-like instrument) or using an ultrasonic probe that emulfsies (breaks up into small pieces) the fat and then removes it with suction.

Persons with localized fat may decide to have liposuction to remove fat from that area. Liposuction is a procedure for shaping the body and is not recommended for weight loss.

Liposuction may be performed on the abdomen, hips, thighs, calves, arms, buttocks, back, neck, or face. A liposuction procedure may include more than one site, for instance, the abdomen, back, and thighs all on the same day.

Liposuction is also used to reduce breast size in men with large breasts (gynecomastia) or to remove fat tumors (lipomas) but it is most commonly used for cosmetic body shaping.

### *Who performs liposuction and where is liposuction performed?*

Many liposuction surgeries are performed by plastic surgeons or by dermatologists. Any licensed physician may perform liposuction.

"Liposuction Information," Center for Devices and Radiological Health, U.S. Food and Drug Administration (FDA), August 2002.

While some physicians' professional societies may recommend training before performing liposuction surgery, no standardized training is required. As a result, there will be differences in experience and training in physicians performing liposuction. You can ask your physician to tell you whether he or she has had specialized training to do liposuction and whether they have successfully done liposuction before. But remember, even the best screened patients under the care of the best trained and experienced physicians may experience complications as a result of liposuction.

Liposuction may be performed in the following locations:

- a doctor's office

- a surgical center

- a hospital

Because liposuction is a surgical procedure, it is important that it be performed in a clean environment. Emergencies may arise during any surgery and access to emergency medical equipment or a nearby hospital emergency room is important. These are things that you should ask your physician before the liposuction.

### *How can I find the right doctor for me?*

The FDA (Food and Drug Administration) cannot recommend physicians to you. However, there are some things that you may consider:

- **Ask questions:** If you decide to take the step to talk to a doctor about liposuction, be sure that you ask questions and understand what happens during the liposuction procedure and what you can expect. Your physician should also answer any and all questions you have about potential problems with liposuction. Remember that you are purchasing a service when you pay a physician to do a liposuction procedure and you shouldn't feel embarrassed to ask hard questions about the procedure or about the physician's experience in performing liposuction.

- **Advertising:** Be wary of advertisements that say or imply that you will have a perfect appearance after liposuction. Remember that advertisements are meant to sell you a product or service, not to inform you of all the potential problems with that service.

- **Don't base your decision simply on cost** and remember that you don't have to settle for the first doctor or procedure you investigate. The decision you make about liposuction surgery is an important one but not one that you must make right away.

- **Read:** You should learn as much as you can about liposuction. It is important for you to read the patient information that your doctor provides.

- **Don't be pressured:** Do not feel that because you speak to a physician about this procedure that you must go through with it. Take your time to decide whether liposuction is right for you and whether you are willing to take the risks of undergoing liposuction for its benefits.

## *What does the FDA regulate?*

In the United States, the Food and Drug Administration (FDA) regulates the sale of medical devices, such as the equipment (cannulas, pumps, collecting containers, ultrasound probes), and drugs (anesthesia) used for liposuction.

Before a medical device can be legally sold in the U.S., the person or company that wants to sell the device must seek approval from the FDA. To gain approval, they must present evidence that the device is reasonably safe and effective for a particular use, the "indication." Once a device is approved, other similar devices may be cleared by the FDA for use. This requires less information since an equivalent device has already been shown to be safe and effective. In some cases, devices that were on the market before FDA started regulating medical devices may be cleared. Once the FDA has approved or cleared a medical device, a doctor may decide to use that device for other indications if the doctor feels it is in the best interest of a patient. The use of an approved or cleared device for other than its FDA-approved indication is called "off-label use."

The FDA does not have the authority to do the following:

- Regulate a doctor's practice. In other words, FDA does not tell doctors what to do when running their business or what they can or cannot tell their patients.

- Set the amount a doctor can charge for liposuction surgery.

- "Insist" that patient information be provided to the potential patient.

- Make recommendations for individual doctors, clinics, or liposuction centers. FDA does not maintain nor have access to lists of doctors performing liposuction.

251

- Recommend a physician to you.

- Conduct or provide a rating system on medical devices it regulates.

## When is liposuction not for me?

You are probably not a good candidate for liposuction surgery if:

- You are not a risk taker. Certain complications are unavoidable in a percentage of patients, and there are no long-term data available for current procedures.

- Cost is an issue. Most medical insurance will not pay for cosmetic liposuction. The cost for liposuction may be significant.

- You are overweight or obese and trying to lose weight. Liposuction is a procedure for shaping the body and is not recommended for weight loss.

- You have a disease or are on medication that affects wound healing. These include current infection or past medical history of bleeding, emboli, thrombophlebitis, edema, or if you are taking medications that may affect your wound healing or blood clotting (such as aspirin, nonsteroidal anti-inflammatory agents, warfarin, heparin, or other anticoagulants) or are taking medication that may interact with the drugs used during liposuction.

- Your skin elasticity is not adequate. Your doctor will evaluate the skin at the site where you are considering liposuction to determine if skin is elastic enough to shrink after liposuction. If it is not, it will be baggy after liposuction.

## What are the alternatives to liposuction?

Liposuction is usually cosmetic surgery so is not considered medically necessary (there are rare exceptions to this). Because of this, it is you who will decide whether or not you will undergo this procedure. You may decide that liposuction is not right for you. You may make this decision without consulting a physician or after consulting with a physician. A consultation with a physician does not obligate you to have liposuction if you decide that you do not want to.

Here are some of the alternatives to liposuction:

- Change diet to lose some excess body fat

- Exercise

- Accept your body and appearance as it is

- Use clothing or makeup to downplay or emphasize body or facial features

### What are the risks or complications associated with liposuction?

**Risks:** Most patients are pleased with the outcome of their liposuction surgery. However, like any other medical procedure, there are risks involved. That's why it is important for you to understand the limitations and possible complications of liposuction surgery. Before you have liposuction, you should be aware of these risks and should weigh the risks and benefits based on your own personal value system. Try to avoid being influenced by friends that have had the procedure or doctors encouraging you to do so. Decide for yourself whether you are willing to take the risks involved in liposuction.

Take your time deciding if you are willing to accept the risks inherent in liposuction. Because it is usually a cosmetic procedure, and not medically necessary, there is no reason to rush. Gather as much information as you can so that you make an informed decision about whether liposuction is right for you. Don't believe that complications "only happen to other people." It is important for you to understand what the risks are and decide if you are willing to accept the possibility that it might happen to you.

**Complications:** Complications include the following:

- **Infections:** Infections may happen after any surgery and may occur after liposuction. Some physicians prescribe an antibiotic to all patients undergoing liposuction but other physicians do not. It is important to keep the wounds clean but even if you do, infections may sometimes occur from the surgery. Sometimes, infections may be serious or life threatening such as in cases of necrotizing fasciitis (bacteria eat away at the tissue) or with toxic shock syndrome, a serious, sometimes fatal infection caused by a bacteria, that is associated with surgery (you may have heard of toxic shock syndrome occurring in women using tampons, also).

- **Embolism:** Embolism may occur when fat is loosened and enters the blood through blood vessels ruptured (broken) during liposuction. Pieces of fat get trapped in the blood vessels, gather in the lungs, or travel to the brain. The signs of pulmonary emboli (fat clots in the lungs) may be shortness of breath or difficulty breathing. If you have the signs or symptoms of fat emboli after liposuction, it is important for you to seek emergency medical care at once. Fat emboli may cause permanent disability or, in some cases, be fatal.

- **Visceral perforations** (puncture wounds in the organs): During liposuction, the physician is unable to see where the cannula or probe is. It is possible to puncture or damage internal organs during liposuction. This may happen, for instance, if the intestines are punctured during abdominal liposuction. When organs are damaged, surgery may be required to repair them. Visceral perforations may also be fatal.

- **Seroma:** After liposuction, there may be a pooling of serum, the straw colored liquid from your blood, in areas where tissue has been removed.

- **Nerve compression and changes in sensation:** You may experience "paresthesias" which is an altered sensation at the site of the liposuction. This may either be in the form of an increased sensitivity (pain) in the area, or the loss of any feeling (numbness) in the area. If these changes in sensation persist for a long period of time (weeks or months) you should inform your physician. In some cases, these changes in sensation may be permanent.

- **Swelling:** Swelling or edema may occur after liposuction. In some cases, swelling may persist for weeks or months after liposuction.

- **Skin necrosis** (skin death): The skin above the liposuction site may become necrotic or "die." When this happens, skin may change color and be sloughed (fall) off. Large areas of skin necrosis may become infected with bacteria or microorganisms.

- **Burns:** During ultrasound assisted liposuction, the ultrasound probe may become very hot and can cause burns.

- **Fluid imbalance:** Fat tissue, which contains a lot of liquid, is removed during liposuction. Also, physicians may inject large amounts of fluids during liposuction. This may result in a fluid imbalance. While you are in the physician's office, surgical center or hospital, the staff will be watching you for signs of fluid imbalance. However, this may happen after you go home and can result in serious conditions such as heart problems, excess fluid collecting in the lungs, or kidney problems as your kidneys try to maintain fluid balance.

- **Toxicity from anesthesia:** Lidocaine, a drug that numbs the skin, is frequently used as a local anesthetic during liposuction. You may have had a similar drug, novocaine, to numb your mouth at the dentist. Large volumes of liquid with lidocaine may be injected during liposuction. This may result in very high doses of lidocaine. The signs of this are lightheadedness, restlessness, drowsiness, tinnitus (a ringing in the ears), slurred speech, metallic taste in the mouth, numbness of the lips and tongue, shivering, muscle twitching and convulsions. Lidocaine toxicity may cause the heart to stop. Of course, this can be fatal. In general, any type of anesthesia may cause complications and is always considered a risk during any surgery.

- **Fatalities related to liposuction:** There are numerous reports of deaths related to the liposuction procedure. Although it is difficult to be sure how often death from liposuction happens, there are several studies that estimate how often patients undergoing liposuction die during the procedure or as a result of it. None of the studies is perfect so the results are just estimates. Some of the studies indicate that the risk of death due to liposuction is as low as 3 deaths for every 100,000 liposuction operations performed. However, other studies indicate that the risk of death is between 20 and 100 deaths per 100,000 liposuction procedures. One study suggests that the death rate is higher in liposuction surgeries in which other surgical procedures are also performed at the same time. In order to understand the size of the risk, one paper compares the deaths from liposuction to that for deaths from car accidents (16 per 100,000). It is important to remember that liposuction is a surgical procedure and that there may be serious complications, including death.

## *What can I expect before, during, and after liposuction?*

**Before:** Before you undergo liposuction, you should undergo a complete physical exam so that your doctor can determine if you are an acceptable candidate for liposuction. It is important for you to discuss any medical conditions that you have and to tell your doctor about any medications that you are taking including any herbal or other non-prescription ones. If your doctor decides that you can have liposuction, discuss the procedure thoroughly with him or her before deciding if you want to go through with the procedure. Just because a physician says that you may have liposuction does not mean that you must decide to have liposuction. You may still change your mind even after discussing the procedure with a physician.

Your physician should be able to answer any questions that you have about liposuction including questions about what to expect during and after liposuction and the complications or problems that sometimes occur with liposuction. Some physicians will provide written information about liposuction. You may also take information from this website to your appointment to discuss with your physician.

You may want to have someone drive you to your appointment for liposuction. You may be tired or uncomfortable after liposuction and unable to drive yourself home. Discuss this with your physician before the day of your procedure.

Your physician may prescribe an antibiotic drug for you to take before and after the surgery. This is to prevent infections.

**During:** On the day of the liposuction surgery, the physician will mark your body with a pen to indicate where the fat is to be removed. Then you will receive anesthesia, which is medicine that prevents you from feeling pain. Some physicians use only local anesthesia, that is, anesthesia that they inject with a syringe or pump into the area where they will do the liposuction. The anesthesia medicine is injected along with a lot of fluid, usually buffered salt water and epinephrine, a drug to reduce bleeding. Large volumes of liquid may be injected, until the skin is very firm. If your physician uses only this kind of local anesthesia, also sometimes called tumescent anesthesia, then you will be awake during the procedure. Other physicians use local anesthesia and a sedative that can be taken by mouth or injected from a syringe. Still others prefer to use general anesthesia that is to use anesthesia that will put you to sleep during the procedure. This is usually done in a hospital.

Once the anesthesia is working, the physician will make an incision (cut) in the area where the liposuction will be performed. A cannula, a hollow tube that is about the size and shape of a skinny pen, will be inserted into the incision. The physician moves this cannula back and forth to suction out the fat. The fat, and liquid that has been injected, are collected in a flask. The physician will monitor the amount of fluid and fat that are removed. Because you will be losing liquid and fat from your body, it may be necessary to replace some of that fluid. This is done with an intravenous (IV) line for the replacement of fluid.

**After:** Depending upon the amount of fat removed and the location of the surgery (doctor's office, surgical center, hospital), you may leave the doctor's office soon after the surgery or you may spend the night in the surgical center or hospital. Ask your doctor how long it will be before you should be able to return to your normal level of activity or if you will need to miss work after liposuction.

The cuts where the doctor inserted the cannula may be leaky or drain fluids for several days. In some cases, the doctor may insert a drainage tube to drain fluid away from the wound.

You will wear special tight garments to keep your skin compressed after the liposuction procedure. Your doctor will tell you how long to wear these, usually for weeks. Some doctors provide these garments but others will tell you where to purchase them before your surgery.

Your doctor will also probably give you some after-surgery instructions. This will include information about wearing compression garments, taking an antibiotic if that has been prescribed, and the level of activity that is safe for you after your liposuction procedure. You should also have information about signs of problems that you should be aware of, for instance the signs of infections or other problems that you need to know about.

When the anesthesia wears off, you may have some pain. If the pain is extreme or of a long duration, you should contact your physician. You will also have some swelling after the surgery. In some cases, this swelling will remain for weeks or even months. If you have pain and swelling, this may be the sign of infection and you should contact your physician.

You will have scars, usually small, where the physician cuts your skin and inserts the cannula to remove fat tissue.

## Will I look the way I want after liposuction?

While medical complications are important, the reason that people have liposuction surgery is for cosmetic reasons. The cosmetic effect after liposuction may be very good and many patients report being satisfied. However, it is possible that the cosmetic effect will not be what you expected. In other words, your appearance after liposuction may not be what you expected or wanted. Some physicians counsel their patients that reasonable expectations are important. It may be difficult to have reasonable expectations after reading advertisements and looking at pictures of women and men who have had liposuction. Remember that advertising is made to make you want to purchase a product or service. Advertisements do not usually tell you about problems or shortcomings of the product or service. If you want to know more about advertising ethics, or want to report on false advertising, explore the following websites:

- www.ftc.gov/bcp/menu-ads.htm
- www.ftc.gov/bcp/menu-health.htm

Some cosmetic shortcomings after liposuction include:

- There may be scars at the site where the doctor made the cut to insert the liposuction cannula. These scars are usually small and fade with time but in some people, scars may be larger or more prominent.

- The liposuction site may have a wavy or bumpy appearance after liposuction.

- Liposuction results may not be permanent. If you gain weight after liposuction surgery, the fat may return to sites where you had liposuction or to other sites.

- Results may be less dramatic than what you were expecting and this can be disappointing.

## Liposuction Surgery Checklist

- Know what makes you a poor candidate for liposuction
    - **Medical conditions:** Do you have any medical conditions that could interfere with healing after liposuction?
    - **Medications:** Are you taking any medications, including herbal remedies or non-prescription medications, that can increase your risk for complications or that may interfere with healing?
    - **Cost:** Can you really afford this procedure?
    - **Weight loss:** Are you considering liposuction as a way to lose weight? Consider changing your diet and exercise regimen if you are trying to lose weight. Liposuction is not a good way to lose weight.
- Know all the risks and procedure limitations
    - **Risks:** Do you understand that complications could happen to you and that some of the complications from liposuction can be serious and even occasionally fatal?

- **Liposuction outcomes:** Do you understand that although many people will be satisfied with the outcome after liposuction, that some people will not have the outcome that they wished for?

- Understand all the answers to your questions about liposuction

  - **Questions answered:** Have you read about and do you understand what liposuction is? Has your doctor answered all of your questions to your satisfaction?

  - **Read and understand the informed consent:** Has your doctor given you an informed consent form to take home and read?

- Know what to before during and after the liposuction operation

  - **Have a thorough medical exam:** Have you had a thorough medical examination and are fit for liposuction?

  - **Arrange for transportation to and from appointment:** Can someone drive you home after surgery?

  - **Plan to take a few days to recover:** Can you take time off if necessary to recover?

  - **Expect some pain/discomfort:** Do you know how much pain to expect?

  - **Know when to seek help:** Do you know what the signs are for different complications after liposuction? Do you know when to seek medical help? Did you receive after care instructions from your doctor telling you what to do if you experience problems after liposuction?

# Chapter 36

# *Breast Enlargement (Augmentation Mammoplasty)*

## *Breast Augmentation*

Breast augmentation, also know as augmentation mammoplasty, surgically enhances—or enlarges—a woman's breasts. Typically, breast augmentation is for women who wish to improve the way they look, to balance out a difference in the size of their breasts, or to reconstruct the natural volume of their breasts after pregnancy. After breast implantation, a woman's bustline may be increased by one or more bra cup sizes.

**Techniques:** Currently, most surgical breast augmentation uses saline-filled implants. Silicone gel implants are also available for certain cases of breast augmentation. Many factors should be discussed with your physician, such as: the size and shape of implants, the location of surgical incisions, and whether the implants should be placed on top of or underneath the chest muscle.

**Anesthesia:** Breast augmentation is performed under general anesthesia.

---

This chapter begins with "Breast Augmentation," reprinted with permission from http://www.columbiasurgery.org, © Columbia University Department of Surgery. Additional text under the heading "Facts about Breast Implants," is excerpted from *FDA Breast Implant Consumer Handbook*, U.S. Food and Drug Administration (FDA), 2004. The complete text of this document, including references, is available online at http://www.fda.gov/cdrh/breastimplants/indexbip.pdf.

**Before surgery:** Avoid taking aspirin, Advil, Motrin, or other aspirin-containing products for two weeks. If you are a smoker, stop smoking to aid in healing.

### *Recovery*

- You will be sore and will need to rest for the first few days.
- Most women are able to resume normal activity after a few days.
- You will need to wear a surgical bra or another non-underwire bra for several weeks, by which time the swelling will subside.
- Fertility and pregnancy are unaffected.
- Breastfeeding is usually possible afterward.

## *Facts about Breast Implants*

### *Device Description*

Breast implants may vary in shell surface (smooth versus textured), shape (round or shaped), profile (how far it sticks out), volume (size), and shell thickness. The primary parts of most breast implants are a shell (otherwise known as the envelope or lumen), a filler, and a patch to cover the manufacturing hole.

With respect to the shell design, while most breast implants are single lumen (just the shell), some breast implants are double lumen (one shell inside another shell). With respect to the filler, some breast implants are manufactured with a fixed volume of filler, some are filled during the operation, and some allow for adjustments of the filler volume after the operation.

It should be noted that tissue expanders, which are silicone shells filled with saline, are regulated by the U.S. Food and Drug Administration (FDA) in a different way than breast implants. This is because tissue expanders are intended for general tissue expansion for a maximum of six months, after which, they are to be removed. Because of this, the design specifications (for example, thinner shell) and preclinical testing recommendations are different for tissue expanders than for breast implants. Tissue expanders are not to be confused with the third type of double lumen silicone gel-filled breast implants (described below). The third type of double lumen silicone gel-filled breast implant is a permanent implant (not intended to be removed) that allows for limited tissue expansion but is regulated by FDA as a breast implant.

**Saline-filled breast implants:** The three types of saline-filled breast implants are as follows:

- One type is a single lumen implant that is filled during the operation with a fixed volume of saline through a valve. There are no adjustments of the saline volume after the operation.

- A second type is a single lumen implant that is filled during the operation with saline through a valve. This type of implant allows for adjustments of the saline volume after the operation.

- A third type is a single lumen implant that is prefilled by the manufacturer with a fixed volume of saline. There are no valves for filling during the operation or for adjustments of the saline volume after the operation.

**Silicone gel-filled breast implants:** The three types of silicone gel-filled breast implants are as follows:

- One type is a single lumen implant that is prefilled by the manufacturer with a fixed volume of silicone gel.

- A second type is a double lumen implant with (1) an inner lumen prefilled by the manufacturer with a fixed volume of silicone gel and (2) an outer lumen that is filled during the operation with a fixed volume of saline through a valve.

- A third type is a double lumen implant with (1) an outer lumen prefilled by the manufacturer with a fixed volume of silicone gel and (2) an inner lumen that is filled during the operation with saline through a valve. This type of implant allows for adjustments of the saline volume after the operation.

**Alternative breast implants:** An alternative breast implant typically has a silicone rubber shell with a filler other than saline or silicone gel. The filler material may or may not be a gel. An alternative breast implant may also have an alternative shell other than one made from silicone rubber.

## Complications

The Institute of Medicine (IOM) completed an independent review of past and ongoing scientific research of silicone [both saline-filled and silicone-gel filled] breast implant safety in June 1999. Below are some of the major findings from the IOM report:

- Local complications (that is, complications that occur in the breast or chest area) are the primary safety issue with breast implants because they are frequent enough to be a concern.

- Local complications accumulate over the lifetime of the implant, and they have not been well studied.

- Information on local complications is crucial for women deciding whether or not they want breast implants.

Key points to consider whether you are undergoing breast augmentation, reconstruction, or revision include the following:

- Breast implants will not last a lifetime. Either because of rupture or other complications, you will likely need to have the implants removed.

- You are likely to need additional doctor visits and re-operations because of one or more complications over the course of your life.

- You are likely to have the implants removed, with or without replacement, because of one or more complications over the course of your life.

- Many of the changes to your breast following implantation may be cosmetically undesirable, as well as irreversible (cannot be undone).

- If you later choose to have your implants removed, you may experience unacceptable dimpling, puckering, wrinkling, loss of breast tissue, or other undesirable cosmetic changes of the breast.

Potential local breast implant complications are bulleted below. You may need nonsurgical treatments or re-operations (including removal of your implant) to treat any of these local complications. Potential local complications include, but are not limited to the following:

- **Asymmetry:** Uneven appearance between a woman's breasts in terms of size, shape, or breast level.

- **Breast pain:** Pain in the nipple or breast area.

- **Breast tissue atrophy:** Thinning and shrinking of the skin.

- **Calcification/calcium deposits:** Hard lumps under the skin around the implant. These can be mistaken for cancer during mammography, resulting in additional surgery, either to biopsy the lumps or to remove the implant.

- **Capsular contracture:** Scar tissue or capsule that normally forms around the implant, which tightens or squeezes the implant. There are four grades of capsular contracture ranging from grade I (breast is normally soft and looks natural) to grade IV (breast is hard, painful, and looks abnormal).

- **Chest wall deformity:** When the chest wall or underlying rib cage appears deformed following removal of the implants and breast tissue.

- **Delayed wound healing:** Incision site fails to heal normally or takes longer to heal.

- **Extrusion:** Skin breakdown with the implant appearing through the skin.

- **Galactorrhea:** Inappropriate breast milk production that may occur after breast implant surgery. In some cases, the milk production stops by itself or after receiving medicine to stop milk production. In other cases, the implant(s) may need to be removed to treat this complication.

- **Granuloma:** Non-cancerous lumps that can form when certain body cells surround foreign material, such as silicone. Like any lump, it should be evaluated to distinguish it from a lump that might be cancerous.

- **Hematoma:** Collection of blood inside a body cavity. Swelling, pain, and bruising may result. If a hematoma occurs, it will usually be soon after surgery; however, it can also occur at any time after injury to the breast. While the body absorbs small hematomas, large ones may require the placement of surgical drains for proper healing. A small scar can result from surgical draining.

- **Iatrogenic injury/damage:** Injury/damage to the tissue or implant due to surgical instruments either during the operation, during a reoperation, during implant removal, or during breast procedures while the implant is in place (for example, cyst aspiration or hematoma drainage).

- **Infection** (including toxic shock syndrome): Can occur with any surgery when wounds are contaminated with microorganisms such as bacteria or fungi. Most infections resulting from

265

surgery appear within a few days to weeks after the operation. However, infection is possible at any time after surgery. Infections with an implant present are harder to treat than infections in normal body tissues. If an infection does not respond to antibiotics, the implant may have to be removed. Another implant may be placed after the infection is gone.

- **Inflammation/irritation:** Swelling of the breast area, usually with redness.

- **Malposition/displacement:** When the implant is placed incorrectly during the initial surgery or when the implant has moved/shifted from its original position. Shifting can be caused by many factors, such as gravity, trauma, poor initial placement, and capsular contracture.

- **Necrosis:** Formation of dead tissue around the implant. Factors associated with increased necrosis include infection, use of steroids in the surgical breast pocket, smoking, chemotherapy/radiation, and  excessive heat or cold therapy.

- **Nipple/breast sensation changes:** An increase or a decrease in the sensation in the nipple or breast. This change can vary in degree and may be temporary or permanent. It may affect comfort while nursing or sexual response.

- **Palpability/visibility:** Palpability is when the implant can be felt through the skin. Visibility is when the implant can be seen through the skin, such as the valve on a saline-filled breast implant or the edge of an implant.

- **Ptosis:** Sagging/drooping of the breast.

- **Redness/bruising:** Bleeding at operative site that causes discoloration and varies in degree and length of time. This is expected following breast implant surgery or breast procedures.

- **Rupture/deflation:** Hole or tear in the shell of the implant that allows for loss of the filler material from the shell.

- **Scarring:** Formation of tissue at the incision. All wounds heal by the formation of a scar. The degree of scarring varies from person to person, and skin type is an important factor for the development of scars. If the scarring becomes irregular and raised, it is called hypertrophic scarring. This may leave a visible, permanent scar. The keloid, a severe type of hypertrophic scar, generally does not fade or flatten with time.

- **Seroma:** Collection of the watery portion of the blood around the implant or around the incision. Swelling, pain, and bruising may result. While the body absorbs small seromas, large ones will require the placement of surgical drains for proper healing. A small scar can result from surgical draining.

- **Unsatisfactory style/size:** Patient or doctor is not satisfied with the overall look based on the style or size of implant used.

- **Wrinkling/rippling:** Wrinkling of the implant that can be felt or seen through the skin.

## *Diseases*

Some women with breast implants have reported health problems that they believe are related to their implants, but most studies of these diseases have failed to show an association with breast implants. There also have been concerns about possible, but unproven, effects on health. Most of the health concerns about breast implants are related to the body reacting to a foreign material, such as silicone gel. These diseases are discussed below.

**Connective tissue diseases (CTDs) and related disorders:** These are a group of diseases and disorders related to the immune system and to the connective tissue of the body (for example, muscle, tendon, bone, etc.) that supports body structures and binds body parts together. The body's immune system is the network of cells that protect against infectious diseases. Antibodies are one type of substance the body produces to fight off infectious agents. The cause of CTDs is unknown. Some CTDs have autoimmune characteristics in that a woman's immune system attacks her own cells as if they were foreign. CTDs with autoimmune characteristics include the following:

- lupus
- rheumatoid arthritis
- polymyositis
- dermatomyositis
- progressive systemic sclerosis or scleroderma

CTDs without autoimmune characteristics include fibromyalgia and chronic fatigue syndrome.

Some women with breast implants have experienced the diseases or disorders mentioned above, as well as a variety of signs and symptoms

267

that could be related to the immune system or to the connective tissues of the body. However, these signs and symptoms are not considered a defined disease or disorder. These signs and symptoms include the following:

- pain and swelling of joints
- tightness
- redness or swelling of the skin
- swollen glands or lymph nodes
- unusual or unexplained fatigue
- swelling of the hands and feet
- excessive hair loss
- memory problems
- headaches
- muscle weakness or burning

Signs and symptoms, such as those bulleted above, may be present in women without CTD or related disorders or in women without breast implants. Individual cases alone cannot scientifically prove or disprove a connection between CTDs and related disorders and breast implants.

Some doctors and women have thought that these signs and symptoms are part of a new disease which is related to silicone and have called the disease "human adjuvant disease," "silicone related syndrome," "atypical disease," or other names. The IOM report stated "The diagnosis of this condition could depend on the presence of a number of symptoms that are nonspecific and common in the general population. Thus, there does not appear to be even suggestive evidence of a novel [new] syndrome in women with breast implants." So, it is unclear at this time whether or not the signs and symptoms experienced by these women are related to their implants. In some cases, women have reported fewer symptoms after the implants were removed. In other cases, there was no change in signs and symptoms after the implants were removed.

Studies have shown that some women with silicone gel-filled breast implants produced antibodies to their own collagen (a connective tissue protein), but we do not know how often these antibodies occur in the general population, and there are no data that show these antibodies cause CTDs and related disorders. There are reports of women with implants who have a variety of autoantibodies. (Autoantibodies are antibodies that your body makes that accidentally target your own tissues.) However, the presence of these autoantibodies does not mean that a woman has an increased risk of actually developing a CTD or related disorder.

When considered together, these studies indicate that the risk of developing a typical or defined CTD or related disorder due to having a breast implant is low. However, these studies have not been large enough to resolve the question of whether or not breast implants slightly increase the risk of CTDs or related disorders. Researchers must study a large group of women without breast implants who are of similar age, health, and social status and who are followed for a long time (such as 10–20 years) before a relationship between breast implants and these diseases can conclusively be made.

There have been reports of women with fibromyalgia following breast implants, and a preliminary study conducted by FDA found an association between self-reported fibromyalgia and extracapsular rupture diagnosed by MRI (magnetic resonance imaging). However, this association has not been repeated in a similar study based on a large group of Danish women and the weight of the epidemiological evidence published in the literature does not support an association between fibromyalgia and breast implants.

**Cancers:** The IOM report indicates that breast cancer is no more common in women with breast implants than those without breast implants. While not conclusive, cancer rates have been reported to be slightly higher for some types of cancers. Cancers rates that have been higher in more than one study are lung and vulva. Because these cancers may be related to other factors that were not examined in these studies (such as smoking) these studies are not conclusive. More information on cancer and breast implants is available at the National Cancer Institute website (www.cancer.gov).

**Neurological symptoms/diseases:** Some women with breast implants have reported that they have neurological symptoms (such as difficulties with vision, sensation, muscle strength, walking, balance, thinking or remembering things) or diseases (such as multiple sclerosis) related to their implants. Several studies have indicated that women with implants are not at an increased risk of being hospitalized with neurological disease compared to other women. The IOM report found no basis for thinking that women with implants were more likely to have neurological diseases or symptoms.

Since the IOM report, an additional follow-up study was published of a Danish group of 1,653 women with cosmetic breast implant surgery at private clinics in Denmark compared to a comparison group of 1,736 women who underwent other types of cosmetic procedures. No increased risks for neurological disorders were found in the breast implant patients. However, it should be noted that these studies are limited in that rare disorders cannot be addressed.

## *Mammography Concerns*

Women with breast implants who are in an age group where routine mammograms are recommended should be sure to have these examinations at the recommended regularly scheduled times. Some women who undergo breast reconstruction will have some breast tissue remaining, and some have all of their breast tissue removed. It is important that a woman with remaining breast tissue continue to have mammography of that breast, as well as of the other breast, to detect breast cancer. (Those who have had breast cancer surgery on both breasts should ask their doctors whether mammograms are still necessary.)

Women should be aware that breast implants may interfere with the detection of cancer and that breast compression (hard pressure) during mammography may cause implant rupture/deflation.

Interference with mammography by breast implants may delay or hinder the early detection of breast cancer either by hiding suspicious lesions (wounds or injuries or tumors) or by making it more difficult to include them in the image (x-ray, ultrasound). Implants increase the difficulty of both taking and reading mammograms.

Mammography requires breast compression, which could contribute to implant rupture. According to the FDA adverse event database, there were 41 reported cases of breast implant rupture during mammography reported between 1992 and 2002. An additional 17 cases of rupture during mammography were reported in the medical literature.

In addition to special care taken by the radiological technologist to reduce the risk of implant rupture during this compression, other techniques are used to maximize what is seen of the breast tissue during mammography. These techniques are called breast implant displacement views, Eklund displacement views, or Eklund views, named for the radiologist who developed the techniques. These special implant displacement views are done in addition to those views done during routine mammograms.

Because of the extra views and time needed, women with implants should always inform the receptionist or scheduler that they have breast implants when making an appointment for mammography. They should also tell the radiological technologist about the presence of implants before mammography is performed. Then, the radiological technologist will use these special displacement techniques and take extra care when compressing the breasts to avoid rupturing the implant.

The displacement procedure involves pushing the implant back and pulling the breast tissue into view. Several factors that may affect the success of this special technique in imaging the breast tissue in women with breast implants include the location of the implant, the hardness of the capsular contracture, and the amount of the breast tissue compared to the implant size.

Also, when reading the mammogram, the radiologist may find it difficult to distinguish calcium deposits in the scar tissue around the implant from a breast tumor. Occasionally, it is necessary to remove and examine a small amount of tissue (biopsy) to see whether or not it is cancerous. Frequently, this can be done without removing the implant. As a last note, FDA does not consider mammograms an adequate means of detecting implant rupture/deflation for silicone gel-filled breast implants. FDA believes that MRI is currently the best method for detecting implant rupture for silicone gel-filled breast implants.

### Breastfeeding Concerns

Women of childbearing age should know that they may not be able to breastfeed after breast implantation. Some women who undergo breast augmentation can successfully breastfeed and some cannot. Women who undergo a mastectomy will be unable to breastfeed on the affected side due to loss of breast tissue and glands that produce milk. The IOM report said that women with either silicone gel-filled or saline-filled breast implants showed lactation insufficiency (not enough milk) ranging from 28–64%. The periareolar approach (incision cite is around the nipple) was the factor most associated with lactation insufficiency.

Having a breast implant may also influence a woman's decision about whether or not she will try to breastfeed, particularly if she has capsular contracture or is worried about problems with the implants.

## Choosing an Implant

You should consider the following when you and your surgeon are discussing implant options.

**Implant status:** Whether or not an implant is premarket-approved (PMA) or investigational (not PMA-approved) should be something you. An implant that is investigational means you will need to be part of a clinical study to get these implants. In addition, the surgeon of your choice may work with only specific breast implants.

**Shape and size:** Depending on the desired shape and size you wish to achieve, you and your surgeon may choose a round or contoured implant shape of appropriate size (volume). You should be aware that contoured implants that are placed submuscular (under the pectoralis major muscle) may assume a round shape after implantation. Your surgeon will also evaluate your existing tissue to determine if you have enough to cover the breast implant.

**Implant surface:** Textured surface implants were designed to reduce the chance of capsular contracture. Some studies with small numbers of women suggest that surface texturing reduces the chance of severe capsular contracture. However, other studies of a large number of women with saline-filled implants show no difference in the likelihood of developing capsular contracture with textured implants when compared to smooth-surfaced implants.

**Implant palpability/visibility:** The following may cause implants to be more palpable (more easily felt) or more visible: textured implants; larger implants; subglandular placement; and smaller amount of skin/tissue available to cover the implant.

## Choosing the Surgical Incision Site

The three common incision sites for breast augmentation are under the arm (transaxillary), around the nipple (periareolar), or within the breast fold (inframammary).

- **Transaxillary:** This incision is less concealed than periareolar but associated with less difficulty than the periareolar incision site when breast feeding.

- **Periareolar:** This incision is most concealed but is associated with a higher likelihood of inability to successfully breast feed, as compared to the other incision sites.

- **Inframammary:** This incision is less concealed than periareolar but associated with less difficulty with breast feeding than the periareolar incision site.

## Questions to Ask Your Surgeon about Breast Augmentation

The following list of questions may help you to remind you of topics to discuss with your surgeon. You may have additional questions as well.

- What are the risks and complications associated with having breast implants?

- How many additional operations of my implanted breast(s) can I expect over my lifetime?

- How will my breasts look if I choose to have the implants removed without replacement?

- What shape, size, surface texturing, incision site, and placement site is recommended for me?

- How will my ability to breastfeed be affected?

- How can I expect my implanted breasts to look over time?

- How can I expect my implanted breasts to look after pregnancy? After breastfeeding?

- What are my options if I am dissatisfied with the cosmetic outcome of my implanted breasts?

- What alternate procedures or products are available if I choose not to have breast implants?

- Do you have before and after photos I can look at for each procedure and what results are reasonable for me?

Chapter 37

# *Breast Lift (Mastopexy)*

Loss of skin elasticity, gravity and other factors such as weight loss, pregnancy and breast-feeding ultimately affect the shape and firmness of your breasts. Patients who are generally satisfied with the size of their breasts can have a breast lift to raise and firm them, resulting in a more youthful breast contour. Some patients may be unhappy that they have lost a significant amount of breast volume over time. In such cases, implants inserted in conjunction with a breast lift can increase breast size at the same time as the shape and position of the breasts are enhanced.

### *Am I a good candidate for a breast lift?*

You may be a good candidate for breast lift surgery if you have one or more of the following conditions:

- breasts that are pendulous, but of satisfactory size

- breasts that lack substance or firmness

- nipples and areolas that point downward, especially if they are positioned below the breast crease

Sometimes these conditions may be inherited traits. In certain cases, the breasts may have developed differently so that one breast is firm and well positioned while the other is not. There may be differences in the size of your breasts as well as their shape. Breasts that are large and heavy can be lifted, but the results may not be as long-lasting as when the procedure is done on smaller breasts.

A breast lift can be performed at any age, but plastic surgeons usually recommend waiting until breast development has stopped. Pregnancy and breast-feeding may have significant and unpredictable effects on the size and shape of your breasts. Nevertheless, many women decide to undergo breast lift surgery before having children and feel that they can address any subsequent changes later. Since the milk ducts and nipples are left intact, breast lift surgery usually will not affect your ability to breast-feed; however, you should discuss this with your plastic surgeon.

### What happens during the personal consultation?

During the consultation, you will be asked about your desired breast shape and size. Your plastic surgeon will discuss with you how your nipples and areolas will be repositioned. You should mention anything else about your breasts that you would like to see improved. This will help your surgeon to understand your expectations and determine whether they realistically can be achieved.

### How will my plastic surgeon evaluate me for breast lift surgery?

Your plastic surgeon will examine your breasts, taking measurements and perhaps photographs for your medical record. The size and shape of your breasts, the quality of your skin, and the placement of the nipples and areolas will be carefully evaluated.

You should come to the consultation prepared to discuss your medical history. This will include information about any medical conditions, drug allergies, medical treatments you have received, previous surgeries including breast biopsies, and medications that you currently take. It is important for you to provide complete information.

You should tell your plastic surgeon if you plan to lose a significant amount of weight, particularly if you have noticed that your breasts sag or become smaller with weight loss. Your surgeon may recommend that you stabilize your weight before having surgery.

### Will my insurance help cover the cost of surgery?

Breast lift surgery, as an aesthetic (cosmetic) procedure, generally is not covered by insurance.

Under certain circumstances, however, insurance coverage may be available. For example, if a breast reconstruction after mastectomy is performed, the opposite breast may need to be modified for symmetry. Many factors determine your eligibility for coverage, including the specific terms of your insurance policy. A letter of predetermination may be required by your insurance company prior to surgery. Your plastic surgeon or a staff member in your surgeon's office will discuss these matters with you.

### How is a breast lift is performed?

Individual factors and personal preferences will determine the specific technique selected to lift your breasts.

Incisions following the breast's natural contour define the area of excision and the new location for the nipple and areola. Skin in the shaded area is removed, and the nipple and areola are moved to a higher position.

### Where are the incisions placed?

A common method of lifting the breasts involves three incisions. One incision is made around the areola. Another runs vertically from the bottom edge of the areola to the crease underneath the breast. The third incision is horizontal beneath the breast and follows the natural curve of the breast crease.

After the plastic surgeon has removed excess breast skin, the nipple and areola are shifted to a higher position. The areola, which in a sagging breast may have been stretched, can be reduced in size. Skin that was formerly located above the areola is brought down and together beneath it to reshape the breast.

The nipples and areolas remain attached to underlying mounds of tissue, and this usually allows for the preservation of sensation and the ability to breast-feed.

### What are some variations to the common breast lifting technique?

There are many variations to the design of the incisions for breast lift surgery. The size and shape of your breasts, size of your areolas, and extent of sagging are factors that will help your plastic surgeon determine the best technique for you.

In some instances, it may be possible to avoid the horizontal incision beneath the breast. Sometimes a technique may be used that avoids this horizontal incision as well as the vertical incision that runs from the bottom edge of the areola to the breast crease.

If you are a good candidate for a modified technique, your plastic surgeon will discuss this with you.

If you and your plastic surgeon have decided that it is desirable to enlarge your breasts at the same time as they are lifted, this will require insertion of breast implants. If this is an option that you wish to consider, your surgeon will review the necessary information with you and may provide you with a brochure on breast augmentation.

### What are the risks?

Fortunately, significant complications from breast lifts are infrequent. Every year, many thousands of women undergo successful breast lift surgery, experience no major problems and are pleased with the results. Anyone considering surgery, however, should be aware of both the benefits and risks.

### I understand that every surgical procedure has risks, but how will I learn more so that I can make an informed decision?

The subject of risks and potential complications of surgery is best discussed on a personal basis between you and your plastic surgeon, or with a staff member in your surgeon's office.

Some of the potential complications that may be discussed with you include bleeding, infection and reactions to anesthesia. Following a breast lift, sometimes the breasts may not be perfectly symmetrical or the nipple height may vary slightly. Minor adjustments often can be made at a later time. Permanent loss of sensation in the nipples or areas of breast skin may occur rarely. Revisionary surgery may sometimes be helpful in certain instances where incisions may have healed poorly.

You can help to lessen certain risks by following the advice and instructions of your plastic surgeon, both before and after surgery.

### Is the surgical experience uncomfortable?

The goal of your plastic surgeon and the entire staff is to make your surgical experience as easy and comfortable for you as possible.

## *How should I prepare for surgery?*

Depending on your age, or if you have a history of breast cancer in your family, your plastic surgeon may recommend a baseline mammogram before surgery and another mammographic examination some months after surgery. This will help to detect any future changes in your breast tissue. Following a breast lift, you will still be able to perform breast self-examination. Breast lift surgery will not increase your risk of developing breast cancer.

If you are a smoker, you will be asked to stop smoking well in advance of surgery. Aspirin and certain anti-inflammatory drugs can cause increased bleeding, so you should avoid taking these medications for a period of time before surgery. Your surgeon will provide you with additional preoperative instructions.

Breast lift surgery is usually performed on an outpatient basis. If this is the case, be sure to arrange for someone to drive you home after surgery and to stay with you at least the first night.

## *What will the day of surgery be like?*

Your breast lift surgery may be performed in a hospital, freestanding ambulatory facility or office-based surgical suite.

Medications are administered for your comfort during the surgical procedure. Often, a general anesthetic is administered, so that you will be asleep throughout the procedure.

Alternatively, a breast lift may be performed using local anesthesia and intravenous sedation. When surgery is completed, you will be taken into a recovery area where you will continue to be closely monitored. Sometimes, small drain tubes will have been placed in your breasts to help avoid the accumulation of fluids. Gauze or other dressings may be placed on your breasts and covered with an elastic bandage or surgical bra.

You may be permitted to go home after a few hours, unless you and your plastic surgeon have determined that you will stay in the hospital or surgical facility overnight.

## *How will I look and feel initially?*

The day after surgery, you will be encouraged to get out of bed for short periods of time. After several days, you should be able to move about more comfortably. Straining, bending and lifting must be avoided, however, since these activities might cause increased swelling or even bleeding. You may be instructed to sleep on your back to avoid pressure on your breasts.

Any surgical drains will be removed within a few days of surgery, at which time your dressings may also be changed or removed. You may be instructed to wear a support bra for a few weeks, until the swelling and discoloration of your breasts diminish. Generally, stitches will be removed in stages over a period of approximately three weeks, beginning about one week after surgery.

You may notice that you feel less sensation in the nipple and areola areas. This is usually temporary. It may, however, take weeks, months or even more than a year before sensation returns to normal. Your breasts may also require some time to assume a more natural shape. Incisions will initially be red or pink in color. They will remain this way for many months following surgery.

## When can I resume my normal activities?

After breast lift surgery, it is often possible to return to work within a week or so, depending on your job. In many instances, you can resume most of your normal activities, including some form of mild exercise, after several weeks. You may continue to experience some mild, periodic discomfort during this time, but such feelings are normal. Severe pain should be reported to your doctor.

Any sexual activity should be avoided for a minimum of one or two weeks, and your plastic surgeon may advise you to wait longer. After that, care must be taken to be extremely gentle with your breasts for at least the next several weeks.

## What are the results of a breast lift?

Breast lift surgery will make your breasts firmer and more uplifted. The position of your areolas and nipples will be enhanced, and the size of your areolas will be aesthetically pleasing.

The incisions from your breast lift surgery will heal and fade over time. It is important to realize, however, that the incision lines will be permanently visible. In some instances, they will eventually be only faint lines. Certain individuals may have incision lines that are more noticeable. Fortunately, the incisions for your breast lift are in locations easily concealed by clothing, even low-cut necklines.

## How long will the results last?

Unless you gain or lose a significant amount of weight or become pregnant, your new breast shape should remain fairly constant. However, gravity and the effects of aging will eventually alter the size and shape of virtually every woman's breasts. If, after a period of years, you again become dissatisfied with the appearance of your breasts, you may choose to undergo a second breast lift procedure to restore their more youthful contour and appearance.

### *Should I maintain a relationship with my plastic surgeon*

You will return to your plastic surgeon's office for follow-up care at prescribed intervals, at which time your progress will be evaluated. Once the immediate postoperative follow-up is complete, many surgeons encourage their patients to come back for periodic checkups to observe and discuss the long-term results of surgery.

Please remember that the relationship with your plastic surgeon does not end when you leave the operating room. If you have questions or concerns during your recovery, or need additional information at a later time, you should contact your surgeon.

# Chapter 38

# *Breast Reduction (Reduction Mammoplasty)*

Patients who undergo breast reduction surgery frequently are seeking relief from physical symptoms caused by the excessive weight of large breasts. Breast reduction usually can solve these problems as well as improve the size and shape of your breasts. Following breast reduction, your breasts will be more proportional to the rest of your body, and clothes will fit you better.

### *Am I a good candidate for breast reduction?*

You may be a good candidate for breast reduction if you have one or more of the following conditions:

- breasts that are too large in proportion to your body frame
- heavy, pendulous breasts with nipples and areolas that point downward
- one breast is much larger than the other
- back, neck, or shoulder pain caused by the weight of your breasts
- skin irritation beneath your breasts
- indentations in your shoulders from tight bra straps

- restriction of physical activity due to the size and weight of your breasts

- dissatisfaction or self-consciousness about the largeness of your breasts

Breast reduction can be performed at any age, but plastic surgeons usually recommend waiting until breast development has stopped. Childbirth and breast-feeding may have significant and unpredictable effects on the size and shape of your breasts. Nevertheless, many women decide to undergo breast reduction before having children and feel that they can address any subsequent changes later. If you plan to breast-feed in the future, you should discuss this with your plastic surgeon.

During the consultation, you will be asked about your desired breast size as well as anything else about your breasts that you would like to see improved. This will help your plastic surgeon to understand your expectations and determine whether they realistically can be achieved.

### How will my plastic surgeon evaluate me for breast reduction surgery?

Your plastic surgeon will examine your breasts, taking measurements and perhaps photographs for your medical record. The size and shape of your breasts, the quality of your skin, and the placement of the nipples and areolas will be carefully evaluated.

You should come to the consultation prepared to discuss your medical history. This will include information about any medical conditions, drug allergies, medical treatments you have received, previous surgeries including breast biopsies, and medications that you currently take. It is important for you to provide complete information.

You should tell your plastic surgeon if you plan to lose a significant amount of weight, particularly if you have noticed that your breasts become smaller with weight loss. Your surgeon may recommend that you stabilize your weight before having surgery.

### Will my insurance help cover the cost of surgery?

Insurance coverage is sometimes available for breast reduction surgery. Many factors determine your eligibility, including the specific terms of your insurance policy and the amount of breast tissue to be removed. A letter of predetermination may be required by your insurance company prior to surgery. Your plastic surgeon or a staff member in your surgeon's office will discuss these matters with you.

### How is breast reduction performed?

Individual factors and personal preferences will determine the specific technique selected to reduce the size of your breasts.

### Where are the incisions placed?

The most common method of reducing the breasts involves three incisions. One incision is made around the areola. Another runs vertically from the bottom edge of the areola to the crease underneath the breast. The third incision follows the natural curve of the breast crease.

After the surgeon has removed excess breast tissue, fat and skin, the nipple and areola are shifted to a higher position. The areola, which in large breasts usually has been stretched, also is reduced in size. Skin that was formerly located above the nipple is brought down and together to reshape the breast. Liposuction may be used to improve the contour under the arm.

Usually, the nipples and areolas remain attached to underlying mounds of tissue, and this allows for the preservation of sensation. The ability to breast-feed may also be preserved by this method, although this cannot be guaranteed.

### What are some variations to the common breast reduction technique?

There are many variations to the design of the incisions for breast reduction. The size and shape of your breasts, as well as the desired amount of reduction, are factors that will help your plastic surgeon determine the best technique for you.

In some instances, it may be possible to avoid the vertical incision that runs from the bottom edge of the areola to the breast crease or the horizontal incision underneath the breast.

Rarely, if your breasts are extremely large, the nipples and areolas may need to be completely detached before they are shifted to a higher level. In such a case, you will need to have made the decision to sacrifice sensation and the possibility of breast-feeding in order to achieve your desired breast size.

## What are the risks?

Fortunately, significant complications from breast reduction are infrequent. Every year, many thousands of women undergo successful breast reduction surgery, experience no major problems and are pleased with the results. Anyone considering surgery, however, should be aware of both the benefits and the risks.

### I understand that every surgical procedure has risks, but how will I learn more so that I can make an informed decision?

The subject of risks and potential complications of surgery is best discussed on a personal basis between you and your plastic surgeon, or with a staff member in your surgeon's office.

Some of the potential complications that may be discussed with you include bleeding, infection and reactions to anesthesia. Rarely, a patient may require a blood transfusion during the operation. This usually can be anticipated in advance, and your plastic surgeon may, under certain circumstances, advise you to donate your own blood in preparation for surgery.

Following reduction, sometimes the breasts may not be perfectly symmetrical or the nipple height may vary slightly. If desired, minor adjustments can be made at a later time. Permanent loss of sensation in the nipples or breasts may occur rarely. Revisionary surgery is sometimes helpful in certain instances where incisions may have healed poorly. In the unlikely event of injury to or loss of the nipple and areola, they usually can be satisfactorily reconstructed using skin grafts.

You can help to lessen certain risks by following the advice and instructions of your plastic surgeon, both before and after surgery.

## How should I prepare for surgery?

Depending on your age, or if you have a history of breast cancer in your family, your plastic surgeon may recommend a baseline mammogram before surgery and another mammographic examination some months after surgery. This will help to detect any future changes in your breast tissue. Following breast reduction, you will still be able to perform breast self-examination. Breast reduction surgery will not increase your risk of developing breast cancer.

If you are a smoker, you will be asked to stop smoking well in advance of surgery. Aspirin and certain anti-inflammatory drugs can cause increased bleeding, so you should avoid taking these medications for a period of time before surgery. Your surgeon will provide you with additional preoperative instructions.

Breast reduction surgery may be performed on an inpatient or outpatient basis. If you are to stay in the hospital or surgical facility, it will most likely be for only one night. Whether you are released the day of surgery or the following day, you will need someone to drive you home and to stay with you for the next day or two.

### Is the surgical experience uncomfortable?

The goal of your plastic surgeon and the entire staff is to make your surgical experience as easy and comfortable for you as possible.

### What will the day of surgery be like?

Your breast reduction surgery may be performed in a hospital, freestanding ambulatory facility or office-based surgical suite.

Usually, a general anesthetic is administered, so that you will be asleep throughout the procedure. When surgery is completed, you will be taken into a recovery area where you will continue to be closely monitored. In many instances, small drain tubes will have been placed in your breasts to help avoid the accumulation of fluids. Gauze dressings will be placed on your breasts and covered with an elastic bandage or surgical bra.

### How will I look and feel initially?

The day after surgery, you will be encouraged to get out of bed for short periods of time. After several days, you will be able to move about more comfortably. Straining, bending and lifting must be avoided, however, since these activities might cause increased swelling or even bleeding. You may be instructed to sleep on your back to avoid pressure on your breasts.

Any surgical drains will be removed a day or two after surgery, at which time your dressings may also be changed or removed. You will be instructed to wear a support bra for a few weeks, until the swelling and discoloration of your breasts diminishes. Generally, stitches will be removed in stages over a period of approximately three weeks, beginning about one week after surgery.

You may notice that you feel less sensation in the nipple and areola areas. This usually is temporary. It may, however, take weeks, months or even more than a year before sensation returns to normal.

Your breasts may also require some time to assume a more natural shape. Incisions will initially be red or pink in color. They will remain this way for many months following surgery.

### *When can I resume my normal activities?*

After breast reduction surgery, it is often possible to return to work within just a couple of weeks, depending on your job. In many instances, you can resume most of your normal activities, including some form of mild exercise, after several weeks. You may continue to experience some mild, periodic discomfort during this time, but such feelings are normal. Severe pain should be reported to your doctor.

Any sexual activity should be avoided for a minimum of one week, and your plastic surgeon may advise you to wait longer. After that, care must be taken to be extremely gentle with your breasts for at least the next six weeks.

### *How long will the results last?*

Unless you gain or lose a significant amount of weight or become pregnant, your breast size should remain fairly constant. However, gravity and the effects of aging will eventually alter the size and shape of virtually every woman's breasts. If, after a period of years, you become dissatisfied with the appearance of your breasts, you may choose to undergo a breast "lifting" procedure to restore their more youthful contour.

### *What are the results of breast reduction?*

Breast reduction surgery will make your breasts smaller and firmer. Without the excessive weight of large breasts, you may find greater enjoyment in playing sports and engaging in physical activity.

The incisions from your breast reduction surgery will heal and fade over time. It is important to realize, however, that the incision lines will be permanently visible, more so in some individuals than others. Fortunately, the incisions for breast reduction are in locations easily concealed by clothing, even low-cut necklines.

Breast reduction often makes a dramatic change in your appearance. For this reason, it may take some time to adjust to your new body image. Most women, however, eventually become comfortable with their smaller breasts and feel very pleased with the results of surgery. In fact, the level of patient satisfaction resulting from breast reduction is among the highest of any plastic surgery procedure.

### *Should I maintain a relationship with my plastic surgeon?*

You will return to your plastic surgeon's office for follow-up care at prescribed intervals, at which time your progress will be evaluated. Once the immediate postoperative follow-up is complete, many surgeons encourage their patients to come back for periodic checkups to observe and discuss the long-term results of surgery.

Please remember that the relationship with your plastic surgeon does not end when you leave the operating room. If you have questions or concerns during your recovery, or need additional information at a later time, you should contact your surgeon.

# Chapter 39

# *Male Breast Reduction (Gynecomastia Surgery)*

## *Is Gynecomastia Surgery for You?*

Gynecomastia is a condition in which male breasts are enlarged. Abnormal growth of male breast tissue usually occurs during puberty, between the ages of 13–17, or after the age of 50. Sixty-five percent of males aged 14–15 have this condition, usually due to hormonal changes that occur during puberty. This enlargement can occur in one or both breasts.

Regardless of when the condition occurs, many men feel uncomfortable or embarrassed about having enlarged breasts. For most men with gynecomastia, ultrasound assisted liposuction of the breasts is an efficient method of treatment that corrects the problem. The procedure removes fat and/or glandular tissue from the breasts, resulting in a chest that is flatter, firmer, and better contoured.

The following gives an overview of this procedure. A one-on-one appointment with your plastic surgeon is the best way to find out if this surgery is right for you.

## *Determining Your Candidacy*

Surgery to correct gynecomastia can be performed on healthy, emotionally stable men of any age. The best candidates for surgery have firm, elastic skin that will reshape to the new contours of the body.

Surgery may be postponed for obese men, or for overweight men who have not first attempted to correct the problem with exercise or weight loss. Also, individuals who drink alcoholic beverages in excess or smoke marijuana are usually not considered good candidates for surgery. Middle-aged men who have this condition need to be evaluated to determine whether the condition is caused by a medical condition.

## Potential Risks

As with any surgery, there are risks; however, when male breast-reduction surgery is performed by a qualified plastic surgeon, complications are rare.

Possible complications can include infection, skin injury, excessive bleeding, adverse reaction to anesthesia, and excessive fluid loss or accumulation. The procedure may also result in noticeable scars, permanent pigment changes in the breast area, or slightly mismatched breasts or nipples ("asymmetry"). If asymmetry is significant, a second procedure may be performed to remove additional tissue.

The temporary effects of breast reduction include loss of breast sensation or numbness, which may last up to a year.

## Planning Your Surgery

In your initial consultation with your surgeon, you will be asked for a complete medical history. Also, your surgeon will examine your breasts and check for causes of the gynecomastia, such as impaired liver function, use of estrogen-containing medications, or anabolic steroids. If such a medical problem is the suspected cause, you will be referred to an appropriate specialist.

Because it is possible for men to have breast cancer, your plastic surgeon may also recommend a mammogram, or breast x-ray as a precautionary measure.

Treatment of gynecomastia may be covered by medical insurance, but policies vary greatly. Check with your insurance carrier. If you are covered, make certain you get written pre-authorization for the treatment recommended by your surgeon.

### Pre-Surgery

You will be given pre-and postoperative instruction including guidelines on eating, drinking, and taking certain vitamins and medications.

Smokers should plan to stop smoking for a minimum of one or two weeks before surgery and during recovery. Smoking decreases circulation, and interferes with proper healing. Therefore, it is essential to follow all of your surgeon's instructions.

### *Surgical Facility*

Surgery for gynecomastia is most often performed as an outpatient procedure. The surgery itself usually takes about an hour and a half to complete. However, more extensive procedures may take longer.

### *Anesthesia Options*

Correction of enlarged male breasts will likely be performed under local anesthesia plus sedation. You'll be awake, but very relaxed and insensitive to pain. Correction that is more extensive may be performed under general anesthesia, which allows the patient to sleep through the entire operation. Your surgeon will discuss which option is recommended for you, and why this is the option of choice.

## Surgical Description

If excess glandular tissue is the primary cause of the breast enlargement, it will be removed by excision or liposuction. In a typical procedure, an incision is made in an inconspicuous location, either on the edge of the areola or in the under arm area. Working through the incision, the surgeon cuts away the excess glandular tissue, fat, and skin from around the areola and from the sides and bottom of the breast. Major reductions that involve the removal of a significant amount of tissue and skin may require larger incisions that result in scars that are more conspicuous. If liposuction is used to remove excess fat, a slim hollow tube, called a cannula is usually inserted through the existing incisions.

If your gynecomastia consists primarily of excessive fatty tissue, your surgeon will likely use ultrasound assisted liposuction to remove the excess fat. A small incision, less than half-inch in length, is made around the edge of the areola—the dark skin that surrounds the nipple. Alternatively, the incision may be placed in the underarm area. Then, a cannula, which is attached to a vacuum pump, is inserted into the incision. Using deliberate strokes, the surgeon moves the cannula through layers beneath the skin, breaking up the fat and suctioning it out. Patients may feel a vibration or some friction during the procedure, but generally no pain.

In extreme cases where large amounts of fat or glandular tissue have been removed, skin may not adjust well to the new smaller breast contour. In these cases, excess skin may have to be removed to allow the remaining skin to readjust to the new breast contour.

Sometimes, a small drain is inserted through a separate incision to draw off excess fluids. Once closed, the incisions are usually covered with a dressing. The chest may be wrapped to keep the skin firmly in place.

## Post-Surgery

There will be some discomfort for a few days after surgery, which can be controlled with medications prescribed by your surgeon. In any case, you will need to have someone drive you home after surgery and to help you out for a day or two, if needed.

You will be swollen and bruised for a while. To help reduce swelling, you'll probably be instructed to wear an elastic pressure garment continuously for a week or two, and for a few weeks longer at night. Although the worst of your swelling will dissipate in the first few weeks, it may be three months or more before the final results of your surgery are apparent.

In the meantime, it is important to begin getting back to normal by walking around on the day of surgery. You can return to work when you feel well enough, which could be as early as a day or two after surgery. Any stitches will generally be removed about 1–2 weeks following the procedure.

Your surgeon may advise you to avoid sexual activity for a week or two, and heavy exercise for about three weeks. You will be told to stay away from any sport or job that risks a blow to the chest area for at least four weeks. In general, it will take about a month before you are back to all of your normal activities.

You should also avoid exposing the resulting scars to the sun for at least six months. Sunlight can permanently affect the skin's pigmentation, causing the scar to turn dark. If sun exposure is unavoidable, use a strong sun block.

## Your New Look

The effects of the procedure are significant and permanent. Most men who undergo this procedure are very satisfied with the results.

# Chapter 40

# *Tummy Tuck (Abdominoplasty)*

Are sit-ups just not giving you the taut tummy you desire? If you've got a little too much flab or excess skin in your abdomen that won't diminish with diet or exercise, you may want to consider an abdominoplasty, popularly referred to as a tummy tuck. This procedure flattens your abdomen by removing extra fat and skin, and tightening muscles in your abdominal wall.

However, this is a major surgery, so if you're considering it, please take the time to educate yourself, thoroughly analyze your own situation, and do not rush to make the final decision. A tummy tuck should be the last resort for people who have exhausted all other measures, and the procedure should not be used as an alternative to weight loss.

### *Who are the best candidates for a tummy tuck?*

A tummy tuck is suitable for both men and women who are in good general health.

A tummy tuck should not be confused with a liposuction (the cosmetic surgery used to remove fat deposits), although your surgeon may elect to perform liposuction as part of a tummy tuck. Women who have muscles and skin stretched by multiple pregnancies may find the procedure

"Tummy Tuck (Abdominoplasty)," © 2007 The Cleveland Clinic Foundation, 9500 Euclid Avenue, Cleveland, OH 44195, www.clevelandclinic.org. Additional information is available from the Cleveland Clinic Health Information Center, 216-444-3771, toll-free 800-223-2273 extension 43771, or at http://www.clevelandclinic .org/health.

useful to tighten those muscles and reduce that skin. A tummy tuck is also an alternative for men or women who were obese at one point in their lives, and still have excessive fat deposits or loose skin in the abdominal area.

### When should you avoid the surgery?

If you're a woman who is still planning to have children, then you may want to postpone a tummy tuck until you're through bearing children. Here's why: During surgery, your vertical muscles are tightened. Future pregnancies can separate these muscles and cause a hernia.

Are you still planning to lose a lot of weight? Then you do not want to consider a tummy tuck until your weight has stabilized.

It's important to note that a tummy tuck causes scarring on the abdomen. This scar is usually long and might be prominent. If this is something you don't want, you may want to reconsider. Your doctor will discuss all these options with you when you go for the consultation.

### How is a tummy tuck done?

Depending on your desired results, this surgery can take anywhere from one to five hours. The complexity of your particular situation also will determine whether you have it completed as an inpatient or outpatient procedure. You will receive general anesthesia, which will put you to sleep during the operation. It's important to have someone with you who can drive you home. If you live alone, you also will need someone to stay with you at least the first night after the surgery, if you're sent home after the procedure.

- **Complete abdominoplasty:** This option is for those patients who require the most correction. The incision will be made low on the abdomen, at about the same level as your pubic hair and usually extends from hip bone to hip bone. Your surgeon will then manipulate and contour the skin and muscle as needed. You will have an incision around your belly button if you undergo this procedure, because it's necessary to free your navel from surrounding tissue. Drainage tubes may be placed under your skin; these will be removed in a few days as your surgeon sees fit.

- **Partial or mini-abdominoplasty:** You and your surgeon will discuss your desired results, and he or she will determine the appropriate procedure during your consultation. Mini-abdominoplasties are often performed on patients whose fat deposits are located below the navel and require shorter incisions. During this procedure, your belly button most likely will not be moved. Your skin will be separated between the line of incision and your belly button. This type of surgery may also be performed with an endoscope (small camera on the end of a tube). This procedure may only take up to two hours, again, depending on your own personal situation and the complexity of your needs. As with the complete abdominoplasty, you may have drainage tubes after surgery.

Whether you're having a partial or complete tummy tuck, your incision site will be stitched and bandaged. Your surgeon may have you wear a special garment after surgery. It's very important that you follow all of your surgeon's instructions on wearing this garment (if you are given one) and caring for the bandage in the days following surgery. Your surgeon will also instruct you on how to best position yourself while sitting or lying down to help ease pain.

If you are an exceptionally physically active person, beware: You will have to severely limit strenuous exercise for at least six weeks. Your doctor will advise you on this as you go through the healing process. You may need to take up to one month off work after the surgery to ensure proper recovery. Again, your doctor will help you determine this based on your personal situation.

### *How should I prepare for a tummy tuck?*

If you smoke, you will have to stop for a certain period as determined by your doctor. It is not enough to just cut down on smoking; you must stop completely, at least for two weeks prior to surgery and for two weeks after. You must stop the use of all nicotine gum and nicotine patches at least two weeks before and after surgery. Smoking can increase the risk of complications and delay healing.

Make sure you eat well-balanced, complete meals and do not try to diet excessively before the surgery. Proper nutrition plays a key role in healing properly.

Your surgeon may instruct you to stop taking some of your medications and dietary supplements for a certain period before and after the surgery. Your surgeon will determine this as part of your pre-operative consultation.

Your home recovery area should include:

- Supply of loose, comfortable clothing that can be taken on and off very easily;

- Telephone within reaching distance;

- Hand-held shower head and bathroom chair.

You know yourself personally, so make sure you set up the safest, most comfortable recovery area before you undergo the surgery to meet your personal needs.

### What are the complications and side effects with a tummy tuck?

As expected, you will have pain and swelling in the days following surgery. Your doctor can prescribe a painkiller if needed, and will instruct you on how to best handle the pain.

Soreness may last for several weeks or months. You may also experience numbness, bruising, and overall tiredness for that same time period.

As with any surgery, there are risks. Remember, this surgery affects a very crucial part of your body. Though they're rare, complications can include infection, bleeding under the skin flap, or blood clots. You may carry an increased risk of complications if you have poor circulation, diabetes, heart, lung, or liver disease, or if you are a smoker.

You may experience insufficient healing, which can cause more significant scarring or loss of skin. If you do heal poorly, you may require a second surgery. As we mentioned before, the scars from a tummy tuck are fairly prominent, and though they may fade slightly, they will never completely disappear. Your surgeon may recommend certain creams or ointments to use after you've completely healed to help with the scars.

### How will returning to living affect me?

Generally, most people love the new look after they've undergone this procedure; however, you may not feel like your normal self for months after the surgery. You've gone through a tremendous amount to make this happen. It is a big commitment, emotionally, physically, and financially. It is very important that you follow proper diet and exercise to maintain your new look.

### Does insurance cover a tummy tuck?

Be warned: Insurance carriers generally do not cover elective, cosmetic surgery. But your carrier may cover a certain percentage if you have a hernia that will be corrected through the procedure, or if you have had surgery for weight loss. It's extremely important that you begin communicating with your insurance company early on, and that you discuss your insurance concerns with your surgeon. In most cases, your surgeon will write a letter to your insurance carrier, making the case for medical necessity, if it applies to you. It's also very important to realize that insurance may only cover certain portions of the surgery, so make sure you get details. With any cosmetic surgery, this may affect future insurance coverage for you, and your premiums may increase.

# Chapter 41

# *Arm Lift (Brachioplasty)*

### *What is brachioplasty?*

Brachioplasty is surgery to remove excess skin from the arms.

### *Who is a candidate?*

Patients after massive weight loss who have hanging, redundant skin are candidates. Candidates also include individuals who have arms that are disproportionate to the rest of their body. Individuals are asked to stop smoking if they are considering this surgery.

### *How is brachioplasty done?*

In the standard technique, an incision is made along the underarm and down the arm, from the underarm to the elbow. The scar looks like a "T." Skin and fat are removed. A drain might be placed under the skin. If so, the drain would be removed about a week after surgery. In cases where excess skin extends from the arm onto the side of the chest, the incision may be extended to cross beyond the underarm to the side of the chest.

---

### Is there an option other than this to contour the arm while limiting the scar?

There are modified techniques. Some patients may be candidates for a technique where the incision is limited to the underarm, which could be well hidden. This is for individuals who have a borderline excess of skin. Some patients may do fine with liposuction alone. Your surgeon will need to discuss your potential options with you as well as the pros and cons of the different procedures.

### Does brachioplasty include liposuction?

Brachioplasty does not include liposuction, but it may be combined with liposuction. This will need to be discussed with your surgeon.

### Do I stay in the hospital after surgery?

If brachioplasty is combined with other procedures, you may stay in the hospital. If performed alone, brachioplasty is an outpatient procedure.

### What is recovery like after surgery?

You may be able to use your hands, but you cannot perform exertional activity with your arms for at least one month. You may have compressive dressings around the arm for several weeks. There may be swelling or numbness along the incisions or in the hands. This swelling or numbness is temporary. A plan to take three to four weeks off of work is reasonable—more time may be needed if lifting is required in your job.

### What are the risks of surgery?

Possible risks include discomfort, bleeding, infection, scar, and difficulty healing. Other risks include numbness and swelling in the hands and arms (this is often temporary). The scar associated with the procedure may be thickened and visible for up to a year after the surgery. For some reason, arms tend to scar more than other areas on the body.

### What is the cost of surgery?

Generally, brachioplasty can run from $4,000 to $8,000 (with less cost for lesser procedures). Cost may be higher if brachioplasty is combined with other procedures, such as liposuction.

# Part Five

# Reconstructive Procedures for Congenital Concerns

# Chapter 42

# *Birthmarks: An Overview*

Birthmarks are apparent in over 10 percent of all children born.

These may sound familiar—stork bites, angel kisses, strawberry marks, port wine stains, moles, café au lait spots, and lentigines. Birthmarks are either vascular (related to blood vessels) or pigmented (related to melanin). Find out what characterizes the different blemishes and what treatment options you have.

Vascular birthmarks, hemangiomas, are made up of blood vessels clustered together in the skin and can be flat, raised, pink, red, or bluish in color. Stork bites are small, faint, red stains that usually appear on the nape of the neck. Angel kisses are similar marks that appear on the child's forehead, eyelids, nose, and upper lip. Stork bites and angel kisses often lighten considerably with age or fade altogether. Strawberry marks are a collection of dilated capillaries that appear as bumpy, red blemishes. This type of birthmark will increase in size for a time, then shrink gradually and often disappear altogether by the time the child is seven. In cases where hemangiomas are not decreasing in size, steroids may be injected or given by mouth. Long-term or repeated treatment may be necessary. Lasers may also be a consideration for removal or to control the growth.

Port wine stains, another common hemangioma, are enlarged blood vessels under the skin that produce reddish to purplish discoloration,

"Skin Blemishes, Birthmarks... Embrace, Conceal, or Remove," *Facial Plastic Surgery Today*, Volume 20, Number 1, 2006. Reprinted with permission from the American Academy of Facial Plastic and Reconstructive Surgery, www.aafprs.org.

most often on the face. Port wine stains are present at birth (occurring in three percent of births), and deepen in color and increase in size with age. These birthmarks can affect a person emotionally and socially, especially when they are noticeable on the face. Treatment may include camouflage makeup or laser surgery.

The second type of birthmark is the pigmented birthmark, i.e., moles, café au lait spots, and lentigines. Unlike hemangiomas, these are composed of abnormal clusters of pigmented cells and not clusters of blood vessels. Moles usually appear after birth and may be tan or brown in color. Those that appear at birth have a higher risk of becoming skin cancer, especially if it covers a sizable area.

If you have pigmented birthmarks that are rather large, you should have a physician check them on a regular basis. Any sudden color change, pain, or bleeding, should warrant a visit to your doctor. Surgical removal of the lesion is the preferred treatment in cases where the mole has a high risk of becoming malignant. Laser surgery, surgical scraping, and cryotherapy (freezing) are not permanent solutions. The lesion will reappear eventually. Medical treatment is not necessary if the birthmark degenerates over time.

If your birthmark is desired and admired, it is still a good idea to have it checked out. If not, make an appointment with your facial plastic surgeon to discuss your aesthetic and medical concerns and the best mode of concealment.

# Chapter 43

# *Pigmented Lesions (Nevi)*

Nevi (singular: nevus) are pigmented lesions (colored "birthmarks" or "moles") that may be congenital (present at birth) or acquired (appearing some time after birth). There are many different types of nevi, and nevi may occur anywhere from head to toe.

### *Does the nevus cause my child any pain?*

Usually nevi are not painful. However, some nevi may become ulcerated or irritated, causing discomfort. These nevi are typically removed surgically.

### *What are the different types of nevi?*

As noted above, there are many different types of nevi. They may be congenital or acquired. Certain types of nevi are more commonly treated with surgical biopsy or excision. These include the giant congenital nevi ("giant hairy nevi") and the nevus sebaceous of Jadassohn. There is an increased risk of melanoma forming within a giant congenital nevus, although this risk is still small. There is about a 10–15% risk of basal cell skin cancer occurring in the nevus sebaceous after puberty; therefore, excision of these nevi is recommended before that time.

---

### Who gets nevi?

Nevi can occur in any child. There are some inherited conditions in which nevi are present. Also, nevi are associated with sun exposure.

### What causes nevi?

Nevi are caused by an overgrowth of specific types of skin cells. As noted above, heredity and sun exposure can play a role in the formation of nevi.

### What are the main issues related to nevi?

The primary issue with a nevus is whether or not it will become a skin cancer of some sort. Most nevi are not worrisome at all and will never cause a problem. However, other types of nevi are more concerning, such as the giant congenital nevus and nevus sebaceous of Jadassohn mentioned above. While a plastic surgeon or dermatologist can usually be quite confident about whether or not a particular nevus is concerning, the definitive diagnosis can only be determined after the nevus is excised and sent to a pathologist for study.

### Are there other problems that occur commonly with nevi?

Nevi on the face or large nevi on other parts of the body can be unsightly and be a source of psychosocial stress for the child.

When giant congenital nevi occur on the head or over the spine, there is a small risk of neurocutaneous melanosis, or involvement of the central nervous system (brain and spinal cord) with melanoma or melanoma precursors. In addition, giant congenital nevi that involve the full circumference of an arm or leg can sometimes restrict the growth of the affected limb.

### What is the treatment for babies and children with nevi?

Nevi can be observed with regular examinations or surgically excised. For small nevi, such surgical treatment can be done as a minor outpatient procedure. Giant congenital nevi may require multiple complex surgical procedures for excision, depending upon the size and location of the nevus. If surgery is appropriate, your surgeon will design a surgical treatment plan specifically for your child after discussing all of the options with you.

# Chapter 44

# *Vascular Anomalies*

Vascular anomalies are abnormal formations or growths of the components of the vascular system: capillaries, venules, arteries, veins, and lymphatics. These anomalies can be broadly categorized as hemangiomas and vascular malformations.

Hemangiomas are tumor-like growths that generally arise soon after birth and then grow rapidly during the first year of the baby's life. Usually, by one year of age, they stop growing and then, over several years time, they regress completely.

Vascular malformations are abnormal collections of arteries, veins, lymphatics, capillaries or combinations of these types of vessels. These lesions are present at birth and grow proportionately with the child. They do not resolve spontaneously.

### *Do vascular anomalies cause my baby any pain?*

Most of the time, these anomalies are not painful. However, in some cases they can be painful, for example if they grow to a large size or if the overlying skin becomes ulcerated. Pain is more often associated with vascular malformations than hemangiomas.

### *What are the different types of vascular anomalies?*

As noted above, vascular anomalies are broadly categorized as hemangiomas or vascular malformations.

Hemangiomas are classically bright red and tense while they are growing, although the color may be more bluish if the hemangioma is in the deeper tissues rather than right beneath the skin. As they gradually regress, their color changes to a gray-purple, and they become softer. Hemangiomas may disappear completely, or leave behind some excess skin and fibrofatty tissue after they have resolved. Approximately 80% of hemangiomas are solitary lesions, while in 20% of cases there is more than one hemangioma present.

Vascular malformations may have a variety of appearances depending on the exact composition of the malformation (capillary, arterial, venous, lymphatic, or combined). There is a great variety of vascular malformations. Some only involve the skin, while others are very extensive and may involve deep structures and even the internal organs and bones.

### Who gets vascular anomalies?

- Hemangiomas occur in 2.6% of newborns and in 12% of Caucasian children by one year of age; they are more common in very small premature babies. Girls are affected three times more often than boys. Hemangiomas are more common in Caucasians than in other racial or ethnic groups.

- Vascular malformations occur equally in boys and girls, and there seems to be no racial predilection.

- Hemangiomas and vascular malformations are not inherited or "genetic" conditions.

### What causes vascular anomalies?

A great deal of research is being done to determine why hemangiomas and vascular malformations occur. However, currently, no clearly defined causes of these lesions have been determined.

### What are the main issues related to vascular anomalies?

Most hemangiomas cause no problems at all. However, some patients with hemangiomas will have problems such as very rapid growth with ulceration of the skin and damage to surrounding tissues; in addition, hemangiomas in the head and neck region can grow large enough to obstruct or interfere with vision, hearing, breathing, or feeding. In rare cases, very large or multiple hemangiomas may be associated with bleeding problems or with cardiac and circulatory problems.

Vascular malformations are so varied that it is difficult to generalize about them. Many of these lesions do not cause any problems. However, depending on the type of lesion, its size, location, and composition, there may be various problems such as pain, limitation of function (for example, if the malformation is in the hand), distortion of surrounding tissues including bones, bleeding, and circulatory problems.

### Are there other problems that occur commonly with vascular anomalies?

Usually, hemangiomas are solitary lesions that are not associated with any other problems. Vascular malformations may occur as isolated problems or as part of a number of different syndromes with many different types of associated abnormalities. Your surgeon will tell you if he/or she thinks that your child may have one of these syndromes and explain it in detail.

### What is the treatment for babies with vascular anomalies?

The vast majority of hemangiomas are not treated in any way. Occasionally, after they have regressed, a minor surgical procedure may be done to remove any excess skin or fibro-fatty tissue left behind. In some cases, when the hemangioma is growing very rapidly, steroids may be given to slow the growth. Surgical removal of a hemangioma is only rarely necessary.

Most vascular malformations can be treated just with observation or with the use of compression garments to prevent swelling. Several different treatment options are available for the different types of vascular malformations. These options include laser treatment, sclerotherapy (injection of a chemical substance directly into the malformation to shrink it), embolization (blocking off the supply of blood to the malformation), and surgery. Surgery may be to just reduce the size of the malformation or, in some cases, to remove the malformation altogether if possible. Because there is such a variety of vascular malformations, the treatment is really customized for each individual patient.

### What is done after my baby is born?

You will often meet with your surgeon soon after your baby is born. Your surgeon will examine your baby and may order x-rays or other images of the affected part of the body. Your baby will be examined at regular intervals in the clinic. The treatment plan and the details of the surgical procedures, if any, will be carefully explained to you by your surgeon. Sometimes compressive garments may be prescribed to keep pressure on areas that are swollen. If necessary, your surgeon may refer you to see other specialists as well.

### What sorts of specialists will be involved in my baby's care?

Your child will be treated by the plastic surgeon. In some cases, other specialists, such as dermatologists, interventional radiologists, ophthalmologists, otolaryngologists (ENT), and general surgeons may be involved depending upon the specific details of the case.

### Will we get to know our surgeon?

Ideally, you will meet your surgeon soon after your baby is born. Your surgeon will see your child regularly in the clinic as he or she grows over a period of months or years. During this process, you will have ample opportunity to ask questions and to get to know your surgeon quite well.

# Chapter 45

# *Cleft Lip and Palate*

Oral-facial clefts are birth defects in which the tissues of the mouth or lip don't form properly during fetal development. In the United States, clefts occur in one in 700 to 1,000 births, making it the one of the most common major birth defects. Clefts occur more often in children of Asian, Latino, or Native American descent.

The good news is that both cleft lip and cleft palate are treatable birth defects. Most kids who are born with these conditions can have reconstructive surgery within the first 12 to 18 months of life to correct the defect and significantly improve facial appearance.

## What Is Oral Clefting?

Oral clefting occurs when the tissues of the lip and/or palate of a fetus don't grow together early in pregnancy. Children with clefts often don't have enough tissue in their mouths, and the tissue they do have isn't fused together properly to form the roof of their mouths.

A cleft lip appears as a narrow opening or gap in the skin of the upper lip that extends all the way to the base of the nose. A cleft palate is an opening between the roof of the mouth and the nasal cavity.

This information was provided by KidsHealth, one of the largest resources online for medically reviewed health information written for parents, kids, and teens. For more articles like this one, visit www.KidsHealth.org, or www. TeensHealth.org. © 2005 The Nemours Foundation. This document was reviewed September 2005 by Barbara P. Homeier, MD.

Some children have clefts that extend through both the front and rear part of the palates, while others have only partial clefting.

There are generally three different kinds of clefts:

- cleft lip without a cleft palate
- cleft palate without a cleft lip
- cleft lip and cleft palate together

In addition, clefts can occur on one side of the mouth (unilateral clefting) or on both sides of the mouth (bilateral clefting).

More boys than girls have a cleft lip, while more girls have cleft palate without a cleft lip.

Because clefting causes specific visible symptoms, it's easy to diagnose. It can be detected through a prenatal ultrasound. If the clefting has not been detected prior to the baby's birth, it's identified immediately afterward.

## What Causes Oral Clefting?

Doctors don't know exactly why a baby develops cleft lip or cleft palate, but believe it may be a combination of genetic (inherited) and environmental factors (such as certain drugs, illnesses, and the use of alcohol or tobacco while a woman is pregnant). The risk may be higher for kids whose sibling or parents have a cleft or who have a history of clefting in their families. Both mothers and fathers can pass on a gene or genes that cause cleft palate or cleft lip.

## Complications Related to Oral Clefting

A child with a cleft lip or palate tends to be more susceptible to colds, hearing loss, and speech defects. Dental problems—such as missing, extra, malformed, or displaced teeth, and cavities—also are common in children born with cleft palate.

Many children with clefts are especially vulnerable to ear infections because their eustachian tubes don't drain fluid properly from the middle ear into the throat. Fluid accumulates, pressure builds in the ears, and infection may set in. For this reason, a child with cleft lip or palate may have special tubes surgically inserted into his or her ears at the time of the first reconstructive surgery.

Feeding can be another complication for an infant with a cleft lip or palate. A cleft lip can make it more difficult for a child to suck on a nipple, while a cleft palate may cause formula or breast milk to be accidentally taken up into the nasal cavity. Special nipples and other devices can help make feeding easier; you will probably be given information on how to use them and where to buy them before you take your baby home from the hospital. And in some cases, a child with a cleft lip or palate may need to wear a prosthetic palate called an obturator to help him or her eat properly.

If you're experiencing problems with feeding, your doctor may be able to offer other suggestions or feeding aids to help you and your baby.

## Treating Clefts

The good news is that there have been many medical advancements in the treatment of oral clefting. Reconstructive surgery can repair cleft lips and palates, and in severe cases, plastic surgery can address specific appearance-related concerns.

A child with oral clefting will need to see a variety of specialists who will work together as a team to treat the condition. Treatment usually begins in the first few months of an infant's life, depending on the health of the infant and the extent of the cleft.

Members of a child's cleft lip and palate treatment team usually include:

- a geneticist;
- a plastic surgeon;
- an ear, nose, and throat physician (otolaryngologist);
- an oral surgeon;
- an orthodontist;
- a dentist;
- a speech pathologist (often called a speech therapist);
- an audiologist;
- a nurse coordinator;
- a social worker and/or psychologist.

The team specialists will evaluate your child's progress regularly, examining your child's hearing, speech, nutrition, teeth, and emotional state. They will share their recommendations with you, and can forward their evaluation to your child's school, and any speech therapists that your child may be working with.

In addition to treating your child's cleft, the specialists will work with your child on any issues related to feeding, social problems, speech, and how you approach the condition with your child. They'll provide feedback and recommendations to help you through the phases of your child's growth and treatment.

## Surgery for Oral Clefting

Surgery is usually performed during the first 12 to 18 months to repair cleft lip and/or cleft palate. Both types of surgery are performed in the hospital under general anesthesia.

Cleft lip often requires only one reconstructive surgery, especially if the cleft is unilateral. The surgeon will make an incision on each side of the cleft from the lip to the nostril. The two sides of the lip are then sutured together. Bilateral cleft lips may be repaired in two surgeries, about a month apart, and usually requires a short hospital stay.

Cleft palate surgery involves drawing tissue from either side of the mouth to rebuild the palate. It requires two or three nights in the hospital, with the first night spent in the intensive care unit. The initial surgery is intended to create a functional palate, reduce the chances that fluid will develop in the middle ears, and help the child's teeth and facial bones develop properly. In addition, this functional palate will help your child's speech development and feeding abilities.

The necessity for more operations depends on the skill of the surgeon as well as the severity of the cleft, its shape, and the thickness of available tissue that can be used to create the palate. Some children with a cleft palate require more surgeries to help improve their speech. Additional surgeries may also improve the appearance of the lip and nose, close openings between the mouth and nose, help breathing, and stabilize and realign the jaw. Subsequent surgeries are usually scheduled at least six months apart to allow a child time to heal and to reduce the chances of serious scarring.

It's a good idea to meet regularly with your child's plastic surgeon to determine what's most appropriate in your child's case. Final repairs of the scars left by the initial surgery may not be performed until adolescence, when facial structure is more fully developed. Surgery is designed to aid in normalizing function and cosmetic appearance so that the child will have as few difficulties as possible.

## Dental Care and Orthodontia

Children with oral clefting often undergo dental and orthodontic treatment to help align the teeth and take care of any gaps that exist because of the cleft.

Routine dental care may get lost in the midst of these major procedures, but healthy teeth are critical for a child with clefting because they're needed for proper speech.

A child with oral clefting generally needs the same dental care as other children—regular brushing supplemented with flossing once the child's 6-year molars come in. Depending on the shape of your child's mouth and teeth, your child's dentist may recommend a toothette, a soft sponge that contains mouthwash, rather than a toothbrush. As your child grows, you may be able to switch to a soft children's toothbrush. The key is to make sure that your child brushes regularly and well.

Children with cleft palate often have an alveolar ridge defect. The alveolus is the bony upper gum that contains teeth, and defects can:

- displace, tip, or rotate permanent teeth;
- prevent permanent teeth from appearing;
- prevent the alveolar ridge from forming.

These problems can be fixed by grafting bone matter onto the alveolus, which allows the placement of your child's teeth to be corrected orthodontically.

Orthodontic treatment usually involves a number of phases, with the first phase beginning as the permanent teeth start to come in. In the first phase, which is called an orthopalatal expansion, the upper dental arch is rounded out and the width of the upper jaw is increased. A device called an expander is placed inside the child's mouth. The widening of the jaw may be followed by a bone graft in the alveolus.

Your child's orthodontist may wait until the remainder of your child's permanent teeth come in before beginning the second phase of orthodontic treatment. The second phase may involve removing extra teeth, adding dental implants if teeth are missing, or applying braces to straighten teeth.

In about 25% of children with a unilateral cleft lip and palate, the upper jaw growth does not keep up with the lower jaw growth. If this occurs, your child may need orthognathic surgery to align the teeth and help the upper jaw to develop.

For these children, phase-two orthodontics may include an operation called an osteotomy on the upper jaw that moves the upper jaw both forward and down. This usually requires another bone graft for stability.

## Speech Therapy

A child with oral clefting may have trouble speaking—the clefting can make the voice nasal and difficult to understand. Some will find that surgery fixes the problem completely.

Catching speech problems early can be a key part of solving them. It's a good idea to take your child to a speech therapist between the ages of 18 months and two years. Many speech therapists like to talk with parents at least once during the child's first six months to provide an overview of the treatment and suggest specific language- and speech-stimulation games to play with the baby.

Shortly after the initial surgery is completed, the speech pathologist will see your child for a complete assessment. The therapist will evaluate your child's developing communication skills by assessing the number of sounds he or she makes and the actual words your child tries to use, and by observing interaction and play behavior.

This analysis helps determine what, if any, speech exercises your child needs and if further surgery is required. The speech pathologist will often continue to work with your child through additional surgeries. Many children who have clefts work with a speech therapist throughout their grade-school years.

## Dealing with Emotional and Social Issues

Our society often focuses on people's appearances, and this can make childhood—and, especially, the teen years—very difficult for someone with a physical difference. Because a child with oral clefting has a prominent facial difference, your child may experience painful teasing, which can damage self-esteem. Part of the cleft palate and lip treatment team includes psychiatric and emotional support personnel.

Ways that you can support your child include:

- Try not to focus on your child's cleft and do not allow it to define your child as an individual.

- Create a warm and supportive home environment, where each person's individual worth is openly celebrated.

- Let your child know that you feel good about who he or she is by showing acceptance and by not trying to make your child into your idea of who he or she should be.

- Encourage your child to develop friendships with people from diverse backgrounds. The best way to do this is to lead by example and to be open to all people yourself.

- Point out positive attributes in others that do not involve physical appearance.

- Encourage autonomy by giving your child the freedom to make decisions and take appropriate risks, letting your child's own accomplishments lead to a sense of personal value. By providing opportunities for your child to make decisions early on—like picking out what clothes to wear—he or she can gain more confidence and the ability to make bigger decisions down the road.

You might also consider encouraging your child to present information about clefting to his or her class with a special presentation that you arrange with the teacher. Or perhaps your child would like you to talk to the class. This can be especially effective with young children.

If your child does experience teasing, encourage discussions about it and be a patient listener. Give your child the tools to confront the teasers by asking what he or she would like to say and then practicing those statements.

If your child seems to have ongoing self-esteem problems, you may want to consult with a child psychologist or social worker for support and information. Together with the members of your child's treatment team, you can help your child through tough times.

Also, it's important to keep the lines of communication open as your child approaches adolescence so that you can address any concerns he or she may have about appearance.

# Chapter 46

# *Craniofacial Anomalies*

## *Craniofacial Syndromes*

The craniofacial dysostosis syndromes are a group of similar, in-herited, congenital anomalies that affect the skull, face, and some-times the limbs. Typically, there is fusion of the coronal sutures of the skull (bicoronal synostosis), that creates a skull that is short from front to back, wide, and tall. In addition, the bones of the midface—from the orbits (eye sockets) down to and including the upper jaw—do not grow forward normally, resulting in a retruded or concave face, with an "underbite." Finally, depending upon the particular syndrome, a variety of hand (and sometimes foot) abnormalities can occur, such as webbed fingers and underdeveloped thumbs.

### *Is this condition painful?*

In general, craniosynostosis is not a painful condition. However, if there is increased pressure upon the brain, this can cause headaches, irritability, nausea, and vomiting. Occasionally, in cases where the fin-gers are tightly webbed together (Apert syndrome), infections around the nails or skin breakdown can occur, causing some discomfort. If the orbits (the bony eye sockets) are really shallow, the corneas may be-come dry and irritated, which can also cause discomfort.

This chapter includes "Craniofacial Syndromes," "Craniosynostosis," "Plagio-cephaly," "Hemifacial Microsomia," and " Microtia," © 2006 University of Missouri Children's Hospital. Reprinted with permission.

321

## What are the different types of craniofacial dysostosis syndromes?

The more common of these syndromes include Apert syndrome, Crouzon syndrome, and Pfeiffer syndrome. However there are several others, such as Nager syndrome, Carpenter syndrome, Jackson-Weiss syndrome, and Saethre-Chotzen syndrome. In Apert syndrome, there is bicoronal synostosis, midface retrusion, and symmetric syndactyly (webbing of the digits) in both the hands and feet. Crouzon syndrome is characterized by bicoronal synostosis and midface retrusion, but normal hands and feet. Pfeiffer syndrome is also characterized by bicoronal synostosis, and midface retrusion, with broad, angulated thumbs and broad great toes. The other syndromes represent variations on this general theme.

## Who gets these syndromes?

The craniofacial dysostosis syndromes are inheritable. The gene mutation for each syndrome has been identified. Almost all of the syndromes are inherited in an autosomal dominant fashion, meaning that there is a 50% likelihood of recurrence of the syndrome in the offspring of the affected individual. Often, the parents of these children are not affected, and the gene mutation arises spontaneously during development. However, the severity of the syndrome may vary from one generation to the next, so that it may not have been detected in a parent, for example, until a more severely-affected child was born.

## What causes these syndromes?

As mentioned previously, these syndromes are caused by genetic mutations. The fibroblast growth factor receptor genes are primarily affected.

## What are the main issues related to the craniofacial dysostosis syndromes?

The most important issue related to craniosynostosis is the potential for increased pressure on the brain. When there is excessive pressure on the brain, problems with neural development, including visual problems can occur. These may be subtle or mild, such as learning disabilities, or more severe, such as mental retardation and loss of vision. Most children never develop such severe symptoms. However, because we cannot predict which children will have these problems, treatment of craniosynostosis is recommended to prevent the possible increased intracranial pressure.

In addition, there are problems associated with the poor growth of the midface in these patients. These patients tend to have an underbite, and can also have problems with their eyes if the orbits (eye sockets) are very shallow. Obstructive sleep apnea can be a problem for these children because of the midface retrusion, which can cause narrowing of the airway.

### Are there other problems that occur commonly with these syndromes?

Depending upon the particular syndrome, there may be problems in other parts of the body, particularly the hands, as mentioned previously. Some of these children also have cleft palates.

In addition, in some cases, the muscles of the eyes do not function normally and may require surgery, and there may be abnormalities of the upper eyelids, such as drooping. There may be abnormalities of the cervical spine in some patients. Because such associated conditions can occur, all children with these syndromes are evaluated by a multidisciplinary group of specialists who can detect these problems.

### What is the treatment for babies with craniofacial dysostosis?

While every patient is treated individually, with treatment plans made specifically for him or her, some generalizations are possible. Treatment usually begins with the craniosynostosis. Treatment for craniosynostosis is surgical. Babies with craniosynostosis are examined early in life by members of the craniofacial treatment team: a pediatrician who specializes in treating infants with craniofacial anomalies, a geneticist, a craniofacial surgeon, a neurosurgeon, and an ophthalmologist. Depending on the particular case, other specialists may be involved also. A computerized tomography scan (CT scan)—a special type of x-ray—is performed to study the bones of the skull and the brain. If there are no signs of increased intracranial pressure by physical examination or by CT scan, then most children will have their surgery at approximately one year of age. If there is increased intracranial pressure, then surgery is performed sooner.

The surgery is performed jointly by the craniofacial surgeon and the neurosurgeon. The skull is enlarged, or expanded, by removing and reshaping the bones of the skull to give the brain room to grow and also to correct the abnormal shapes that occur as a result of the various types of craniosynostosis. While this is a very specialized and complex surgical procedure, it is now performed safely and effectively with modern anesthetic and surgical techniques.

Other surgical procedures are dependent upon the unique features in each syndrome. The child may need to have a surgical procedure to move the midface forward to correct problems such as a severe underbite and sleep apnea. More than one jaw surgery is usually required to achieve a normal relationship of the upper and lower teeth. Cleft palate repair is required in some cases, and a variety of hand surgery procedures may be required in certain syndromes.

### What is done between the time my baby is born and the first surgery?

After the initial craniofacial team evaluation, described earlier, the child is evaluated periodically to ensure that he or she is growing and developing normally and that there is no sign of increased intracranial pressure. The CT scan may be repeated at some point before the surgery. Your surgeons will meet with you several times to examine your baby and to ensure that all of your questions about the surgery are answered and that you feel comfortable with the whole process.

### What sorts of specialists will be involved in my baby's care?

The optimal treatment of children with these complex syndromes is achieved in a multidisciplinary setting. As noted above, these children may have a number of other medical issues that must be addressed. Usually, the specialists involved include the craniofacial surgeon (a plastic surgeon who has done additional specialized training), a neurosurgeon, a pediatric ophthalmologist, a developmental pediatrician, a geneticist, the craniofacial nurse, and an orthodontist.

### Will we get to know our surgeon?

Because children with craniofacial syndromes are followed closely before, during, and after their surgery, you will become very familiar with your surgeons. Treatment is not finished after the surgery, because it is important to continue to monitor your child's growth and development over the long term. This long-term surveillance involves physical examinations and periodic CT scans to ensure that there are no signs of any problems. Your surgeons will guide you and help you through the surgery and postoperative period. In addition, children with these syndromes require multiple surgical procedures throughout their childhood and adolescence, so they and their families often develop a close bond with their surgeon.

## Craniosynostosis

The skull is made up of several flat bones that fit together like the pieces of a jigsaw puzzle. The joints between these bones usually remain loose and open during growth and development to allow the brain to grow and expand. These joints are called "sutures." Craniosynostosis is the condition in which these sutures grow together or become fused prematurely. When that happens, the skull can no longer stretch and expand to accommodate the growing brain in the area where the sutures have fused. In some cases, the result is increased pressure on the growing brain.

### Is this condition painful?

In general, craniosynostosis is not a painful condition. However, if there is increased pressure upon the brain, this can cause headaches, irritability, nausea, and vomiting.

### What are the different types craniosynostosis?

There are multiple different cranial sutures. There can be fusion of one suture or multiple sutures. Each type of suture fusion is associated with a particular type of head shape. Fusion of the metopic suture causes a triangular forehead shape, or trigonocephaly. Fusion of the sagittal suture causes a long, narrow head shape, or scaphocephaly. Coronal suture fusion causes flattening of the forehead on the affected side, called anterior plagiocephaly. When both coronal sutures are fused, the skull becomes tall and short from front-to-back; this is called brachycephaly, or turribrachycephaly. Fusion of the lambdoid sutures is causes flattening of the back of the head on the side of the affected suture; this is caused by posterior plagiocephaly.

### Lots of babies have slightly abnormal head shapes; how do I know when it is something to worry about?

Abnormal head shapes in babies are quite common. In general, abnormal head shapes can be caused by either craniosynostosis or by external forces that push on the skull to deform it. The latter condition is much more common and is called deformational plagiocephaly. Deformational plagiocephaly does not cause any increased pressure on the brain and is not associated with any danger to the neural development of the child. The most common form of deformational plagiocephaly is flattening of the back of the head, caused by repetitive sleep positioning.

If your baby has an abnormal head shape, you should raise this concern with your pediatrician. Often the pediatrician will be able to distinguish whether your child has the much more common deformational plagiocephaly or the much less common craniosynostosis. If the pediatrician in unsure, then you should be referred to see a craniofacial surgeon, who can usually make the diagnosis by physical exam.

### Who gets craniosynostosis?

Craniosynostosis can occur in any newborn infant. Some cases are "sporadic," meaning that there is no family history. However, other cases may have a family history or be part of a syndrome. Metopic and sagittal synostosis are more common in boys than in girls.

### What causes craniosynostosis?

There are three main theories that have been proposed to explain craniosynostosis. Most likely, as with many other congenital anomalies, multiple factors can contribute to this condition. Craniosynostosis can be caused by a genetic mutation, as in some syndromes like Apert syndrome. Alternatively, there is evidence that mechanical forces can create suture fusion; for example, when the brain is very small and is not expanding or growing normally, the cranial sutures can fuse prematurely because there is no force from the brain keeping them open. Finally, there is the theory that there is some intrinsic biochemical abnormality of the sutures themselves that causes them to fuse prematurely.

### What are the main issues related to craniosynostosis?

The most important issue related to craniosynostosis is the potential for increased pressure on the brain. When there is excessive pressure on the brain, problems with neural development, including visual problems can occur. These may be subtle or mild, such as learning disabilities, or more severe, such as mental retardation and loss of vision. Most children never develop such severe symptoms. However, because we cannot predict which children will have these problems, treatment of the craniosynostosis is recommended to prevent the possible increased intracranial pressure.

### Are there other problems that occur commonly with craniosynostosis?

Some types of craniosynostosis occur as part of a syndrome, or a collection of abnormalities that affect different parts of the body. Most commonly, these other abnormalities affect the face and hands. Specifically, the face may not grow forward normally, and appear retruded, flat, or dish-like. In addition, the hands may have webbed fingers (syndactyly), extra digits (thumbs usually), small thumbs, large thumbs, and other types of abnormalities. Most of these syndromes have a genetic basis, and some of these genetic abnormalities can now be identified by testing.

### What is the treatment for babies with craniosynostosis?

While every patient is treated individually, with treatment plans made specifically for him or her, some generalizations are possible. Treatment for craniosynostosis is surgical. Babies with craniosynostosis are examined early in life by members of the craniofacial treatment team: a pediatrician who specializes in treating infants with craniofacial anomalies, a geneticist, a craniofacial surgeon, a neurosurgeon, and an ophthalmologist. Depending on the particular case, other specialists may be involved also. A computerized tomography scan (CT scan)—a special type of x-ray—is performed to study the bones of the skull and the brain. If there are no signs of increased intracranial pressure by physical examination or by CT scan, then most children will have their surgery at approximately one year of age. If there is increased intracranial pressure, then surgery is performed sooner; also, patients with sagittal synostosis usually are treated at an earlier age.

The surgery is performed jointly by the craniofacial surgeon and the neurosurgeon. The skull is enlarged, or expanded, by removing and reshaping the bones of the skull to give the brain room to grow and also to correct the abnormal shapes that occur as a result of the various types of craniosynostosis. While this is a very specialized and complex surgical procedure, it is now performed safely and effectively with modern anesthetic and surgical techniques.

### What is done between the time my baby is born and the surgery?

After their initial craniofacial team evaluation, described previously, the child is evaluated periodically to ensure that he or she is growing and developing normally and that there is no sign of increased intracranial pressure. The CT scan may be repeated at some point before the surgery. Your surgeons will meet with you several times to examine your baby and to ensure that all of your questions about the surgery are answered and that you feel comfortable with the whole process.

### What sorts of specialists will be involved in my baby's care?

The optimal treatment of children with craniosynostosis is achieved in a multidisciplinary setting. As noted earlier, these children may have a number of other medical issues that must be addressed, especially if they have a syndrome. Usually, the specialists involved include the craniofacial surgeon (a plastic surgeon who has done additional specialized training), a neurosurgeon, a pediatric ophthalmologist, a developmental pediatrician, a geneticist, the craniofacial nurse, and an orthodontist.

## Plagiocephaly

Plagiocephaly is a term that is derived from the Greek *plagio*—slanted or oblique—and *kephale*—head. Literally, it means slanted, or crooked head. In general, this term is applied to an abnormally-shaped head. Plagiocephaly can be caused by premature fusion of the cranial sutures (see craniosynostosis) or, much more commonly, by external forces that deform the malleable infant skull. These external forces may be due to pressure on the skull in utero, pressure from repetitive sleep positioning, or related to abnormal head posture that is secondary to a problem with the eyes or the muscles of the neck. Posterior deformational plagiocephaly (flattening of the back of the head) has become quite common since the American Academy of Pediatrics recommended that infants be positioned on their backs to sleep.

### Is this condition painful?

No, deformational plagiocephaly causes no symptoms.

### Are there different types deformational plagiocephaly?

In general, plagiocephaly can affect the forehead (anterior plagiocephaly) or the back of the head (posterior plagiocephaly). Posterior plagiocephaly is much more common because babies are usually positioned on their backs to sleep.

### Lots of babies have slightly abnormal head shapes; how do I know when it is something to worry about?

Abnormal head shapes in babies are quite common. In general, abnormal head shapes can be caused by either craniosynostosis (premature fusion of the cranial sutures), which is described elsewhere in this website, or by deformational plagiocephaly, which is much more common. Deformational plagiocephaly does not cause any increased pressure on the brain and is not associated with any danger to the neural development of the child. The most common form of deformational plagiocephaly is flattening of the back of the head (posterior plagiocephaly), caused by repetitive sleep positioning.

If your baby has an abnormal head shape, you should raise this concern with your pediatrician. Often the pediatrician will be able to distinguish whether your child has the much more common deformational plagiocephaly or the much less common craniosynostosis. If the pediatrician is unsure, then you should be referred to see a craniofacial surgeon, who can usually make the diagnosis by physical exam.

### Who gets deformational plagiocephaly?

Deformational plagiocephaly can occur in any infant. Anterior plagiocephaly (flattening of the forehead) occurs most commonly on the left side, because the left occiput anterior position is the most common intra-uterine fetal head position. The heads of babies with anterior plagiocephaly often engage in the maternal pelvis rather early. Deformational plagiocephaly is also more common in multiple pregnancies, in which there is less space for the growing skull. Moreover, there may be molding of the skull that occurs from compressive forces during normal vaginal delivery.

Post-natally, repetitive sleep positioning can cause deformational plagiocephaly. If the baby sleeps in the same position repeatedly, the skull will become flattened on the side on which the baby sleeps. In addition, some eye muscle imbalances cause infants to tilt their heads to achieve binocular vision, and this head tilt can also result in deformation from repetitive positioning. Similarly, torticollis (tightness of the sternocleidomastoid muscle in the neck) can cause a head tilt with the same result.

### What are the main issues related to deformational plagiocephaly?

Deformational plagiocephaly is essentially a cosmetic deformity. There are no issues related to the growing brain or to intellectual ability. However, as noted previously, there may be underlying causes of deformational plagiocephaly, such as ocular problems or torticollis that must be investigated and addressed. In severe cases, the deformity may become a source of psychosocial stress for the child as he or she grows.

### What is the treatment for babies with deformational plagiocephaly?

Most babies can be treated with modification of their sleep positioning. The goal is to relieve pressure on the flat area of the head. By using positioning devices, such as foam wedges, and by changing the orientation of the child's crib, pressure can be relieved and the shape of the skull will gradually correct itself. In infants with ocular problems, eye muscle surgery may be required to correct the head tilt. For infants with torticollis, usually a physical therapy program of stretching will correct the head tilt; in some cases, surgical release of the tight neck muscle is required.

When it seems that these maneuvers are ineffective, molding helmet therapy can be used to treat deformational plagiocephaly. The baby is fitted for a helmet that gently reshapes the skull. The helmet is adjusted at regular intervals, and must be worn twenty-three hours per day for several months. Helmet therapy is most effective if it is instituted before approximately ten months of age.

In extremely rare cases of very severe deformities, surgical reconstruction of the deformed skull is performed.

### What sorts of specialists will be involved in my baby's care?

Babies with deformational plagiocephaly are seen primarily by the craniofacial surgeon and the neurosurgeon. When molding helmet therapy is used, the baby is seen frequently by the orthotist, who makes the helmet and modifies it as needed.

## Hemifacial Microsomia

In general, hemifacial microsomia (HFM) refers to under-development of one side of the face, with resulting asymmetry. Specifically, the skull, ear, upper and lower jaws, and soft tissues, including the nerves that help move the facial muscles, may be affected. HFM occurs on a spectrum of deformity, from very mild, with only subtle changes, to very severe, with all of these parts of the face and skull being affected. HFM may also be called Goldenhar syndrome, oculo-auriculo-vertebral sequence, and first and second branchial arch syndrome.

Typically, patients with HFM have a small or absent ear (microtia) and a small upper and lower jaw on the affected side of the face. This causes a slanted or crooked smile, slanting upward toward the affected side.

### Is this condition painful?

No, HFM does not cause your child any discomfort.

### How common is HFM?

HFM is one of the most common craniofacial anomalies, occurring in approximately one out of 5,500 newborns.

### What are the different types of HFM?

As mentioned above, there is a spectrum of deformity in HFM. This may range from a small, abnormally-shaped, or absent ear only or just a minor facial asymmetry to involvement of all of the bones and soft tissues on the affected side of the face. The facial nerve, which is responsible for the movement of the face, may also be affected in more severe cases.

Because there is such a spectrum of deformity, it can sometimes be difficult to diagnose HFM. That is why evaluation by a multidisciplinary craniofacial team is important, so that the craniofacial surgeon, geneticist, and other specialists can all provide their opinions. Special x-rays of the facial skeleton and computerized tomography (CT or CAT) scans are usually obtained to help with diagnosis and treatment planning.

### What causes HFM?

HFM may occur sporadically—that is, as a new diagnosis with no family history—or it may be inherited ("genetic"). When it is inherited,

HFM may occur as an autosomal dominant condition, in which there is a 50% chance of having a child with HFM; as an autosomal recessive condition, in which there is a 25% chance; or as a multifactorial condition, in which environmental factors as well as genetics play a role. Even in inherited cases, the severity of HFM is not constant, because there is a spectrum of deformity; one relative may be severely affected while another has only a very subtle manifestation. This phenomenon is known as variable expression.

Ultimately, it is thought that the blood supply to the affected side of the face may be damaged or disrupted in utero, and that this is the cause of the underdevelopment on the affected side.

### What are the main issues related to HFM?

Most commonly, patients with HFM have the following problems:

- facial asymmetry
- orthognathic (dental and jaw) problems due to the asymmetry
- microtia (small or absent ear)

### Are there other problems that occur with HFM?

Because there is such a spectrum of deformity with HFM, other problems may arise. These can include under-development of the orbit (the eye socket), under-development of the cheek bone, facial paralysis, and severe thinning of the soft tissues of the cheek.

### What is the treatment for children with HFM?

While every patient is treated individually, with treatment plans made specifically for him or her, some generalizations are possible. Usually, treatment for HFM must address the asymmetry of the jaws, the small or absent ear, and occasionally the soft tissues of the cheek. The exact nature and timing of the procedures depends upon the severity of deformity in each specific case.

When the jaw deformity is very severe, a rib bone and cartilage graft can be used to reconstruct the deficient side of the mandible. In less severe cases, the deficient side of the mandible can be stretched or lengthened by the technique of distraction osteogenesis, in which the bone is cut and a device is place on the bone to slowly lengthen it. In either of these situations, a repeat jaw surgery will be required in adolescence to achieve a normal relationship of the teeth of the upper an lower jaws. In the mildest cases, an operation is done in adolescence on the upper and lower jaws to correct the facial slant and the jaw asymmetry.

Ear reconstruction is begun after the age of six. The child's own rib cartilages are used to build an ear, which is then placed in the appropriate position on the side of the head. This complex reconstruction is done in three or four staged procedures.

A variety of methods may be used to correct asymmetry of the soft tissues of the cheek. These can vary from simple interventions, such as the placement of soft tissue fillers as are used in cosmetic surgery, to very complex procedures that involve transplantation of tissue from another part of the body to the face.

### What sorts of specialists will be involved in my child's care?

The optimal treatment of children with HFM is achieved in a multidisciplinary setting. As noted above, these children may have a number of issues that must be addressed. Usually, the specialists involved include:

- the geneticist, who helps assign a diagnosis and counsels the family regarding the possibility for recurrence in future children;

- the craniofacial surgeon (a plastic surgeon who has done additional specialized training), who does most of the operations;

- an orthodontist, who helps to assess facial growth and development of the teeth, and aligns the teeth;

- an otolaryngologist (ENT), who can address hearing problems or perform middle ear surgery if necessary;

- a pediatric ophthalmologist, who can assess vision and movement of the eye;

- a developmental pediatrician, who can follow the child's physical and mental development;

- and the craniofacial nurse, who is instrumental in coordinating care and counseling and educating families.

## Microtia

Microtia refers to an under-developed or absent ear. This can occur as part of hemifacial microsomia (HFM) and in some cases may be the only manifestation of HFM. Microtia occurs more commonly on the right side, and occurs on both sides in 10% of cases. Boys are more commonly affected than girls.

### Is this condition painful?

No, microtia does not cause any pain or discomfort.

### Are there different types of microtia?

Yes, microtia can occur on a spectrum from mild deformity to complete absence of the cartilaginous framework of the ear. Usually, some remnant of the earlobe is present, although in an abnormal position and orientation.

### What causes microtia?

Please see the discussion of causes of hemifacial microsomia (HFM).

### What are the main issues related to microtia?

The appearance of the ear and hearing in the affected ear are the primary issues for microtia patients. Almost all patients with significant microtia have abnormalities of the ear canal or middle ear, and have abnormal hearing in the affected ear. Children with microtia are evaluated by an otolaryngologist who works with the craniofacial treatment team to decide whether any surgery should be done specifically to improve hearing or whether a hearing aid would be beneficial.

### Are there other problems that occur with microtia?

Since microtia is part of the spectrum of HFM, patients with microtia may have any of the associated anomalies that occur with HFM.

### What is the treatment for children with microtia?

The craniofacial surgeon (plastic surgeon) and the otolaryngologist ("ENT") will decide together on the timing of any surgery on the ear canal or middle ear for hearing. Reconstruction of the external ear is a staged process; that is, a series of procedures is required. The child must be at least six years of age before beginning this process, so that enough growth has taken place to allow an adequate reconstruction.

The reconstruction is done using the child's own tissues: cartilage taken from the ribs is used to build an ear, and then implanted beneath the soft tissues on the side of the head. Usually, either three or four operations are required to complete the reconstruction. The whole process takes about a year. The most extensive procedure is the first procedure, in which the rib cartilages are used to construct the ear framework. The remaining procedures are relatively minor in comparison, and can be done on an outpatient basis.

### What sorts of specialists will be involved in my child's care?

The optimal treatment of children with microtia is achieved in a multidisciplinary setting. As noted previously, these children may have a number of issues that must be addressed. Usually, the specialists involved include:

- the geneticist, who helps assign a diagnosis and counsels the family regarding the possibility for recurrence in future children;

- the craniofacial surgeon (a plastic surgeon who has done additional specialized training), who does most of the operations;

- an otolaryngologist (ENT), who can address hearing problems or perform middle ear surgery if necessary;

- a developmental pediatrician, who can follow the child's physical and mental development;

- and the craniofacial nurse, who is instrumental in coordinating care and counseling and educating families.

# Chapter 47

# *Congenital Hand Anomalies*

## *Syndactyly*

Syndactyly, the most common congenital hand anomaly, is an abnormal connection of fingers or toes to one another—the digits are "webbed," and have failed to separate normally during development. It most commonly involves the middle and ring fingers. In about 50% of cases, both hands are involved. Syndactyly may occur alone, or with other anomalies as part of a syndrome.

### *Does syndactyly cause my baby any pain?*

Typically, syndactyly is not painful. However, in some very severe cases, in which the nails might dig into the joined fingertips, minor infections and wounds can cause some discomfort.

### *What are the different types of syndactyly?*

Syndactyly may occur in different forms. Complete syndactyly occurs when the digits are joined all the way to their tips, while in incomplete syndactyly, the digits are joined only for part of their length. Simple syndactyly means that the digits are joined by the skin and soft tissue only, while complex syndactyly means that the bones of the digits are fused together.

---

This chapter includes "Syndactyly," "Polydactyly," "Cleft Hand," "Amniotic Band Syndrome," and "Radial Dysplasia," © 2006 University of Missouri Children's Hospital. Reprinted with permission.

### Who gets syndactyly?

Syndactyly can occur in any newborn infant. Overall, syndactyly occurs in approximately one out of 2,500 newborns. In up to approximately 40% of cases, there is a family history of syndactyly. If syndactyly occurs alone, it is inherited as an autosomal dominant condition; that is, the children of an affected individual will have a 50% chance of having syndactyly. However, syndactyly is not the same from one generation to the next, and can be more or less severe than in the affected parents. Syndactyly is more common in Caucasians than in other ethnicities, and affects boys twice as often as girls.

### What causes syndactyly?

When the hands and feet are developing in the womb, they start out as flat "paddles" that then normally separate into five digits. Syndactyly occurs when there is a failure of this separation process. This may be caused by a genetic abnormality or by environmental influences.

### What are the main issues related to syndactyly?

The primary issue in syndactyly is function of the hand and digits. Syndactyly causes limitation of function, because the involved digits cannot move completely independently. In very severe cases, with multiple digits involved in complex syndactyly, there can be problems with infections and skin breakdown.

### Are there other problems that occur commonly with syndactyly?

Some children with syndactyly will have other congenital abnormalities or syndromes. Syndactyly may occur as part of several different syndromes. For example, in the craniofacial dysostosis syndromes, such as Apert syndrome, in addition to very severe, symmetric syndactyly of the hands and feet, there are also significant head and face abnormalities.

### What is the treatment for babies with syndactyly?

While every patient is treated individually, with treatment plans made specifically for him or her, some generalizations are possible. Syndactyly is treated surgically, with an operation that separates the digits using skin from the digits and, usually, skin grafts from the lower abdomen to cover the separated fingers. When the small finger or thumb is involved, this operation is done at about six months of age, to avoid distortion of the adjacent ring or index finger with growth, since the thumb and small finer are shorter than their neighboring digits. Otherwise, syndactyly release is usually done at about eighteen months of age. Before this age, the incidence of wound healing complications and skin graft failures is significantly higher. In special cases with very complex syndactyly—or complicated syndactyly—such as in Apert syndrome), surgery may begin earlier, and multiple procedures may be required in a staged sequence to achieve separation of all the digits.

## Polydactyly

Polydactyly literally means "extra digits." There may be an extra thumb, small finger, or, less commonly, an extra digit in the central part of the hand. Polydactyly is one of the most common congenital hand anomalies.

### Does polydactyly cause my baby any pain?

No, typically there is no pain associated with polydactyly.

### What are the different types of polydactyly?

Radial, or pre-axial polydactyly means that there is an extra thumb; there are several different types of radial polydactyly. Ulnar, or post-axial polydactyly means that there is an extra small finger; there may be a well-formed extra small finger, or just a poorly-formed extra digit attached by a thin stalk of soft tissue. Central polydactyly means that the extra digit is in the central part of the hand, between the thumb and small finger.

### Who gets polydactyly?

Polydactyly can occur in any newborn infant. Most types of radial polydactyly are not inherited. Postaxial polydactyly with a small, poorly-formed extra digit is ten times more common in African-Americans than in Caucasians and is inherited as an autosomal dominant trait (that is, there is a 50% chance of polydactyly in the children of an affected individual). However, postaxial polydactyly with a well-formed extra digit is equally common in all ethnicities. Central polydactyly is inherited as an autosomal dominant condition with variable expression, meaning that it may be more or less severe from one generation to the next.

### *What causes polydactyly?*

When the hands and feet are developing in the womb, they start out as flat "paddles" that then normally separate into five digits. Polydactyly occurs when this separation process is excessive, and an extra "segment" is created. This may be caused by a genetic abnormality or by environmental influences.

### *What are the main issues related to polydactyly?*

The primary issue in most types of polydactyly is function of the hand and digits; appearance of the hand is also an issue, but is secondary to function.

### *Are there other problems that occur commonly with polydactyly?*

Certain rare types of preaxial polydactyly are associated with other problems, such as blood disorders, heart abnormalities, or craniofacial abnormalities. Postaxial polydactyly in which the extra digit is well-formed is associated with polydactyly of the feet, also.

### *What is the treatment for babies with polydactyly?*

Polydactyly is treated surgically. In preaxial polydactyly, a single thumb must be reconstructed from the two duplicated, or split, thumbs. This procedure involves reconstructing the skin and soft tissues, the tendons, joints, and ligaments to create a single thumb. In postaxial polydactyly, when the extra digit is attached only by a narrow stalk of soft tissue, this may be removed either with a minor operation or, if the stalk is narrow enough, by ligating the stalk in the nursery. When the extra digit is well-formed, the surgery is more involved and may involve reconstruction of soft tissues, tendons, joints, and ligaments as in preaxial polydactyly. Finally, central polydactyly requires a complex surgical procedure to reconstruct the hand. Again, the soft tissues, tendons, ligaments, and joints must be reconstructed. In some of these cases, more than one operation is required.

## Cleft Hand

In cleft hand, there is a central V-shaped gap or cleft in the hand. One or more digits may be absent, but the small finger is always present. There is an extremely wide variety of presentations. Usually both hands and both feet area affected. Often, despite an unusual appearance, these children demonstrate quite good hand function. Cleft hand is a rare congenital hand anomaly. This condition has been known by several other names, such as ectrodactyly, split hand, and lobster claw hand. These terms have now been largely abandoned in favor of "cleft hand."

### Does cleft hand cause my baby any pain?

No, typically there is no pain associated with this condition.

### What are the different types of cleft hand?

The presentation of cleft hand may vary from a simple central gap in the hand to an absence of all the digits except the small finger. Like many of the congenital anomalies, there is a spectrum of deformity with cleft hand.

### Who gets cleft hand?

Cleft hand is inherited as an autosomal dominant condition. This means that there is a 50% chance of cleft hand occurring in the children of an affected individual. The condition may arise as a new genetic mutation, in which case the parents are not affected.

### What causes cleft hand?

The exact cause of cleft hand is not currently known.

### What are the main issues related to cleft hand?

The primary issue in cleft hand is function of the hand and digits; appearance of the hand is also an issue, but is secondary to function. Some of these children with very mild involvement will have almost no functional limitation, while others may have significant functional limitations (for example, when there is only a small finger present).

### Are there other problems that occur commonly with cleft hand?

A number of other anomalies have been observed in association with cleft hand. Some of these include cleft lip and palate, congenital heart disease, anomalies of the anus, anomalies of the eyes, and deafness.

In addition, other bone and joint anomalies in the upper and lower limbs may be present. Therefore, it is critical that all babies with cleft hand be carefully and thoroughly examined by an experienced pediatrician.

### *What is the treatment for babies with cleft hand?*

While every patient is treated individually, with treatment plans made specifically for him or her, some generalizations are possible. The primary goals in surgical treatment of cleft hand are to close the cleft or gap in the hand, to reconstruct a functional thumb and first web space (the space between the normal thumb and index finger), and to enable pinch and grasp. Many different surgical procedures may be used, depending upon the specifics of each patient. The timing and sequence of procedures is unique for each patient. In general, however, the first procedure is usually done at or after one year of age.

## Amniotic Band Syndrome

In amniotic band syndrome, strands of the amniotic sac ensnare parts of the developing body, causing a variety of problems. These may include syndactyly, bands or constriction rings, amputations, swelling, or other deformities. There are several different names for this condition.

### *Does amniotic band syndrome cause my baby any pain?*

No, typically there is no pain associated with this condition. However, occasionally, if there is a very tight band associated with some skin breakdown or infection, there may be minor discomfort.

### *What are the different types of amniotic band syndrome?*

Amniotic band syndrome may present in many different forms. For example, it may cause only a minor groove or indentation in one of the limbs; or it may cause syndactyly of multiple digits on the hand or foot with multiple bands or constriction rings on multiple digits; or amputations of digits or larger parts of the limbs. Each case is unique.

### *Who gets amniotic band syndrome?*

Amniotic band syndrome can occur in any newborn infant. There is no pattern of inheritance. This condition occurs in approximately one in 15,000 newborns.

### What causes amniotic band syndrome?

Although there are many theories, the cause of amniotic band syndrome has not been determined.

### What are the main issues related to amniotic band syndrome?

The primary issue in most types of amniotic band syndrome is function of the hand and digits; appearance of the hand is also an issue, but is secondary to function. When there is syndactyly of the digits (fingers or toes joined together), independent function of the digits is limited. When the digits are short because of growth arrest or intrauterine amputations, function may also be limited.

### Are there other problems that occur commonly with amniotic band syndrome?

The most common problems that are associated with amniotic band syndrome are cleft lip/palate and clubfoot. Associated anomalies may occur in approximately 40–60% of cases. Usually, no there are no abnormalities of the internal organs.

### What is the treatment for babies with amniotic band syndrome?

While every patient is treated individually, with treatment plans made specifically for him or her, some generalizations are possible. Amniotic band syndrome is treated surgically. The exact type, number, timing, and sequence of operations depends upon the specific deformity present in each case. When the fingertips are joined together (acrosyndactyly), the first operation usually is done to release the fingertips so that the fingers may move more independently. This procedure is done in the first three to six months of life. After that, procedures may be done to deepen the web spaces between digits to increase their effective length; these operations may involve the use of skin grafts from the abdomen. Constriction bands are "contoured" by excising them and rearranging the skin and soft tissues on either side of the band to create a smooth, cylindrical shape to the digit or limb. Occasionally, even more complicated procedures may be done to lengthen digits, such as using distraction osteogenesis to stretch the bones or using microsurgery to transfer toes to the hand.

## *Radial Dysplasia*

Radial dysplasia is underdevelopment, abnormal development, or absence of the structures on the radial side (the "thumb side") of the forearm, wrist, or hand. There is a spectrum of involvement, ranging from a slightly small thumb, to complete absence of the thumb, radial wrist bones, and the radius bone itself (the bone on the "thumb side" of the forearm). In some cases, only the radius is involved. The term "radial clubhand" comes from the appearance of the hand and forearm when the radius is very short or absent: the hand is bent at 90 degrees to the forearm, resembling the appearance of a golf club. Radial dysplasia affects only one side in about 50% of cases, and the right side is twice as commonly affected as the left.

### *Does radial dysplasia cause my baby any pain?*

No, typically there is no pain associated with this condition.

### *What are the different types of radial dysplasia?*

There is a spectrum of involvement in radial dysplasia, as in many of the congenital anomalies. Radial dysplasia may involve only the forearm; the forearm, wrist, and thumb; only the thumb; or the thumb and wrist. Moreover, for each involved structure (the radius, the thumb), there is a range of involvement, from mild to severe.

### *Who gets radial dysplasia?*

Radial dysplasia can occur in any newborn infant. There is no pattern of inheritance. This condition is rare, and occurs in approximately one in 30,000 to 1 in 100,000 newborns. Boys are affected slightly more often than girls, and Caucasians are affected more than other races.

### *What causes radial dysplasia?*

Although there are many theories, the cause of radial dysplasia has not been determined.

### *What are the main issues related to radial dysplasia?*

The primary issue in radial dysplasia is function of the hand and digits; appearance of the hand is also an issue, but is secondary to function. Children with an under-developed or absent thumb cannot pinch and grasp objects effectively. This is a significant limitation, because the thumb normally accounts for about 40% of total hand function. If the thumb is only mildly or moderately under-developed, the child will try to use it. However, if the thumb is severely under-developed or absent, the index finger begins to substitute for the thumb: the space between the index and middle fingers gradually widens, the index finger rotates toward the middle finger, and the child tries to pinch between the index and middle fingers.

In addition, if the forearm is short and the hand bent in the "club-hand" position, the child may have difficulty with various tasks, such as reaching for objects or getting the hand into a sleeve.

### Are there other problems that occur commonly with radial dysplasia?

Yes, radial dysplasia may be associated with a number of other problems, some of them potentially very serious. Therefore, it is critical that any baby with radial dysplasia be carefully and thoroughly examined by an experienced pediatrician. Diagnostic tests such as special x-rays and ultrasounds are usually done. The commonly associated problems may be remembered by the acronym VACTERL: V for vertebral, or spine; A for anal or rectal; C for cardiac, or heart; TE for tracheoesophageal (the trachea and esophagus); R for renal, or kidney; and L for limb. In addition, there may be serious anemias and other blood disorders.

### What is the treatment for babies with radial dysplasia?

While every patient is treated individually, with treatment plans made specifically for him or her, some generalizations are possible. When the radial clubhand deformity is present, a regimen of stretching and splinting is begun with the help of a hand therapist to try to keep the wrist supple and allow the hand to be passively straightened on the forearm. In some babies, the elbow is very stiff and does not bend well; in those patients, straightening the hand would be detrimental, because the baby will actually take advantage of the bent position of the hand to reach its mouth. Many different procedures exist to achieve a better posture of the hand on the forearm. Your surgeon will work with your child to determine the best option for him or her.

The most important treatment intervention is to reconstruct a functional thumb. In cases with mild or moderate under-development of the thumb, reconstruction is done using the tissues of the small thumb and borrowing a tendon from other digits on the hand. However, when the thumb is severely under-developed or absent, reconstruction is not possible. Rather, a completely new thumb is created, usually using the index finger, in an elegant operation known as pollicization. In pollicization, the index finger is moved into the thumb position and adjusted in length and posture to look and function like a thumb.

Hand therapy will be an on-going part of the treatment plan, before and after surgery.

# Chapter 48

# *Ambiguous Genitalia*

## *Birth Defects—Ambiguous Genitalia*

Ambiguous genitalia (also known as atypical genitalia) is a birth defect (or birth variation) of the sex organs that makes it unclear whether an affected newborn is a girl or boy. This condition occurs approximately once in every 4,500 births. The baby seems to have a mixture of both female and male parts—for example, they may have both a vulva and testicles. Associated intersex conditions for male babies include hypospadias, where the urethral opening is located in an unusual position such as the underside of the penis.

The causes of ambiguous genitalia include genetic variations, hormonal imbalances, and malformations of the foetal tissues that are supposed to evolve into genitals. Tests (including ultrasound, x-rays, and blood tests) are needed before the baby's sex can be identified. Mild forms of ambiguous genitalia may be characterised by a large (penis-like) clitoris in baby girls or undescended testicles in boys.

## *Sexual Determination during Embryo Development*

A baby's sex is decided at conception. The mother's egg provides an X chromosome and the father's sperm determines the baby's sex by contributing either an X or Y sex chromosome. An XX embryo is female while an XY embryo is male. Both female and male embryos develop in exactly the same way and have identical gonads and genital parts until around the eighth week of gestation. The sexual determination process includes:

- **Girls:** The internal genital parts transform into the uterus, fallopian tubes and vagina. The gonads turn into ovaries which start producing female sex hormones. The lack of male hormones is fundamental in allowing the development of female genitalia.

- **Boys:** The internal genital parts transform into the prostate gland and vas deferens. The gonads turn into testes which start producing male sex hormones. The presence of male hormones allows the penis and scrotum to develop.

### *Different Types of Ambiguous Genitalia*

The different types of ambiguous genitalia include:

- The baby has ovaries and testicles, and the external genitals are neither clearly male nor female.

- The baby has ovaries and a penis-like structure or phallus.

- The baby has undescended testes and external female genitals including a vulva.

### *A Range of Causes*

For typical genital development, the gender 'message' must be communicated from the sex chromosomes to the gonads. The gonads must then manufacture appropriate hormones and the genital tissues and structures have to respond to these hormones. Any deviations along the way can cause ambiguous genitalia. Some specific causes include:

- **Androgen Insensitivity Syndrome (AIS):** A genetic condition characterised by the foetal tissue's insensitivity to male hormones. This affects genital development. For example, a newborn may have some of the female reproductive organs but also have testicles.

- **Congenital Adrenal Hyperplasia (CAH):** An inherited condition that affects hormone production. A child with CAH lacks particular enzymes, and this deficiency triggers the excessive manufacture of male hormones. For example, female genitals are masculinised.

- **Sex Chromosome Disorders:** Instead of having either XX or XY sex chromosomes, a baby may have a mixture of both ('mosaic' chromosomes); or specific genes on the Y chromosome may be inactive; or one of the X chromosomes may have a tiny Y segment attached to it. Research at the University of California at Los Angeles (UCLA) indicates that ambiguous genitalia can be caused by the doubling up of a particular gene (named WNT-4) on the sex chromosome. This variation will interfere with male sexual development so that a genetically male baby will appear female.

- **Maternal Factors:** The pregnant mother may have had an androgen-secreting tumour while pregnant, and the excess of this male hormone affected her baby's genital development. In other cases, the placenta may have lacked a particular enzyme which failed to deactivate male hormones from the baby as a result, both the mother and the female baby were masculinised by the excess of these hormones.

### *Diagnosis Methods*

There are currently no prenatal tests that can detect ambiguous genitalia. American research into the WNT-4 gene suggests that a prenatal test could one day be developed. Tests performed at birth to determine the baby's gender can take about one week and may include:

- Physical examination;
- Hormone tests using blood, urine, or both;
- Genetic tests using blood, urine, or both;
- Ultrasound scan;
- X-rays.

### *Treatment Options*

Treatment options to help assign the baby a definite gender may include:

- **Parental Counselling:** Successful sex assignment and identity for the child depends largely on the attitude of the parents. It is important that both the mother and father are fully informed about their child's condition. Support groups may provide help in this area.

- **Surgery:** For example, an overly large clitoris may be trimmed, or a fused vulva separated, or undescended testicles relocated into the scrotum. However, surgical gender assignment depends heavily on what genital structures the surgeons have to work with. The majority of babies with ambiguous genitalia have been brought up as girls. A few operations may be needed, usually begun in the child's first year. Further surgery might be required during adolescence. Some intersex support groups feel that surgery is not always the answer, particularly when the gender of the child is not clear. Others suggest that surgery should wait until the child is old enough to decide for themselves. However, most medical professionals advocate early surgical and hormonal intervention for the sake of clearly establishing the child's gender and sense of belonging in society.

- **Counselling for the Child:** The child needs to be informed and talked to about their diagnosis in a very careful way.

- **Hormone Therapy:** During their teenage years, the child may need hormone supplementation therapy to help bring on puberty. A child with CAH will need to have daily hormone therapy.

### *Possible Longterm Problems*

Some of the possible problems faced by a person born with ambiguous genitalia may include:

- Infertility;

- Problems with sexual functioning;

- Feelings of insecurity and uncertainty about their gender identity, such as feeling like the opposite gender to the sex that was determined earlier in life.

## *Where to Get Help*

- Your doctor

- Endocrinologist

- Genetic counsellor

- Endocrinology clinic counsellor
- Congenital Adrenal Hyperplasia Support Group Tel. (03) 5227 8405
- AIS Support Group Australia Tel. (03) 9315 8809

## Things to Remember

- 'Ambiguous genitalia' is a birth defect of the sex organs that makes it unclear whether an affected newborn is a girl or boy.
- Causes include genetic variations, hormonal imbalances and malformations of the foetal tissues that would have otherwise evolved into genitals.
- Treatment aims at assigning the baby a specific gender.
- Treatment options include corrective surgery, hormone therapy, peer support and counselling.

This information has been produced in consultation with, and approved by Murdoch Childrens Research Institute.

# Part Six

# Disease-Related and Post-Traumatic Reconstructive Procedures

# Chapter 49

# *Scar Treatment Methods*

Scars result when the skin repairs wounds caused by accident, disease, or surgery. They are a natural part of the healing process. The more the skin is damaged and the longer it takes to heal, the greater the chance of a noticeable scar.

Typically, a scar may appear redder and thicker at first, then gradually fade. Many actively healing scars that seem unsightly at three months may heal nicely if given more time.

The way a scar forms is affected by an individual's age and the location on the body or face. Younger skin makes strong repairs and tends to overheal, resulting in larger, thicker scars than does older skin. Skin over a jawbone is tighter than skin on the cheek and will make a scar easier to see. If a scar is indented or raised, irregular shadows will be seen, giving the skin an uneven appearance. A scar that crosses natural expression lines or is wider than a wrinkle, will be more apparent because it will not follow a natural pattern nor look like a naturally occurring line.

Any one, or a combination of these factors may result in a scar that, although healthy, may be improved by dermatologic surgical treatment.

## What Can and Cannot Be Done for Scars

Several techniques can minimize a scar. Most of these are done routinely in the dermatologist's office. Only severe scars, such as burns over a large part of the body may require general anesthesia or a hospital stay.

Surgical scar revision can improve the way scars look by changing the size, depth, or color. However, no scar can ever be completely erased; and no magic technique will return the scar to its normal uninjured appearance. Surgical scar revision typically results in a less obvious mark. Because each scar is different, each will require a different approach.

The most important step in the treatment of scars is careful consultation between the patient and the dermatologic surgeon—finding out what bothers a patient most about a scar and deciding upon the best treatment.

## Scar Treatment

**Surgical scar revision:** Based on the ability of the skin to stretch with time, surgical scar revision is a method of removing a scar and rejoining the normal skin in a less obvious fashion. The surgical removal of scars is best suited for wide or long scars, those in prominent places, or scars that have healed in a particular pattern or shape. Wide scars can often be cut out and closed, resulting in a thinner scar, and long scars can be made shorter. A technique of irregular or staggered incision lines, rather than straight-line incisions, to form a broken-line scar that is much more difficult to recognize may be used. Sometimes, a scar's direction can be changed so that all or part of the scar that crosses a natural wrinkle or line falls into the wrinkle, making it less noticeable. This method can also be used to move scars into more favorable locations, such as into a hairline, or a natural junction (for instance, where the nose meets the cheek). Best results are obtained when the scar is removed and wound edges are brought together without tension or movement (pull) on the skin.

**Dermabrasion:** Dermabrasion is a method of treating acne scars, pockmarks, some surgical scars, or minor irregularities of the skin's surface. An electrical machine is used by a dermatologist to remove the top layers of skin to give a more even contour to the surface of the skin. While it can offer improvement for certain scars, it cannot get rid of the scar entirely. Patients can usually return to work within a week. If defects are minor, only one dermabrasion will be needed. Several abrasions may be required if defects are deep and extensive, as in deep acne scars.

**Laser resurfacing and pulsed dye:** Another method of improving acne and chicken pox scars is laser skin resurfacing. High-energy light is used to remove unwanted, damaged skin. Patients can return to work or regular activity within one week, but skin may stay pink for several weeks or months. Several different lasers are available depending on the skin defect requiring improvement. A pulsed dye laser, for example, uses yellow light to remove scar redness and to flatten out raised scars (hypertrophic scars or keloids). This laser can also improve itching and burning sensations in the scar. Hypertrophic scars or keloids typically need two or more pulsed dye laser treatments every two months. Acne scars or other indented (atrophic) scars can also be improved with laser skin resurfacing.

**Soft tissue fillers** (collagen injections or fat transfer): Injectable collagen, a natural animal protein, is a substance used to elevate indented, soft scars. The amount of collagen injected will vary with the size and firmness of the scar. Patients with a personal history of certain collagen diseases or "autoimmune" diseases cannot safely receive injectable bovine collagen. Patients are always tested on the forearm and observed prior to treatment to ensure that they are not allergic to the collagen. Allergic patients or those with collagen vascular diseases may not use human collagen or other related filler materials. Improvement is immediate but is not permanent. Collagen injections typically need to be repeated every three to six months. The patient's own fat or injectable donated fascia can be used in full-thickened deep depressed scars. New research may develop more permanent substances to inject into scars.

**Punch grafts and punch excisions:** Punch grafts are small pieces of normal skin used to replace scarred skin. A tiny instrument is used to punch a hole in the skin and remove the scar. The area is then filled in with a matching piece of unscarred skin, usually taken from the skin behind the ear. The "plugs" are taped into place for five to seven days as they heal. Punch excisions, on the other hand, involve the use of stitches to close the holes produced by the tiny skin punch. The stitches are removed in five to seven days. Even though the punch grafts and excisions form scars of their own, they provide a smoother skin surface which is less visible than depressed scars. Deep or "pitted" acne scars are best treated by punch grafts or excisions.

**Chemical peels:** This procedure involves the use of a chemical to remove the top layer of the skin in order to smooth depressed scars and give the skin a more even color. It is most helpful for shallow superficial scars.

The chemical is applied to the skin with an ordinary cotton-tipped applicator beginning on the forehead and moving over the cheeks to the chin. Different chemicals can be used for different depth peels. Light peels require no healing time while deeper peels can require up to two weeks to heal. The amount of scarring and color change determines the type of peel selected.

### Other Scar Treatment Methods

Pressure bandages and massages can flatten some scars if used on a regular basis for several months.

Silicone-containing gels, creams, and bandages have also been helpful in reducing scar thickness and pain. They must also be used regularly and results are variable.

Cryosurgery involves freezing the upper skin layers which causes blistering of the skin. This can sometimes cause scars to diminish in size. This technique has been used on raised acne scars.

Cortisone (steroid) injections or tapes are effective in softening very firm scars (or keloids) causing them to shrink and flatten. This is usually the treatment of choice for hypertrophic scars and keloids.

Silicone impregnated gels can be used by the patient at home to remodel elevated scars in addition to injections of scar tissue.

Interferon is a chemical that can be given by injection and may help improve the hardness and cosmetic appearance of the scar.

Cosmetics applied correctly can be very good at covering up scars. Physicians encourage patients to wear make-up after scar treatments. Make-up will improve the appearance while nature completes the healing process.

# Chapter 50

# Post-Mastectomy: Facts about Breast Protheses and Reconstruction

## Breast Prostheses and Post-Mastectomy Products

### What is a breast prosthesis?

An external breast prosthesis is an artificial breast form that can be worn after the breast has been surgically removed. There are several different types of prostheses. They may be made from silicone gel, foam, fiberfill, or other materials that feel similar to natural tissue. Most are weighted so that they feel the same as the remaining breast (if only one breast has been removed). Some adhere directly to the chest area while others are made to fit into pockets of post-mastectomy bras (see description below). Different types of prostheses may also have different features, such as a mock nipple or special shape. In many cases, a woman will be fitted for a prosthesis so that it can be custom-made for her body. Partial prostheses, called equalizers or enhancers, are also available for women who have had part of their breasts removed.

This chapter includes "Breast Protheses and Post-Mastectomy Products" and "Breast Reconstruction." This information is reprinted with permission from www.imaginis.com. © 2006 Imaginis Corporation. All rights reserved. Additional text under the heading "Choices in Reconstructive Procedures," is excerpted from *FDA Breast Implant Consumer Handbook*, U.S. Food and Drug Administration (FDA), 2004. The complete text of this document is available online at http://www.fda.gov/cdrh/breastimplants/indexbip.pdf.

### What is a mastectomy and a post-mastectomy bra?

A mastectomy is a common treatment for breast cancer that involves surgically removing the breast. A modified radical mastectomy is the most common type of mastectomy performed today. This procedure involves removing the breast, nipple/areolar region, and often the axillary (underarm) lymph nodes. Other types of mastectomies include simple mastectomy (removes the breast, with its skin and nipple, but no lymph nodes) and partial mastectomy (remove a portion of the breast tissue and a margin of normal breast tissue).

After a mastectomy, some women will be able to wear their regular bras with few or no adjustments. If the surgical area is especially sensitive after surgery, a bra extender can help increase the circumference around the body and make wearing a bra feel more comfortable. Bra shoulder pads can help prevent bra straps from digging into the shoulder.

If a woman chooses to wear a breast prosthesis that does not adhere directly to the skin, she will need to wear a special post-mastectomy bra with pockets for the breast form (special swimsuits also hold breast forms). Some women find that special sleep or leisure bras with or without pockets for a prosthesis are comfortable to wear overnight.

### Who should consider a prosthesis and/or post-mastectomy bra?

Any woman who has undergone breast cancer surgery that has removed a significant portion of tissue is a candidate for a breast prosthesis, which often needs to be worn with a post-mastectomy bra. Many women do not wish to have surgical breast reconstruction after breast cancer surgery or decide to wait several months or years before having reconstructive surgery. For these women, breast prostheses and mastectomy bras are viable alternatives.

### When can women begin wearing prostheses?

Usually, a patient's physician will recommend that she wear a camisole (sleeveless undergarment made of soft material) with a non-weighted breast prosthesis after breast cancer surgery until the surgical site is completely healed. This typically takes between four and eight weeks but may be longer or shorter depending on the individual situation. After the chest area has healed, a woman may be fitted for a weighted external breast prosthesis.

### *What are the advantages and disadvantages of wearing a prosthesis?*

The main benefit of wearing a breast prosthesis (versus nothing) is that a weighted prosthesis can help balance the body and anchor the bra, preventing back or neck pain, shoulder sagging, or having a bra "ride up" in the back. Some women find that their prosthesis feels heavy at first since they are not used to wearing it. However, in time, most women feel comfortable with their prosthesis. Breast prostheses can also help protect the chest area and mastectomy scars.

While breast prostheses can provide physical and emotional benefits after breast cancer surgery, some women do not feel satisfied wearing breast forms. For these women, surgical breast reconstruction is a more appropriate decision. Most women who undergo breast cancer surgery are candidates for reconstructive surgery, either during the same surgery as the breast is removed or at a later date. The two main types of reconstructive surgeries are implant insertion and muscle flap reconstruction (the latter involves using the patient's own tissue from another area of the body to reconstruct the breast).

### *Is a prescription necessary in order to purchase a prosthesis or post-mastectomy bra?*

While not required, it is highly recommended that breast cancer patients have their physicians write a prescription for a breast prosthesis and post-mastectomy bra. Many insurance companies will cover some or all of the costs for these products if they are prescribed by a physician. Patients should check with their insurance providers for details about the coverage. It is also important for the physician to specify how many prostheses are necessary and how often they should be replaced. For example, Medicare will cover the cost of a new breast prosthesis every two years and two post-mastectomy bras every six months.

### *How much do prostheses and post-mastectomy bras cost?*

Taking a sufficient amount of time to consider the different types of breast prostheses is important. The prices of prostheses vary significantly and a higher priced prosthesis may not be the most comfortable one. Approximate prices of breast prostheses range from $30 to $400;

approximate prices for post-mastectomy bras and camisoles range from $20 to $80.

### *Will insurance providers cover the cost of a prosthesis or post-mastectomy bra?*

Many insurance companies will cover the cost of a limited number of breast prostheses and post-mastectomy bras if they have been prescribed by a physician. In some cases, additional paperwork or procedures need to be followed to ensure coverage. Breast cancer patients who wish to wear prostheses and/or post-mastectomy bras should contact their insurance providers prior to purchasing these items to determine whether they are covered and what needs to be done to ensure coverage. Since the prices of prostheses and post-mastectomy bras vary significantly depending on the style, type, etc., patients should also determine whether their insurance provider has set a "price limit" for these items.

In some instances, women will need to purchase the prosthesis and post-mastectomy bras themselves and turn in the appropriate paperwork to their insurance providers to receive partial or total reimbursement. Other times, the manufacturer or shop where the items are purchased will bill the patient's insurance company directly. Again, these matters should be worked out with the insurance company prior to making a purchase. Some insurance companies may require patients to order products from a specific manufacturer or shop.

It is also important for women to ask their physicians to note how often the prosthesis will need to be replaced. On average, prostheses need to be replaced every one to two years and additional post-mastectomy bras need to be purchased every three months to a year. For example, breast cancer patients on Medicare receive coverage for one new prosthesis every two years and two post-mastectomy bras every six months.

### *Where can I find additional information about breast protheses and post-mastectomy bras?*

The American Cancer Society provides information on breast prostheses at http://www.cancer.org and The Ted Mann Family Resource Center, a nonprofit organization working in conjunction with the Jonsson Comprehensive Cancer Center at the University of California at Los Angeles, provides information on breast prostheses and post-mastectomy bras at http://cancerresources.mednet.ucla.edu.

# Breast Reconstruction

## Overview

Breast reconstruction is a surgical procedure to rebuild the contour of the breast, along with the nipple and areola (the pigmented area surrounding the nipple) if desired. Recent advances in reconstructive techniques have given patients more choices when it comes to breast reconstruction, including the option to have breast reconstruction during the same operation in which the breast is removed. Being diagnosed with breast cancer is not usually a medical emergency; most women have a sufficient amount of time to research treatment and reconstructive options before having to make any decisions.

Though some women are not interested in breast reconstruction, many breast specialists support reconstructive surgery as an important option for patients to consider. Women are encouraged to weigh both the advantages and disadvantages of breast reconstruction with their plastic surgeons and cancer treatment team and make an informed decision based on their own situation. Breast reconstruction is most often an option for women who have had mastectomy if their entire breast has been removed. Women who undergo lumpectomy (surgical removal of a breast lump and a margin of surrounding tissue) rarely need breast reconstruction.

The goal of breast reconstruction is to create breast symmetry when a woman is wearing a bra. When a woman is nude, the reconstructed breast will look different from the unaffected breast, regardless of the type of reconstruction chosen. However, when a woman is wearing a bra, the size and shape of the reconstructed breast should closely resemble the unaffected breast.

It is a common misconception that women may have to wait a year or longer to begin the reconstructive progress after breast surgery. Though breast cancer patients who receive chemotherapy after mastectomy may have to delay reconstruction until chemotherapy is finished, the majority of women may begin reconstruction soon after the surgery in which the breast is removed (if not during the same operation).

## Types of Breast Reconstruction

There are two main types of breast reconstruction available to most mastectomy patients:

- Saline breast implants
- Muscle flap reconstruction

The insertion of saline (salt-water filled) implants is usually a two-part procedure. The first implant operation involves placing a tissue expander in the intended breast area beneath the skin and chest muscle. The tissue expander is similar to a balloon, and the surgeon will fill the expander with salt-water solution periodically (usually once a week). The procedure to insert the tissue expander into the breast area typically takes about forty-five minutes. After the skin has sufficiently stretched, the surgeon will replace the tissue expander with a permanent saline implant, usually three to four months after the first implant surgery. Occasionally, a woman will not need a tissue expander. If this is the case, then the surgeon will proceed directly to permanent implant surgery. Approximately 50% of saline implants need some type of modification or replacement after five or ten years.

The second main type of breast reconstruction, muscle flap reconstruction, involves using a patient's own tissue to rebuild the contour of the breast. Tissue may be taken from the back, stomach, or buttocks. Muscle flap operations leave scars both from where the tissue was taken and on the reconstructed breast. In a free TRAM (transverse rectus abdominis muscle) flap procedure, the surgeon transfers some abdominal skin, fat, and a small piece of muscle under the skin to the intended breast area. The tissue from abdomen is usually enough to create a breast shape. If not, a saline implant may also be inserted. In a back tissue (latissimus dorsi) reconstructive flap, a surgeon transfers muscle and skin from the patient's back to the intended breast area. This creates a pocket where an implant is usually inserted.

Muscle flap procedures take much longer than implant operations, lasting about four to five hours, and patients typically stay in the hospital three to four days, compared to one day with the implant operation. Though the recovery is slower, the breast usually looks and feels more natural to most women.

Because muscle flap reconstruction involves the blood vessels, women who smoke or have diabetes, vascular, or connective tissue diseases cannot typically undergo this type of breast reconstruction.

Because many breast cancers involve the nipple areolar complex, the surgeon usually removes the nipple during mastectomy. After the breast volume has been rebuilt with a tissue expander or muscle flap procedure, the nipple may be recreated. Most nipple recreation takes place two to six months after the initial breast reconstruction to allow the new breast area ample time to heal. A new nipple may be created from a skin graft from a woman's inner thigh or from the areola (the pigmented region surrounding the nipple) on her natural breast. Occasionally after a skin graft, the skin of the newly created nipple turns white. Some surgeons prefer to tattoo the skin graft of the new nipple to ensure that the color matches the color of the nipple from the natural breast.

## Peg Procedures

A new type of breast reconstruction developed by Dr. Edward Knowlton, M.D., promises to reduce a patient's mastectomy scar. Results of Dr. Knowlton's research were published in the September 1992 issue of *Contemporary Surgery* and also presented in San Diego at the annual meeting of the American Society of Plastic and Reconstructive Surgeons. According to Dr. Knowlton, the peg procedures can recreate both the shape and size of the breast as well as the nipple and areola (darker pigment surrounding the nipple). In one type of peg procedure, the traditional straight-line mastectomy scar is replaced with a circular scar that is hidden within the border of the newly created nipple.

The newest peg procedure (called the pectoralis peg) uses only the remaining breast skin after a mastectomy and relies on the body's own healing processes to create a normal-looking nipple. After the body heals from mastectomy, new blood vessels usually grow into the remaining skin from the pectoralis muscle on the chest wall. The pectoralis peg procedure uses this new blood supply to provide circulation to the newly created nipple and areola. Thus, a skin graft from another portion of the patient's body is not necessary (as it is with most muscle flap reconstructive techniques).

The following are some benefits of peg procedures:

- Camouflaging scars around the reconstructed nipple and areola

- Immediate breast reconstruction can usually be performed in one procedure

- The breast skin envelope is preserved

- A full range of breast sizes and shapes are possible

- Breast symmetry is usually achieved

- Effects of the procedures do not typically change significantly over time

- The procedures can be modified for a variety of accepted techniques including: immediate reconstruction, delayed reconstruction, TRAM flap reconstruction, implant insertion, and repositioning of the breast

The peg procedures are not suitable for all women considering breast reconstruction.

### Finding a Plastic Surgeon

If a woman is contemplating breast reconstruction, she should discuss her options with a plastic surgeon. It is important to make sure that the plastic surgeon is certified by the American Society of Plastic Surgeons and has experience with breast reconstruction.

Women may contact the American Society of Plastic Surgeons (ASPS) at 800-635-0635 to find out if their plastic surgeon is board certified. The ASPS was formed in 1972 and provides women with a list of ASPS certified members in the caller's area. The ASPS website also allows women to search for a plastic surgeon by name, city, state, or zip code.

### Possible Complications with Breast Reconstruction

As with any type of surgery, breast reconstruction has certain risks women should consider before deciding on reconstructive surgery. The most common complication with breast implants is capsular contracture: the scar or capsule around the implant begins to tighten and squeezes down on the soft implant, causing the breast to feel hard. Capsular contracture may be treated with additional surgery to remove the scar tissue. Occasionally, patients with capsular contracture may have to have the breast implant removed and replaced with a new one.

Other rare complications from general surgery may also occur during breast reconstruction, including: bleeding, fluid collection, excessive scar tissue, infection, and problems with anesthesia. Women who smoke may experience a slower rate of healing or more noticeable scars since nicotine often interferes with the body's natural healing process. Rarely, these complications may require additional surgery.

**Note:** It is not possible for women to breast-feed from the reconstructed breast. Even with nipple reconstruction and tattooing of the areola, the breast still lacks the proper glandular tissue and ducts necessary to produce milk. There has been no evidence that breast reconstruction causes a recurrence of breast cancer.

### The Ban on Silicone Gel Implants

In 1992, the U.S. Food and Drug Administration (FDA) imposed a ban on the general use of silicone gel-filled breast implants. Silicone implants may only be used in closely monitored medical trials until they are determined to be safe for widespread use. Questions concerning the safety of silicone implants arose after manufacturing defects and implant misuse led to silicone leakage and rupturing in many patients. When silicone gel is free in breast tissue, it may move to nearby tissues or to the lymph nodes. Some physicians attribute silicone leakage to immune-related disorders and other sicknesses. Many women who experienced silicone leakage reported:

- breast pain
- fatigue
- myalgias (muscle pain)
- arthralgias (joint pain)
- hair loss
- memory loss

There is much controversy surrounding silicone breast implants. Many medical experts doubt silicone implants cause any significant medical disease. Radiologists do worry about the difficulty in detecting breast cancer in breast with implants (saline or silicone).

### Advantages and Disadvantages to Breast Reconstruction

The majority of women diagnosed with breast cancer will undergo some type of breast surgery as part of their treatment. For many simple or modified radical mastectomy patients, breast reconstruction may be possible during the same surgical procedure. However, there are advantages and disadvantages to immediate breast reconstruction:

*Advantages to Immediate Breast Reconstruction*

- Patients do not wake up to the "shock" of losing a breast.
- Patients may avoid additional reconstructive surgery.

- Many doctors agree that the best-looking results occur when the cancer surgeon and the plastic surgeon plan the operation together.

*Disadvantages to Immediate Breast Reconstruction*

- Patients may find it emotionally difficult to weigh all of their breast reconstruction options while also dealing with their recent breast cancer diagnosis and treatment alternatives.

- If surgeons find that the cancer is more advanced than they initially thought, breast reconstruction may interfere with treatment (such as chemotherapy or radiation therapy).

Some doctors recommend that women who need radiation therapy after breast surgery have delayed breast reconstruction. Though radiation after the insertion saline implants or muscle flap procedures may potentially distort the breasts, this is rare. Radiation therapy can usually be administered to patients after breast reconstruction without any significant consequences.

Usually women who have breast reconstruction may choose to have the nipple and areola (the pigmented region surrounding the nipple) reconstructed during additional surgeries. Nipple and areola reconstruction occurs after the breast has had time to settle after the initial reconstructive surgery. Tissue for the nipple can be taken from the newly created breast, the opposite nipple, or even the ear. Tissue for the areola can be taken from the upper inner thigh. To match the other nipple and to create the areola, tattooing may be done.

The American Cancer Society suggests breast cancer patients ask their plastic surgeons the following questions before having breast reconstructive surgery:

- Am I a candidate for breast reconstruction?

- When can I have reconstruction?

- What types of reconstruction are possible for me?

- What is the average cost of each type of reconstruction and does insurance typically cover them?

- What type of reconstruction is best for me? Why?

- How much experience do you (plastic surgeon) have with this procedure?

- What results are realistic for me?
- Will the reconstructed breast match my remaining breast in size?
- How will my reconstructed breast feel to the touch?
- Will I have any feeling in my reconstructed breast?
- What possible complications should I know about?
- How much discomfort will I feel?
- How long will I be in the hospital?
- Will I need blood transfusions? If so, can I donate my own blood?
- How long is the recovery time?
- When can I begin to exercise? Play sports?
- Are there any patients I can speak with who have had the same surgery?
- Will reconstruction interfere with chemotherapy?
- Will reconstruction interfere with radiation therapy?
- How long will the implant last?
- What kind of changes to the breast can I expect over time?
- How will aging affect the reconstructed breast?
- What happens if I gain or lose weight?
- What new reconstruction options should I know about?

### Health Insurance Coverage for Breast Reconstruction

According to the American Society of Plastic and Reconstructive Surgeons, the following are average surgeon fees for breast reconstruction:

- $2,841 implant alone
- $3,413 for a tissue expander
- $5,646 for a back flap procedure
- $7,088 for a TRAM flap procedure
- $9,315 for a microsurgical free flap procedure

These fees do not include bills from anesthesiologists, hospitals, or the cost of implants. Most health insurance companies do cover the cost of breast reconstruction after mastectomy. In 1998, the Women's Health and Cancer Rights Act was passed, which requires all health insurance providers who cover mastectomy procedure to also cover the costs of breast cancer reconstruction for mastectomy patients. Under this legislation, insurance companies who cover the cost of mastectomy must also cover the costs of the following:

- reconstruction on the post-mastectomy breast
- surgery and reconstruction on the other breast to create symmetry
- breast prostheses
- treatment of complications from mastectomy, including lymphedema (chronic swelling) of the arm

Several states also have their own laws that require health plans who cover the costs of mastectomy to also provide the option of reconstruction. The Women's Health and Cancer Rights Act is designed to provide coverage to women whose health plans are not required by state law to cover the costs of breast reconstruction. To view laws for each state regarding breast reconstruction, please visit the Plastic Surgery Information Service website at http://www.plasticsurgery .org/advocacy/brstlaws.htm.

Although the Women's Health and Cancer Rights Act was passed in 1998, there are several issues that still need to be worked out, including questions about retroactive coverage, delayed breast reconstruction, etc. The Department of Labor is expected to address these and other issues in the near future. In the meantime, women who have questions about these issues should call their health insurance provider, the Department of Labor's hotline (202-219-8776), or their State Insurance Commissioner's office.

### Breast Imaging after Reconstruction

It is important for women who have had breast reconstruction to continue receiving yearly mammography on the normal breast. Women who have had breast reconstruction should also practice monthly breast self-examination (BSE) and have yearly clinical breast exam.

Many radiologists do not take screening images of the area where the breast was removed (even if an implant or tissue flap is present) unless there is a clinical concern (for example, a new lump is found). Imaging breasts with implants requires a radiologist to take several special mammography views so he or she may see both the breast tissue and the implant. For this reason, diagnostic mammography is usually performed on women after breast reconstruction. Diagnostic mammography involves pinpointing the exact size and location of breast abnormalities as well as imaging the surrounding breast tissue and lymph nodes.

## Choices in Reconstructive Procedures

The type of breast reconstruction procedures available to you depends on your medical situation, breast shape and size, general health, lifestyle, and goals. You can have your breast reconstructed with a breast implant, a tissue flap (your own tissues), or a combination of the two. If you have breast reconstruction, with or without breast implants, you will probably undergo several reoperations to improve symmetry and appearance.

For example, after your breast has healed from the original implant surgery, you may want to build a new nipple and darken the areola (skin around the nipple). This procedure can usually be performed on an outpatient basis. Ask your doctor to explain the various ways this can be done, such as using a skin graft from the opposite breast or by tattooing the area. Ask your doctor about the pros and cons of each implant technique.

If you decide to have reconstruction for one breast, your doctor may suggest surgery on the other breast to achieve a similar appearance. The following issues should be considered for women with breast cancer:

- The physical and cosmetic results with breast implants may be affected by chemotherapy, radiation therapy, or any other factor that significantly affects the healing process.

- Skin necrosis may occur because blood circulation to the remaining tissue has been changed by a mastectomy. Radiation treatment may also increase skin necrosis.

- It usually takes more than one operation to achieve the desired cosmetic outcome, especially if the reconstruction procedures include building a new nipple.

- Breast reconstruction is an optional procedure and is not needed to treat the cancer.

# Chapter 51

# *Hand and Finger Amputation, Replantation, and Prosthetics*

## *Amputation of the Hand or Finger and Prosthetics*

### *What is amputation?*

Amputation is the complete removal of an injured or deformed body part. An amputation may be the result of a traumatic injury or may be the result of a planned operation where the finger must be removed. Some traumatically amputated fingers may be replanted or reattached, but in some cases, reattachment of the amputated finger is not possible or advisable. Conditions, such as a tumor, may require that a finger be surgically amputated to preserve a person's health.

### *How is an amputation done?*

When an amputation is necessary, the surgeon removes the injured body part and prepares the remaining part for future prosthetic use. This means careful treatment of the skin, muscles, tendons, bones, and nerves, so that a prosthesis can be worn with comfort. The surgeon decides the length of the remaining body part based on medical and prosthetic factors.

## *What can I expect after surgery?*

For the first couple of weeks, you should expect some pain, which is controlled with pain medications. While you are healing, your doctor will tell you how to bandage and care for the surgical site and when to return to the office for follow-up care. You may be given exercises to build your strength and range of motion. You may be asked to touch and move your skin to desensitize it and to keep it mobile.

## *What type of prosthesis will I get?*

The type of prosthesis depends on the location and length of your residual finger or hand and your functional and lifestyle needs. The prosthesis replaces some of the function and the appearance of the missing body part. It is important to communicate to your doctor and prosthetist the activities you feel are most important so that an appropriate prosthesis can be provided for you. Prostheses can restore length to a partially amputated finger, enable opposition between the thumb and a finger, or in the case of a prosthetic hand, stabilize and hold objects with bendable fingers. If your hand is amputated through or above the wrist you may be given a full arm prosthesis with an electric or mechanical hand. Some patients may decide not to use a prosthesis.

## *How is a prosthesis made?*

A prosthesis is fabricated from an impression cast taken from the residual finger or limb and the corresponding part on the undamaged hand. Through this process, an exact match to the details of the entire hand can be achieved. The prosthetic finger or hand is fabricated out of a flexible, transparent silicone rubber. Colors dispersed in the silicone are carefully matched to the individual's skin tones, which give the prosthesis the life-like look and texture of real skin. The finger or hand is usually held on by suction. The flexibility of the silicone permits good range of motion of the remaining body parts. Fingernails can be individually colored before applying them to the fingers so they can be matched almost perfectly. The nails can be polished with any nail polish and the polish can be removed with a gentle-action nail polish remover. Silicones are resistant to staining. Inks wash off easily with alcohol or soap and warm water. With proper care a silicone prosthesis may last three to five years. Creation of your prosthesis usually begins three months after you are completely healed from surgery. This waiting period allows time for swelling to subside and for the remainder of your hand to take its final shape. You may need therapy to learn to use your new prosthesis.

### What kinds of feelings are common following an amputation?

The loss of a body part, especially one as visible as a finger or hand, can be emotionally upsetting. It may take time to adapt to changes in your appearance and ability to function. Talking about these feelings with your doctor or other patients who have had amputations often helps you come to terms with your amputation. You may ask your doctor to recommend a counselor to assist with this process. It is important to remember that with time, you will adapt to your situation by finding new ways of doing your daily activities. A resource that can help is the Amputee Coalition of America www.amputee-coalition .org/index.html. These resources can help you to be strong during the course of recovery. Remember that the quality of life is directly related to your attitude and expectations—not just obtaining and using a prosthesis.

## Replantation

### What is it?

"Replantation" refers to the surgical reattachment of a finger, hand, or arm that has been completely cut from a person's body. The goal of replantation surgery is to give the patient back as much use of the injured area as possible. In some cases, replantation is not possible because the part is too damaged. If the lost part cannot be reattached, a patient may have to use a prosthesis (a device that substitutes for a missing part of the body). In many cases, a prosthesis may give a person without hands or arms the ability to function better than they would without the prosthesis.

Replantation is usually recommended when the replanted part will work at least as well as a prosthesis. Generally, a missing hand or finger would not be replanted knowing that it would not work, be painful, or get in the way of everyday life. Before surgery the doctor, if possible, will explain the procedure and how much use is likely to return following replantation. The patient or family member must decide whether that amount of use justifies the long and difficult operation, time in the hospital, and months or years of rehabilitation.

## How is the procedure done?

There are a number of steps in the replantation process. First, damaged tissue is carefully removed. Then bone ends are shortened and rejoined with pins or plates. This holds the part in place to allow the rest of the tissues to be restored to a normal position. Muscles, tendons, arteries, nerves, and veins are then repaired.

## What kind of recovery can I expect?

The patient has the most important role in the recovery process. Smoking causes poor circulation and may cause loss of blood flow to the replanted part. Allowing the replanted part to hang below heart level may also cause poor circulation. Younger patients have a better chance of their nerves growing back; they may regain more feeling, and may regain more movement in the replanted part. Generally, the further down the arm the injury occurs, the better the return of use of the replanted part to the patient. Patients who have not injured a joint will get more movement back than those with a joint injury. A cleanly cut part usually works better after replantation than one that has been crushed or pulled off. Recovery of use depends on re-growth of two types of nerves: sensory nerves that let you feel, and motor nerves that tell your muscles to move. Nerves grow about an inch per month. The number of inches from the injury to the tip of a finger gives the minimum number of months after which the patient may be able to feel something with that fingertip. The replanted part never regains 100% of its original use, and most doctors consider 60% to 80% of use an excellent result. Cold weather may be uncomfortable and provide reason for frequent complaint even for those with excellent recovery.

## What about therapy and rehabilitation?

Complete healing of the injury and surgical wounds is only the beginning of a long process of rehabilitation. Therapy and temporary bracing are important to the recovery process. From the beginning, braces are used to protect the newly repaired tendons but allow the patient to move the replanted part. Therapy with limited motion helps keep joints from getting stiff, helps keep muscles mobile, and helps keep scar tissue to a minimum. Even after you have recovered, you may find that you cannot do everything you wish to do. Tailor-made devices may help many patients do special activities or hobbies. Talk to your physician or therapist to find out more about such devices. Many replant patients are able to return to the jobs they held before the injury. When this is not possible, patients can seek assistance in selecting a new type of work.

### Are emotional problems common following replantation?

Replantation can affect your emotional life as well as your body. When your bandages are removed and you see the replanted part for the first time, you may feel shock, grief, anger, disbelief, or disappointment because the replanted part simply does not look like it did before. Worries about the look of a replanted part and how it will work are common. Talking about these feelings with your doctor often helps you come to terms with the outcome of the replantation. Your doctor may also ask a counselor to assist with this process. You may find it helpful to talk with someone about it, and work through your feelings so you can move on with your life.

### Will additional surgery be necessary?

After replantation surgery, some patients may need additional surgery at a later time to gain better function of the part. These are some of the more common procedures:

- **Tenolysis:** frees tendons from scar tissue.

- **Capsulotomy:** releases stiff, locked joints.

- **Tendon or muscle transfer:** moves tendons or muscles to another spot so that they can work in an area that needs the tendon or muscle more.

- **Nerve grafting:** replaces a scarred nerve or a gap in the nerves to improve how the nerve works.

- **Late amputation:** removing the part because it does not work well, interferes with use of the hand, or has become painful.

Stay in the flow of life. You have many great gifts. Even with the best medical care, you need to be strong during the course of recovery. Remember that quality of life is directly related to your attitude and expectations—not on just regaining limb use.

# Chapter 52

# *Treating Facial Fractures*

There are a number of possible causes of facial trauma. Sports, accidental falls, motor vehicle accidents, assault, and work related accidents account for the majority of maxillofacial injuries. Oral and maxillofacial surgeons (OMS) are highly trained and skilled in the management of facial injuries and are involved in all aspects of treatment from care of the initial injuries through any necessary reconstruction and implant placement. This chapter describes the types of facial injuries that occur along with a description of the indicated treatment for these injuries. Goals in the treatment of facial injuries include rapid bone healing, a return of normal ocular (eye), masticatory (chewing), and nasal functions, restoration of speech, and an acceptable facial and dental esthetic result.

## *Dentoalveolar Trauma*

Dentoalveolar traumas involve injuries to the teeth and the surrounding bone. Isolated injuries to the teeth are quite common and are usually treated by your general dentist. Sometimes these injuries require the expertise of various dental specialists.

Teeth that have been "knocked out" (avulsed) can be saved if replaced and properly splinted in an timely fashion. In the event of an avulsed tooth one, should find the tooth and rinse it gently in cool water. (Do not scrub it or clean it with soap—just use water). If possible, replace the tooth in the socket and hold it there with clean gauze or a washcloth. If you can't put the tooth back in the socket, place the tooth in a clean container with milk, saliva, or water. Call your dentist immediately to have the tooth replaced and splinted. Time is of the utmost importance; the faster you act, the better chance of saving the tooth.

Dentoalveolar fractures involve the teeth and surrounding bony housing. These injuries usually require the expertise of oral and maxillofacial surgeons. Treatment involves reducing the fracture (placing the involved segment in the proper anatomic position) along with stabilization and immobilization of the bony segments. This requires splinting or wiring the segment to the adjacent uninvolved teeth.

Some dentoalveolar trauma cannot be anticipated or prevented, but if you or your child are involved in sports where collisions can occur an athletic mouth guard should be used. The athletic mouth guard is clearly one of the most effective pieces of equipment available with documented effectiveness against dental trauma and concussion. There are several types of mouth guards available, but the custom-fitted mouth guard is much more desirable in sports with continuous activity such as basketball and soccer.

## Mandible Fractures

Mandible fractures are lower jaw fractures. The specific anatomic location of the fracture is dependent on the mechanism of injury and direction of the traumatic blow. For instance, an impact of the chin region (symphysis) may result in a fracture in that location, but the force may also result in a fracture at a distant sight. Patients commonly present with fractures of both the symphysis and subcondylar area (just below the jaw joint) region. Another common sight for fractures to occur is in the angle region of the mandible through impacted wisdom teeth that have not been previously removed.

One of the most important aspects of surgical correction of mandible fractures is restoration of the pre-injury occlusal (closing bite) relationship. The teeth are first aligned, and then the upper and lower jaws are temporarily wired together establishing the proper occlusion. The devices used to wire the teeth together are termed arch bars and are similar to braces. Once the occlusion has been established, depending on the nature of the fracture, a bone plate is surgically placed across the fracture site (open reduction) aiding in stabilization of the fracture. At this point, the teeth are unwired, and the occlusion is checked for accuracy. When an open reduction is performed most patients do not have to have their teeth wired together (termed intermaxillary fixation) after the operation. There are some fractures that do not require an open reduction and are best treated with placement of arch bars and a period of postoperative intermaxillary fixation. The surgeon will determine which is the best treatment on a case-by-case basis. Postoperative care for mandible fractures is similar to that described in the chapter on orthognathic surgery (see Chapter 53).

## *LeFort I, II, and III Fractures*

The diagram in Figure 52.2 demonstrates the location of LeFort I, II, and III fractures. All LeFort fractures affect the occlusal relationship. Therefore, a primary goal in the treatment of these fractures is the restoration of the occlusal relationship. Principles of treatment are similar to those in the treatment of mandible fractures. All LeFort II and III level fractures involve the bony orbit and can therefore result damage to the eye. Fractures of this type all require careful ophthalmologic evaluation as well. As a general rule, all midface fractures should have an ophthalmologic evaluation prior to surgical intervention.

## *Zygoma (Cheekbone) Fractures*

Patients with fractures of the zygoma often present with pain, difficulty opening the mouth, visual changes, and cosmetic defects. Displaced zygoma fractures can mechanically obstruct the normal

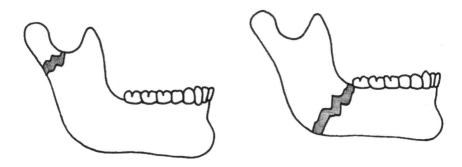

**Figure 52.1.** *Subcondylar Fracture, left; Angle of Mandible Fracture, right.*

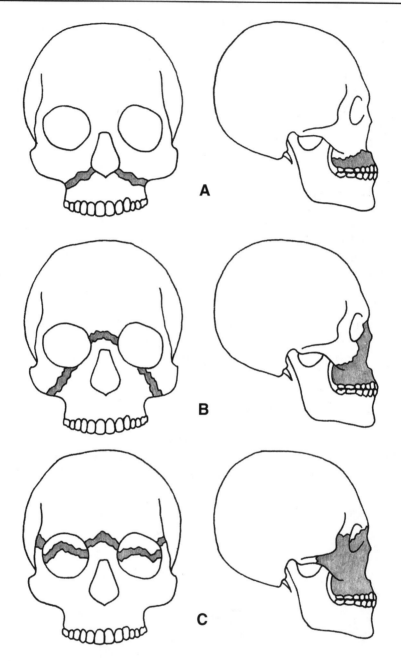

**Figure 52.2.** *(a) LeFort I Fracture, frontal view on the left, lateral view on the right. (b) LeFort II Fracture, frontal view on the left, lateral view on the right. (c) LeFort III Fracture, frontal view on the left, lateral view on the right.*

movement of the mandible, resulting in limited opening. Zygoma fractures involving the orbit and the bony fracture segments can impinge the muscles responsible for movement of the eye resulting in diplopia (double vision) and other visual changes. It is therefore extremely important to obtain precise realignment of the fractured bone to prevent long-term visual changes. Noticeable flattening of the cheekbone occurs with displaced zygoma fractures and can be prevented with precise reduction and fixation of the fracture. Isolated zygoma fractures do not directly involve the occlusion and patients may resume a normal diet after they have been repaired.

## Nasal-Orbital-Ethmoid Fractures

The nasal-orbital-ethmoid area is bordered by the orbital (eye) cavities laterally. Anteriorly, the space is demarcated by the frontal process of the maxilla (upper jaw), the nasal bones, and the frontal process of the frontal bone (forehead). Posteriorly, the boundary is the anterior aspect of the sphenoid bones (at the base of the skull) and the roof is formed by the cribriform plate of the ethmoid bone (by the ears) (see Figure 52.3). Injuries to this region of the facial skeleton

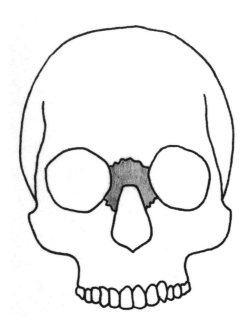

**Figure 52.3.** *Nasal-Orbital-Ethmoid Fractures*

generally occur from a direct frontal force. The diagnosis of fractures in this region is usually made by physical findings aided by a CT (computed tomography) scan. Routine films often fail to demonstrate the degree and location of the disruption. Special considerations of fractures in this region involve assessment of the lacrimal apparatus (tear duct system) and injury to the canthal ligaments (fibrous tissue by the corner of the eye). Disruption of the canthal ligaments can result in traumatic telecanthus (apparent widening of distance between the eyes). Treatment of nasal-orbital-ethmoid injuries must be directed toward the proper reduction of the nasal fractures, the correction of the medial canthal ligament disruption, and the correction of traumatically induced lacrimal system abnormalities.

## Orbital (Eye) Floor Fracture

The classic orbital blowout fracture, by definition, implies an intact orbital rim and a disruption of one of the walls or floor of the orbit (the bony, hollow space that contains the eyeball). If the floor or the orbit is fractured and displaced one may experience prolapse of the orbital tissues into the maxillary sinus. Diplopia, entrapment of

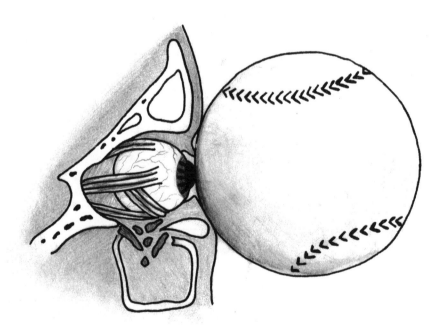

*Figure 52.4. Orbital Floor Fractures (orbital blowout fractures)*

infraorbital tissues (resulting in inability to move the eye) and enophthalmos ("sunken eye") can result when these fractures occur. Again, treatment involves reduction of the fractures, which usually requires an open reduction and repair of the defect with a graft material. The reason for repairing a defect with a graft is to support the orbital contents in the correct anatomical position. There have been many different materials used to repair orbital blowout fractures. Alloplasts are frequently used to reconstruct the orbital floor. Among them have been methyl methacrylate, Teflon, Silastic, and titanium. Autogenous bone grafts are also used for orbital reconstruction but are generally for more complex reconstructions. There are a variety of graft sites available to obtain autogenous bone. If a large quantity of bone is needed hipbone is often used. Other sites include the cranium, tibia, rib, and intraoral sites as well.

# Chapter 53

# *Correcting Orthognathic (Jaw) Abnormalities*

Orthognathic surgery involves a wide variety of surgical procedures performed to place the teeth, jaw bones, and other associated hard and soft tissue structures into their best anatomical positions. This may be necessary as a result of congenital abnormalities, growth disturbances, or trauma. Correction of these abnormalities generally results in improvement in function such as chewing, speaking, and breathing and often enhances facial aesthetics.

Whenever a jaw and bite abnormality is severe enough that orthodontics alone cannot correct the problem, surgery is often necessary. In this type of case the orthodontist moves the upper teeth into their best position in relation to the upper jaw and the lower teeth into the best position in relation to the lower jaw. Surgery is then necessary to correct the position of either the upper jaw, lower jaw, or both. After the jaws are repositioned, the orthodontist is then able to properly finish the bite into the best possible relationship. Surgery may also be helpful as an adjunct to orthodontic treatment to enhance the long term results of orthodontic treatment and to shorten the overall time necessary to complete treatment.

In order to help answer some questions which you may have about surgical treatment, the following information is provided.

"Orthognathic Surgery," © 2007 Drs. Spagnoli, Tucker, Crowley, Galup, Misiek, and Farrell, P.A (University Oral and Maxillofacial Surgery); reprinted with permission. For additional information, visit http://www.universityoralsurgery .com.

## *Why Have Surgery?*

There are several reasons why correction of a jaw abnormality through orthodontics and surgery may be beneficial. Some of these reasons are listed here:

- **When orthodontic treatment alone cannot correct a problem:** There are times when congenital abnormalities, growth disturbances, or previous trauma have resulted in jaw positions that prevent conventional orthodontics from achieving a satisfactory functional and esthetic result.

- **To improve jaw function:** Correcting the bite frequently helps many people chew food more normally and eat things that they have been previously unable to eat.

- **To enhance the long term orthodontic results (stability):** In some cases orthodontic treatment alone can, in fact, produce a good bite relationship during and immediately after the time of orthodontic treatment. However, when an underlying jaw abnormality is responsible for the bite problem, orthodontic movement must sometimes be done in such a way that it will be difficult to maintain the position of the teeth over a period of time after the braces have been removed. Surgery can often improve the long term results in these cases.

- **Reduction in overall treatment time:** In some cases there are several options for treatment including orthodontics alone or a combination of orthodontics and surgery. In some of these cases the combined orthodontic surgical approach can be completed in a shorter period of time since movement of the jaw bone to a better anatomical position may decrease the amount of orthodontic treatment that is necessary.

- **Change in facial appearance:** Placement of jaws in the proper position may often result in a more pleasing facial appearance.

- **Improved breathing:** When surgery is performed on the jaw, the ability to breathe is frequently improved. This type of surgery often greatly improves problems associated with sleep apnea.

- **Improved speech:** Correction of poorly positioned jaws or teeth may have a positive effect on abnormal speech. Jaw surgery may need to be combined with speech therapy to correct speech abnormalities.

**Improvement in jaw pain:** Patients who have jaw joint pain or pain in their jaw muscles may experience some improvement after correction of jaw position. While this pain reduction occurs for many patients, there is no absolute guarantee that correction of jaw positioning will be able to totally eliminate or reduce pain.

## Evaluation and Treatment Sequencing

**Initial evaluation:** During this appointment your physician hopes to discuss your concerns and goals for orthodontic and surgical treatment. Your healthcare provider will do a thorough history and clinical examination and obtain the necessary records for complete treatment planning. These records include the following:

- Photographs of your face and bite
- Special radiographs (x-rays) designed for evaluation of facial bones
- Computerized video images of your face
- Dental impressions of your teeth so that study models can be made

Many of these records may be completed by your orthodontist and, in some cases, these records can be used rather than repeating the process.

**Treatment planning consultation:** At this time the results of your physician's evaluation and treatment recommendations will be presented to you and any family or friends which you feel should be involved in this process. Your photographs, radiographs (x-rays), computerized video images, and/or models may be used to show you what type of treatment will be necessary. You may also be shown illustrations of the type of surgery that is recommended and examples of similar cases. Ask questions. If additional questions arise afterwards, call your healthcare provider's office for a phone discussion or to make another appointment to discuss your surgery in person.

**Insurance preauthorization:** Ask your physician's office for help understanding the requirements of your insurance plan. They may be able to help you by obtaining a predetermination for the insurance coverage on the anticipated surgical treatment plan. This will allow you to anticipate any financial obligation not covered by your insurance.

Contact your insurance company for any insurance-related questions your physician's office is unable to answer.

## Treatment Sequence

**Preoperative preparation** (from now until a few weeks prior to surgery): Prior to the time jaw surgery is completed, the orthodontist will place orthodontic appliances (braces) on your teeth. If it is necessary to remove any teeth to help with this alignment, it will be done at this time. The orthodontist will attempt to align the upper teeth properly in the upper jaw and the lower teeth in the lower jaw prior to surgery. This may not be completely finished before surgery since it may be impossible to finalize the alignment of teeth until the jaws are placed into their proper position.

**Immediate presurgical period** (a few weeks prior to surgery): During this time the orthodontist will place "surgical wires or hooks" on your upper and lower braces. These wires will have small hooks or wire loops which will be used to help place your teeth in the proper position during surgery and to help hook on small elastic rubber bands or wires after surgery.

New records will be taken to formulate the final details of your treatment plan. New photographs, models, radiographs (x-rays), and video images will be completed a few days or weeks prior to surgery.

If you are having upper jaw surgery, we may ask you to donate one unit of your own blood. While the need for transfusion is very rare, should you need a transfusion after surgery you will be able to receive your own blood.

A few days before surgery your physician will complete a final discussion about the details of surgery and answer any of your questions. Your healthcare provider will also perform a complete medical history and physical exam.

## Hospital Routine for Surgery

You will be given a time to go to the hospital, usually very early in the morning on the day of your surgery. Your physician's office will instruct you about procedures for checking in with the hospital's admitting office.

You will then be taken to the operating room where your surgery will be completed.

After surgery you will be taken to the recovery room where you will stay for one to two hours while you wake up.

After leaving the recovery room, you will be taken to your room on the floor in the hospital.

You will be discharged from the hospital one or two days after your surgery. This depends on how you are feeling, how much swelling you have, and whether or not you are taking enough liquid orally so that you do not need your IV. In some cases you may even be discharged the same day of your surgery.

At the time of discharge you will be sent home with following:

- Postoperative instructions

- Medications or prescriptions to pick up your medication

- A postoperative appointment

## The Orthognathic Surgery Team

When undergoing surgical treatment to correct jaw abnormalities, a large team of people is involved:

- The orthodontist and his/her staff

- The surgeon, surgical assistants and office staff

- The anesthesiologist

- Operating room personnel

- Nurses and other health care professionals who work in the hospital

On occasion other dental and medical specialists such as periodontists, endodontists, prosthodontists, plastic surgeons, and otolaryngologists may be consulted for specific needs when indicated. If this is necessary, the reasons will be explained to you and the specialist will be contacted.

## Potential Risks and Complications Associated with Surgery

As with any type of surgical treatment, certain risks must be considered and these should be weighed against the potential benefits. Your surgeon would not likely recommend an operation to you if he or she did not feel that the benefits outweighed any risks associated with surgery. However, it is important for you to understand that the risks associated with orthognathic surgery may include the following:

**Side effects of any surgical procedure:** These actually are not risks but side effects usually associated with any type of surgery:

- Discomfort/postoperative pain as a result of the surgery itself

- Swelling

- Bleeding. Since most jaw surgery is performed through incisions inside the mouth, it is impossible to put a dressing over this area. After surgery some bleeding occurs, just as when teeth are taken out.

**Infections:** Infections with jaw surgery are rare, generally easy to treat, and usually resolved quickly. However, infection may result in more severe consequences such as improper healing and the need for further surgery.

**Structural damage:** Damage to normal structures such as gum tissue, bone, or teeth. Again, this type of problem is extremely rare.

**Numbness or decreased sensation after surgery:** Since jaw surgery is performed to the face, bruising of these nerves sometimes results in some decrease feeling in certain parts of the face. In the case of upper jaw surgery this usually occurs around the nose and upper lip. In lower jaw surgery this occurs around the lower lip and chin. While this may feel strange in the immediate post operative period, this numbness also helps decrease the amount of pain which you will feel after surgery. This decreased feeling is usually temporary. However, in a few patients there may be some permanent loss of feeling.

**Risks associated with anesthesia:** General anesthesia is very safe particularly in elective surgery cases such as orthognathic surgery. The anesthesiologist will discuss all aspects of your anesthetic care prior to your surgery.

## Recovery after Surgery

The speed of surgical recovery depends on several factors including age and the extent of surgery. After the surgical procedure you can expect the following during your recovery.

**Jaw movement:** Most patients undergoing orthognathic surgery will not have their jaws wired together. This will allow some immediate postoperative jaw function. Light elastics (rubber bands) will be used to help your jaw function into a new bite relationship. Over the first two or three weeks you will see significant improvement in jaw movement. Since the jaws are not wired together this makes it easier to speak, drink, eat, and perform oral hygiene.

**Diet:** For the first few days immediately after surgery your diet will be a very soft or blenderized diet. At approximately seven days to two weeks after surgery your diet will consist of foods such as chopped spaghetti, scrambled eggs, or other soft foods which can be eaten without extensive chewing. At two to six weeks after surgery your diet will progress to foods such as ground beef, small pieces of very soft meat such as flaky fish, and other foods which require some chewing.

In most cases your diet will be near normal after six weeks.

**Physical activity:** You should limit your activity for four to five days. This usually means staying around the house with minimal activity.

At about one week after surgery you may be able to return to some limited activity such as slightly restricted work activity, some school activity, and easy leisure activity. For some patients this may be delayed for up to two weeks depending on the type of surgery and how quickly you recover after surgery.

# Chapter 54

# *Septoplasty: Repairing a Deviated Septum*

The septum is the piece of cartilage and bone that gives shape and support to the nose. If it's bent or irregular, it can cause difficulty breathing or make the nose appear crooked.

This surgery (septoplasty) can be performed for a variety of reasons:

- To improve breathing. Septoplasty can be used to relieve nasal airway obstruction. The surgery can remove the malformed cartilage and bony portion of the septum, allowing normal airflow.

- As a secondary operation to a rhinoplasty (nose job). In this instance, a septoplasty is often performed to improve the airway or straighten a crooked nose.

It's important to remember that if you've had a nose injury, you may not be able to undergo septoplasty for at least six months after the injury.

Septoplasty can relieve the following: nasal airway obstruction, which can force you to breathe by your mouth; it can also be part of the surgery for sleep apnea.

"Septoplasty," © 2007 The Cleveland Clinic Foundation, 9500 Euclid Avenue, Cleveland, OH 44195, www.clevelandclinic.org. Additional information is available from the Cleveland Clinic Health Information Center, 216-444-3771, toll-free 800-223-2273 extension 43771, or at http://www.clevelandclinic.org/health.

### *How is a septoplasty done?*

In your pre-surgery consultation, your surgeon will examine your nasal airway and evaluate how air flows from each nostril in order to determine exactly how to handle your situation. Your allergies, medications, and health history will also be reviewed. It is helpful to bring your current medications with you.

Your surgery will usually be done on an outpatient basis under general anesthesia.

During the actual procedure, your surgeon will make an incision internally on one side of the nasal septum. He or she will lift the mucous membrane (mucosa) away from the cartilage, removing the obstructive cartilage and occasionally some bone. Your surgeon will usually use splints inside your nose to support the septum during healing. These splints will then be removed during one of your post-op visits.

### *How should I prepare for a septoplasty?*

You should allow one to two weeks in your schedule when you can be free of work and social commitments. Most patients are comfortable being out in public by two weeks after surgery.

Two weeks prior to surgery, you will need to stop taking aspirin and other medications that can increase your risk of bleeding.

You should have nothing to eat or drink after midnight on the night before your surgery.

On the day of surgery, you should wear a loose button-down blouse or shirt; that is, one that does not need to be pulled over your head or face.

If your procedure is to be done on an outpatient basis, you will need someone to drive you home and stay with you the first twenty-four hours. Your surgeon may need to see you back the morning after your surgery.

We recommend having the following items available:

- Gauze.

- Container to hold water for cool compresses. DO NOT use ice packs.

- Button-down blouses or shirts which do not need to be pulled over your head.

- General painkillers, such as acetaminophen. (Continue to avoid aspirin and other medications like ibuprofen for approximately one week after surgery.)

- Have any prescriptions for pain medications or antibiotics filled before you get home.

- A cool mist humidifier is recommended, but not mandatory.

### *What should I expect after a septoplasty?*

Your surgeon will give you a prescription painkiller and a list of postoperative instructions. It's extremely important to follow these instructions very carefully to make sure your nose heals properly. Your doctor might pack your nose with dressings. Your surgeon will usually remove the packing during the first few days following the surgery. The only person who should remove this packing is your surgeon. Make sure you understand exactly how and why your surgeon packs your nose, and the follow-up care that is required to ensure proper treatment.

If your surgeon has covered your nose with a splint, you can have this removed in just about one week. If you have internal stitches, these will dissolve. If you have external stitches, your surgeon will want to remove these in about one week.

### *What are the possible complications or side effects of a septoplasty?*

- As with any surgery, there is always a risk of infection. Your surgeon may prescribe an antibiotic as a precaution.

- You should expect some nasal drainage with a small amount of bleeding for the first few days after surgery.

- You may experience numbness of the nose, cheeks, and upper lip. Numbness in the tip of the nose may take several months to return to normal. Other areas will resolve more quickly.

- You should expect some bruising and swelling of the nose, eyelids, and upper lip. Most of this will resolve in the first two weeks after surgery.

### *When should I call a doctor?*

When you experience any of the following:

- fever
- excessive bleeding
- difficulty breathing

## *Does insurance cover septoplasty?*

Insurance coverage for septoplasty will depend on two factors: the reason it's being done, and your insurance carrier. It's important that you call your insurance carrier and find out the details of your particular plan. Don't assume it's covered! If septoplasty is required to correct a medical problem (such as difficulty breathing), or due to nose injury, then your insurance carrier will be more likely to cover the procedure. Insurance plans do not provide coverage for elective cosmetic surgery. If you are undergoing a septoplasty along with a rhinoplasty, for cosmetic purposes, make sure you understand all associated costs and what you are expected to pay.

# Chapter 55

# *Bariatric Surgery for the Management of Obesity*

## *Introduction*

Weight loss (bariatric) surgery is a unique field, in that with one operation, a person can be potentially cured of numerous medical diseases including diabetes, hypertension, high cholesterol, sleep apnea, chronic headaches, venous stasis disease, urinary incontinence, liver disease, and arthritis. Bariatric surgery is the only proven method that results in durable weight loss. This proven surgical approach, combined with the dismal failure of dieting, the marked improvement in quality of life, and the quick recovery with minimally invasive techniques, has fueled the surge in the number of bariatric procedures performed annually over the last 10 years.

Weight loss operations can be divided into restrictive procedures and malabsorptive procedures. Malabsorptive procedures reduce the absorption of calories, proteins, and other nutrients. In contrast, restrictive operations decrease food intake and promote a feeling of fullness (satiety) after meals. Some operations are a combination of both. The gastric bypass (open and laparoscopic), the laparoscopic adjustable band and the biliopancreatic diversion (with or without the duodenal switch) are the primary procedures used currently.

---

While the majority of patients who undergo these procedures are very successful, no procedure is perfect. Only through an honest discussion with a bariatric surgeon can patients decide which procedure may be best suited for them. With the development of new techniques and innovative procedures, patients and surgeons must remember the lessons learned from pioneering surgeons.

## Jejunoileal Bypass

The first operations designed solely for the purpose of weight loss were initially performed in the 1950s at the University of Minnesota. The jejunoileal bypass (JIB) induced a state of malabsorption by bypassing most of the intestines while keeping the stomach intact. Although the weight loss with the JIB was good, too many patients developed complications such as diarrhea, night blindness (from vitamin A deficiency), osteoporosis (from vitamin D deficiency), protein-calorie malnutrition, and kidney stones. Some of the most worrisome complications were associated with the toxic overgrowth of bacteria in the bypassed intestine. These bacteria then caused liver failure, severe arthritis, skin problems, and flu-like symptoms. Consequently, many patients have required reversal of the procedure.

The JIB is no longer a recommended bariatric surgical procedure. The lessons learned from the JIB include the crucial importance of long-term follow-up and the dangers of a permanent, severe, and global malabsorption. Long-term follow-up by experienced bariatric surgeons is strongly recommended for all patients who have had a JIB in the past.

## Gastric Bypass

Drs. E.E. Mason and C. Ito initially developed this procedure in the 1960s. The gastric bypass was based on the weight loss observed among patients undergoing partial stomach removal for ulcers. Over several decades, the gastric bypass has been modified into its current form, using a Roux-en-Y limb of intestine (RYGBP). The RYGBP is the most commonly performed operation for weight loss in the United States. In the U.S. approximately 140,000 gastric bypass procedures were performed in 2005, far outnumbering the LAP-BAND®, duodenal switch, and vertical banded gastroplasty procedures.

Initially the operation was performed as a loop bypass with a much larger stomach. Because of bile reflux that occurred with the loop configuration, the operation is now performed as a "Roux-en-Y" with a limb of intestine connected to a very small stomach pouch which prevents the bile from entering the upper part of the stomach and esophagus.

The remaining stomach and first segment of small intestine are bypassed. In the standard RYGBP, the amount of intestine bypassed is not enough to create malabsorption of protein or other macronutrients. However, because the bypassed portion of intestine is where the majority of calcium and iron absorption takes place, anemia and osteoporosis are the most common long-term complications of the RYGBP. Therefore, lifelong mineral supplementation is mandatory. Other clinically important deficiencies that may occur include deficiencies of Vitamin $B_1$ (thiamine) and Vitamin $B_{12}$. Lifelong follow-up with a bariatric program and daily multivitamins are strongly recommended prevent nutritional complications.

The RYGBP has been proven in numerous studies to result in durable weight loss and an improvement in weight-related medical illnesses. Half of the weight loss often occurs during the first six months after surgery; weight loss usually peaks at 18–24 months. The obesity-related comorbidities that may be improved or cured with the RYGBP include diabetes mellitus of the adult onset type (so-called insulin resistant), hypertension, high cholesterol, arthritis, venous stasis disease, bladder incontinence, liver disease, certain types of headaches, heartburn, sleep apnea, and many other disorders. Furthermore, the RYGBP has resulted in marked improvements in quality of life.

Although the most commonly performed RYGBP (sometimes called the proximal gastric bypass) involves little malabsorption, some surgeons modify the RYGBP to incorporate an element of malabsorption for the purpose of augmenting weight loss in special circumstances. This modification is sometimes called a distal gastric bypass, which may result in more severe nutritional complications than the proximal RYGBP. Whether long-term weight loss is superior to the proximal RYGBP or whether the malabsorptive complications are worth the possible improvements in weight loss has not been well established. Many surgeons reserve the distal RYGBP for very select circumstances.

The mechanism in which the RYGBP works is complex. After surgery, patients often experience marked changes in their behavior. Most patients have a reduction in hunger and feel full sooner after eating. Patients often state that they enjoy healthy foods and lose many of their improper food cravings. Rarely do people feel deprived of food. These complex behavioral changes are partially due to alterations in several hormones (ghrelin, GIP, GLP, PYY) and neural signals produced in the GI tract that communicate with the hunger centers in the brain. Another mechanism for weight loss after the RYGBP is referred to as the dumping syndrome. Dumping may result in lightheadedness, flushing, heart palpitations, diarrhea, and other symptoms early (within 10 to 30 minutes) after eating sweets or foods with a high concentration of sugar. Some people remain extremely sensitive to sweets for the rest of their lives; most patients lose some or all of their sweets sensitivity over time.

The risk of dying in the first month after a RYGBP from complications of the operation is about 0.2 to 0.5% in expert centers. Studies have demonstrated that the mortality rate from hospitals with a low experience with the procedure is far higher than that reported by expert centers. The American Society of Bariatric Surgeons fully supports the initiative of the Surgical Review Committee to establish rigid criteria to certify that hospitals with quality programs will be designated as a "Center of Excellence."

### *Advantages of RYGBP*

- Better weight loss than after purely restrictive procedures
- Low incidence of protein-calorie malnutrition and diarrhea
- Rapid improvement or resolution of weight-related comorbidities
- Appetite reduction

### *Complications of RYGBP*

- Early:
  - Anastomotic Leak
  - Pulmonary embolism
  - Wound infection
  - Gastrointestinal hemorrhage
  - Respiratory insufficiency
  - Mortality
- Late:
  - Incisional hernia
  - Bowel obstruction

- Internal hernia
- Stomal stenosis
- Micronutrient deficiencies
- Marginal ulcer

## Laparoscopic Gastric Bypass

Although the open RYGBP can be performed with a relatively low morbidity and mortality, the wound-related complications such as infection and incisional hernia can be troublesome. Wound infection occurs in as many as 8% of patients after open RYGBP and late incisional hernia occurs in as many as 20% of patients. However, some surgeons have reported a much lower rate. The laparoscopic approach to RYGBP was initiated in an effort to improve the early outcomes including a reduction in postoperative complications arising from a large incision in a severely obese patient.

In 1994, Drs. A.C. Wittgrove and G.W. Clark reported the first case series of laparoscopic RYGBP. The primary differences between laparoscopic and open RYGBP are the method of access and method of exposure. Laparoscopic RYGBP is normally performed through five or six small abdominal incisions (0.5–2.0 cm); the peritoneal cavity (abdomen) is insufflated with carbon dioxide gas which creates a space within which to work, allowing exposure of the operative field. In contrast, open RYGBP is performed through a larger incision and abdominal wall retractors are used for exposure. By reducing the size of the surgical incision and the trauma associated with the operative exposure, the surgical insult has been shown to be less after laparoscopic compared to open RYGBP. However, not all patients are candidates for a laparoscopic approach based on body habitus or previous intra-abdominal surgery.

Clinical studies have demonstrated that laparoscopic RYGBP is a safe and effective alternative to open RYGBP for the treatment of morbid obesity. K.D. Higa and colleagues reported the largest laparoscopic RYGBP experience with 1,500 operations. There have been three prospective, randomized trials comparing the outcomes of laparoscopic and open RYGBP. The largest trial was reported by N.T. Nguyen and colleagues in 2001. In 2004, a group from Murcia, Spain published their results. Long-term weight loss after laparoscopic and open RYGBP should not differ, as the primary differences between the two techniques is largely in the method of access and not the gastrointestinal reconstruction.

Despite the advantages of the laparoscopic approach, open bariatric surgery still plays a prominent role in management of morbidly obese patients. Relative contraindications for laparoscopic bariatric surgery include patients with extremely high body mass index, patients with multiple previous upper abdominal surgeries, and patients with prior bariatric surgery. Another limitation of the laparoscopic approach is the steep learning curve of this technically challenging procedure for the surgeon, so it is not an operation for the surgeon who has not been trained specifically in this technique. The advantages and disadvantages of laparoscopic RYGBP are listed below.

### *Advantages of Laparoscopic Compared to Open RYGBP*

- Lesser intraoperative blood loss
- Shorter hospitalization
- Reduced postoperative pain
- Less pulmonary complications (atelectasis)
- Faster recovery
- Better cosmesis
- Fewer wound complications (incisional hernias and infections)

### *Disadvantages of Laparoscopic Compared to Open RYGBP*

- Complex laparoscopic operation associated with a steep learning curve
- Possible increase in the rate of internal hernia

## *Silastic® Ring Gastric Bypass*

The Silastic® ring gastric bypass is a banded pouch RYGBP. A Silastic® ring is placed around the vertically constructed gastric pouch above the anastomosis between the pouch and intestinal Roux limb. The band controls stoma size by prevention of dilatation of the gastric pouch outlet, and is thought to provide better long-term control of the rate of emptying of the pouch and caloric intake. This procedure also includes placement of a gastrostomy tube for decompression of the distal stomach; a radio-opaque ring marker may be placed around the gastrostomy site to facilitate future percutaneous access to the distal stomach. A small percentage (3%) of patients may have band erosion or obstruction, necessitating reoperations and band removal.

## Biliopancreatic Diversion

Dr. Nicola Scopinaro first performed the biliopancreatic diversion (BPD) which was designed to be a safer malabsorptive alternative to the JIB. This operation induces controlled malabsorption without many of the potential side effects caused by bacterial overgrowth associated with the JIB. The malabsorptive operations differ from the RYGBP and the gastric banding, which work mainly through restriction.

Malabsorption is defined by the incomplete uptake of calories and nutrients and occurs via two mechanisms. First, the bile and pancreatic fluids released into the duodenum to digest food and break down fats, carbohydrates, and proteins are diverted away from ingested food—hence the name, biliopancreatic diversion. The digestive enzymes eventually join the ingested food—but at a point in the distal small intestine (ileum) where there is much less chance for complete breakdown and absorption. When food is in the diverted small intestine it is not absorbed as well because of the lack of enzymes to break down the larger fat, protein, and carbohydrate molecules into their smaller building blocks, the actual particles absorbed. Because of the particular digestive aids necessary to absorb fats (bile and lipase are crucial), fat calorie malabsorption predominates. Unfortunately, undigested fats cause gas and loose, foul-smelling bowel movements, called steatorrhea. The second mechanism through which malabsorption occurs is by decreasing the amount of small intestine through which the ingested food passes. With less surface area of intestine with which food is in contact, less nutrients can be absorbed.

Unlike the RYGBP where no stomach is removed (only bypassed), the BPD involves the removal of 70% of the stomach. This procedure is done to decrease the amount of acid produced by the remaining stomach. Gastrin, a hormone produced by G-cells in the antrum, is responsible for stimulating the upper stomach to produce acid. Of note, the portion of the remaining upper stomach is far larger than the small "pouch" created for the RYGBP. This allows patients to eat larger volumes than after a restrictive operation before feeling full (satiety). After entering the upper stomach, food passes through a newly created connection (anastomosis) into the small intestine (alimentary limb). This anatomy is very similar in principle to the standard RYGBP, except that the length of the intestine from the stomach to the colon is much shorter—promoting malabsorption. The bile and pancreatic secretions pass through the bypassed biliopancreatic channel and connect with the alimentary channel (where the food travels)

50–100 cm from the colon. Some of these secretions are reabsorbed in this channel prior to meeting the alimentary tract. The part of the intestines where bile and pancreatic fluids (from the biliopancreatic channel) and food (from the alimentary channel) mix is called the common channel. Surgeons use various formulas to determine the appropriate length of the alimentary channel and the common channel.

The amount of excess weight loss after the BPD has been reported to be around 70 percent—with weight loss in some patients persisting up to 18 years. However, like all weight loss data, this percentage of excess weight lost varies depending on the length of follow-up, the quality of follow-up, the country where the procedure was performed, the surgeon, and the initial weight of the patient. Being a malabsorption operation, however, the BPD requires life-long medical follow-up.

## Duodenal Switch

The duodenal switch (DS) is a modification of the BPD designed to prevent ulcers, increase the amount of gastric restriction, minimize the incidence of dumping syndrome, and reduce the severity of protein-calorie malnutrition. However, the dumping syndrome is also believed by many to be a benefit, rather than a detriment, in that it helps patients avoid eating sugary and high fat foods which would adversely affect weight loss. The DS was first reported by Dr. Doug Hess in 1986.

The DS works through an element of gastric restriction as well as malabsorption. The stomach is fashioned into a small tube, preserving the pylorus, transecting the duodenum and connecting the intestine to the duodenum above where digestive juices enter the intestine. Compared to the BPD, the DS leaves a much smaller stomach that creates a feeling of restriction much like that of a RYGBP. Anatomically, the main difference between the DS and the BPD is the shape of the stomach—the malabsorptive component is essentially identical to that of the BPD. Instead of cutting the stomach horizontally and removing the lower half (such as with the BPD), the DS cuts the stomach vertically and leaves a tube of stomach that empties into a very short (2–4 cm) segment of duodenum.

The duodenum is tolerant of stomach acid and therefore is much more resistant to ulceration compared to the small intestine. Removing part of the stomach also decreases the amount of acid present. Whereas the BPD involves an anastomosis (connection) between the stomach and the intestine, the DS involves an anastomosis between the duodenum and the intestine. The duodenum is cut about 2–4 cm from the stomach (measured from the pyloric valve). The intestine is sewn to the end of the duodenum which remains in continuity with the stomach. The other side of the duodenum will carry all the bile and pancreatic secretions. A theoretical (but clinically unproven) benefit of the DS is an improvement in absorption of iron and calcium in comparison to the BPD. The disadvantage of transecting the duodenum is the large number of vital structures immediately adjacent to the duodenum. Several large blood vessels and the major bile duct are located here. Injury to these structures can be life-threatening.

These procedures have some of the highest reported weight loss in long-term studies, but also have the highest rate of nutritional complications compared to the RYGBP and the purely restrictive procedures. These operations are some of the most complex in bariatric surgery. However, as with most studies of weight loss surgery, there is wide variability in long-term results between different centers. Only multi-center comparative studies can establish definitively the true differences between all these operations.

Some patients and surgeons believe that the DS is a superior operation to the RYGBP and BPD because of the lack of a dumping syndrome, described earlier. The DS and BPD have their own particular side effects. After a meal that is high in fat, people can experience foul smelling gas and diarrhea.

### Advantages of BPD and DS

- Increased amount of food intake compared to the bypass and band

- Less food intolerance

- Possibly greater long-term weight loss

- More rapid weight loss compared with gastric banding procedures

### Complications of BPD and DS

- Diarrhea and foul smelling gas, with an average of three to four loose bowel movements a day

- Malabsorption of fat soluble vitamins (Vitamins A, D, E, and K)

- Vitamin A deficiency, which causes night blindness

- Vitamin D deficiency, which causes osteoporosis

- Iron deficiency—a similar incidence with the RYGBP

- Protein-calorie malnutrition, which might require a second operation to lengthen the common channel

- Ulcers (less frequent with DS)

- Dumping syndrome (less frequent with DS)

### Summary

Both the BPD and the DS can be performed laparoscopically. However, these operations are more demanding technically than the RYGBP and should only be performed in the most experienced hands. Long-term follow up and daily vitamin supplements are crucial to the success of these operations. Life-long monitoring is necessary to prevent nutritional and mineral deficiencies—just as with the RYGBP.

## Gastroplasty

The gastroplasty was designed in the early 1970s to be a safer alternative to the RYGBP and the JIB. The operation itself was made possible by the introduction of mechanical staplers. The gastroplasty was the first purely restrictive operation performed for the treatment of obesity. The original (horizontal) gastroplasty involved stapling the stomach into a small partition—and only leaving a small opening for food to pass from the upper stomach pouch to the lower one, thus the lay term—stomach stapling. This form of gastroplasty resulted in very poor long-term weight loss and, after several attempted modifications, was abandoned eventually.

The vertical banded gastroplasty (VBG) features a pouch based on the lesser curvature of the stomach and a polypropylene mesh band or Silastic® ring around the outlet of the pouch. The advantages of the VBG include a low mortality rate and the virtual absence of micronutrient deficiencies. Also, since no anastomosis is created, there is a lower risk of infectious complications.

However, once a very popular surgical option for obesity, the VBG is being performed much less frequently, because long-term studies have shown a prominent rate of weight regain or exacerbation of severe heartburn. Several randomized, prospective trials have demonstrated superior weight loss with RYGBP compared to VBG. Weight loss for sweets eaters has been shown to be superior with RYGBP compared to VBG, presumably as a result of symptoms of the dumping syndrome with sweets.

## Gastric Banding

Another example of a purely restrictive bariatric procedure is nonadjustable gastric banding. It was first introduced in 1978 by S. Wilkinson, who applied a 2 cm Marlex mesh round the upper part of the stomach and separated the stomach into a small upper pouch and the rest of the stomach. Eventual pouch dilatation resulted in unsatisfactory weight loss.

In 1980, M. Molina described the gastric segmentation procedure, in which a Dacron vascular graft was placed around the upper stomach. The gastric pouch was smaller than Wilkinson's procedure. Because the Dacron graft produced adherence of the liver to the band, it was replaced ultimately by PTFE (Gortex®).

In 1983, L.I. Kuzmak began using a 1 cm Silicone® band to encircle the stomach, creating a 13 mm stoma and a 30–50 mL proximal gastric pouch. This band was later modified to provide adjustability of the band diameter using an inflatable balloon (see "Laparoscopic Adjustable Gastric Banding").

### Advantages of Gastric Banding

- Absence of anemia
- Absence of dumping
- Lack of malabsorption
- Short hospital stay
- Very low mortality rate

### Complications of Gastric Banding

- Gastric perforation
- Incisional hernia
- Stomal stenosis
- Band slippage
- Band erosion into stomach
- Need for reversal or revision

## Laparoscopic Adjustable Gastric Banding

The adjustable band was developed by Kuzmak who devised a Silicone® band lined with an inflatable balloon in 1986. This balloon was connected to a small reservoir that is placed under the skin of the abdomen through which the diameter of the band can be adjusted. Inflation of the balloon functionally tightens the band and thereby increases weight loss, while deflation of the balloon loosens the band and reduces weight loss. These bands can be inserted laparoscopically, thereby reducing the complications and discomfort of an open procedure.

Currently several brands of adjustable bands are available—the LAP-BAND® System, the Swedish Adjustable Band and the Mid-Band. None have yet been shown clearly to be superior to the other. The LAP-BAND® system (Inamed, Santa Barbara, CA) received U.S. FDA approval in 2001.

Since these procedures do not involve an intestinal bypass, laparoscopic adjustable gastric banding (LAGB) is a procedure which induces weight loss solely through the restriction of food intake. For optimal results, strict patient compliance and frequent follow-up for band adjustments are required. The LAP-BAND® is a reversible procedure that does not carry the risks of nutritional and mineral deficiencies of other bariatric procedures. The mortality risk with the LAGB is about 0.1%, which is less than that with the RYGBP.

The LAGB is safe and has a low rate of life-threatening complications. Excess weight loss with the laparoscopic adjustable gastric band is lower than that with the gastric bypass or malabsorptive procedures, varying between 28% and 65% at 2 years and 54% at 5 years. An improvement in weight-related comorbidities has been observed, including Type II diabetes mellitus, dyslipidemia, sleep apnea, gastroesophageal reflux, hypertension, and asthma. However, compared to the gastric bypass, the impact on comorbidities appears to be somewhat less favorable. Remission of diabetes with LAGB is seen in 64–66% at one year and 80% at two years versus 93% at nine years with RYGBP. Long-term results comparing LAGB with gastric bypass or BPD are not yet available.

While some studies have documented weight loss equal to RYGBP with fewer complications, other groups have had disappointing outcomes. Some studies document a substantial number of patients who have required re-operation for long-term complications of the adjustable band (such as for port problems, erosions and slippage, or inadequate weight loss). Conversion of a failed LAGB to another bariatric procedure may be technically more difficult and associated with more complications than with a first time RYGBP or DS operation.

### *Advantages of LAGB*

- Same as gastric banding
- Adjustability of the band
- Reversibility (by band removal)
- Laparoscopic placement

### *Complications after LAGB*

- Intraoperative:
  - Hemorrhage
  - Injury to the spleen, stomach, or esophagus
  - Conversion to open procedure
- Postoperative:
  - Band slippage (stomach prolapse)
  - Leakage of the balloon or tubing
  - Port Infection
  - Band infection
  - Obstruction
  - Nausea and vomiting
- Late complications:
  - Band erosion into the stomach
  - Esophageal dilatation
  - Failure to lose weight

## On the Horizon

Many other procedures are in development. The implantable gastric stimulation device uses small electrodes attached to the stomach which, when stimulated electrically, are supposed to create the feeling of fullness. The intragastric balloon is being reintroduced as a simple procedure that can be placed through an endoscope. The balloon is designed to "take up space" and thereby decrease the amount of food patients can eat. Both of these procedures, while interesting in their simplicity, have not had documented adequate long-term weight loss. However, as these procedures are potentially much safer than other operations, they may have a significant role in the future.

## Staged Procedures

Surgeons are also devising different procedures to decrease the complication rate in high-risk patients—patients who have extreme obesity or severe medical comorbidities. Some surgeons are using a staged approach to bariatric surgery. This approach involves performing a less invasive procedure that reduces weight to a safer level (which in itself is not effective enough on its own) and improves overall medical condition first; then a more complex, definitive procedure is performed once the operative risks of the patient decrease significantly due to the initial weight loss. These less invasive steps have included the "sleeve gastrectomy," the gastric balloon and the adjustable band as an interim step before a RYGBP or DS is performed.

## Summary

Almost all bariatric procedures have resulted in consistent short-term weight loss. Unfortunately there is no perfect operation. The remarkable drive for the obese patient to regain weight cannot be eliminated in all patients. Furthermore, the history of bariatric surgery is replete with procedures that seemed initially to be very promising and safe in theory, but which were later found to be failures. As such, newer procedures should always be viewed with caution. The RYGBP, LAGB, DS, and BPD have withstood appropriate scrutiny through the literature. Only through careful research and discussion with a qualified bariatric surgeon can patients decide which procedure may be the best for them.

# Chapter 56

# *Helping Wounds Heal*

When Darren Benton leaned over to light a homemade firecracker a few days before the Fourth of July in 2000, all he was expecting was a sizzle and a loud noise. But what he got was a flash fire that burned 90 percent of his face.

"I didn't feel anything at first," says Darren. But after looking at himself in the mirror, he got very scared. The 13-year-old's face was completely black, and his right hand and knee also were burned.

Darren's parents rushed him to the hospital. Two days later, after the swelling from his burns went down, surgeons at Children's Hospital in Washington, D.C., anesthetized Darren, scrubbed the dead skin off, and gently applied a wound dressing made of human cells and synthetic material.

For several days afterward, Darren stared out of two small eye slits cut in the bandages that swathed his face to hold the wound dressing in place. He sipped liquid food through a straw poked into another small slit in the bandages.

The surgeons couldn't predict whether his face would be scarred or discolored, says Darren's mother, Patricia Benton. "Children's Hospital hadn't been using [the wound dressing] very long, and they had never used it on a child's face, but they were very positive."

Darren left the hospital after a week, and six months later, he had "completely healed," says Bruce Benton, Darren's father. Except for

"Helping Wounds Heal," by Linda Bren, U.S. Food and Drug Administration (FDA), *FDA Consumer magazine*, May–June 2002 (http://www.fda.gov/fdac).

the loss of a few freckles on the redheaded boy's face and a slightly paler color, "it was as if nothing had happened," he says. "It was a miracle," adds Darren's mother.

The skin covering used on Darren, called TransCyte, is one of several cellular wound dressings approved by the U.S. Food and Drug Administration (FDA). These products are helping to transform the treatment of burns and chronic wounds by decreasing the risk of infection, protecting against fluid loss, requiring fewer skin grafts, and promoting and speeding the healing process.

Each year, about 45,000 Americans are hospitalized for burn treatments and 4,500 deaths occur from fire and burns, according to the American Burn Association (ABA). Twenty years ago, burns covering half the body were routinely fatal, but today, even people with extensive and severe burns have a good chance of survival, says the ABA. Essential to survival is the process of quickly removing dead tissue and immediately covering the wound.

Surgeons discovered many years ago that dead tissue was a breeding ground for bacterial infections, says Charles Durfor, Ph.D., a chemist in the FDA's Plastic and Reconstructive Surgery Devices Branch. "So there was a tremendous advance in surgical care of burns when they started cutting off that dead tissue. All of a sudden the survivability rate went way up."

But once the dead skin has been removed, the blood and fluids that the skin holds within the body start evaporating and weeping, says Phillip Noguchi, M.D., director of the FDA's Division of Cellular and Gene Therapies. "People literally can dehydrate and die from exposure."

This is where the cellular wound dressings come in. "They provide a cover that keeps fluids from evaporating and prevents blood from oozing out," says Noguchi. "And some of these products grow in place and expand much like your own skin would do when you heal."

## *Is It Really Skin?*

As the largest organ of the body, skin protects our internal organs and tissues from toxins, disease-carrying bacteria and viruses, bumps and bruises, and extreme heat and cold. Skin has a sensory function, too. Nerve endings near the surface give us a sense of touch and the ability to feel sensations such as hot and cold.

Two layers make up the skin: the epidermis, which is the thin top layer of tissue, and the dermis, which is the thicker bottom layer. The outermost surface of the epidermis is a tough, protective coating of dead cells called keratinocytes. Underneath these dead cells are live keratinocytes, which divide and replenish the outer layer as the dead cells fall off. Also found within the epidermis are cells that give skin its color (melanocytes) and cells that help protect the body against infection (Langerhans' cells).

The dermis, the lower layer of skin, consists of cells called fibroblasts. These fibroblasts produce collagen, the most common protein in the body, which gives structure and flexibility to the skin. The dermis also contains blood vessels, nerves, hair follicles, and oil and sweat glands.

Cellular wound dressings are sometimes called "artificial skin" or "skin substitutes," but FDA scientists prefer to avoid these labels. "Although they may look and feel like skin, these products do not function totally like skin," says Durfor. "Unlike real skin, they are missing hair follicles, sweat glands, melanocytes and Langerhans' cells."

In some respects, cellular wound dressings try to simulate the two layers of real skin. Some have a synthetic top layer structured like an epidermis. Over time, it peels away or is replaced with healthy skin through skin grafting. The bottom layer usually consists of a scaffold, or matrix, which supports cells that help promote the growth of new skin. Blood vessels, fibroblasts, and nerve fibers from healthy tissue surrounding a burn or wound cross into the matrix to mix with the wound dressing's cells. The matrix eventually disappears as a new dermis forms.

"No one has a full understanding of how these products work," says Durfor. "How they are involved in wound repair is a subject of great scientific interest."

"We do know that they promote a higher rate of healing," says Stephen Rhodes, head of the FDA's Plastic and Reconstructive Surgery Devices Branch. "More patients heal with these devices than with the standard of care, which includes compression bandages and gauze."

## Skin Deep

How a burn is treated and the type of cellular wound dressing used depends on the depth and extent of the burn and the overall health of the person burned.

Traditionally classified as first-, second-, or third-degree, burns are frequently classified by health professionals as superficial, partial thickness, or full thickness, depending on their depth and the amount of tissue damage. Superficial burns, such as a sunburn, redden the skin and damage only the epidermis, making it possible for the body to repair itself. Healthy cells from the dermis reproduce and migrate to the epidermis to heal the damaged skin.

Partial thickness burns cause blisters and damage all of the epidermis and part of the underlying dermis. Although these burns usually heal on their own when treated with cleaning and bandaging, if they are extensive or in a sensitive area, such as the face, they may benefit from the use of cellular wound dressings.

Full-thickness burns completely damage both the epidermis and the dermis, and may even destroy the underlying flesh and bones. The body is unable to heal itself properly because there are no healthy cells to regenerate. These burns require surgery to replace damaged skin with healthy skin, a process known as grafting. If these wounds are not treated, the body attempts to close them by forming scar tissue that contracts over time, leading to disfigurement and loss of motion in nearby joints.

In grafting of burn wounds, surgeons use healthy skin from another part of the person's own body (autografting) as a permanent treatment. But when the skin damage is so extensive that there is not enough healthy skin available to graft initially, surgeons may use cellular wound dressings. These temporary coverings help prevent infection and fluid loss until autografting can be performed. "And these products may allow surgeons to take thinner grafts because not as much dermis in the autograft is required," says Durfor.

An alternative to autografting is to use skin from another person (allograft) or from another species (xenograft) as a temporary covering to protect the wound.

Allografting uses skin from cadaver donors, and xenografting uses skin from animals. "Allografts provide the natural protection of human skin and are used most commonly. Xenografts of pigskin are sometimes used if allografts are not available," says Steven Boyce, Ph.D., director of the department of tissue engineering at Shriners Burns Hospital in Cincinnati. "Xenografts of pigskin are in plentiful supply and it's the closest anatomically to human skin."

Allografts and xenografts are temporary measures because, within several weeks, both types will be rejected and must be replaced with an autograft. "The immune system recognizes that the foreign cells do not belong to the patient," says Boyce. "Immune cells, called T-cells, will attack and destroy foreign cells in the grafts."

Grafts may not be necessary for partial-thickness burns, such as those suffered by Darren Benton; cellular wound dressings are more commonly used. "Almost 80 percent of burns in children are partial thickness," says Martin Eichelberger, M.D., director of emergency trauma and burn services at Children's Hospital in Washington, D.C., where Darren was treated. "The largest volume is from scalding."

Since the introduction of the cellular wound dressing TransCyte, Children's Hospital has used it to treat several hundred children, says Eichelberger. "It's changed our entire paradigm of care for partial thickness burns in children. The mean length of stay used to be 14 days; it's now down to one to two days." Before cellular wound dressings, when gauze was the traditional wound treatment, the pain could be so intense that the patient had to be sedated with morphine or another painkiller just to change the dressing, says Eichelberger. The development of advanced wound dressings such as TransCyte and Integra have changed that. "We're doing fewer skin grafts and we've cut our utilization of morphine by almost 80 percent," he says.

## Types of Cellular Wound Dressings

Biobrane and Integra were the first FDA-approved biologically based wound dressings. Biobrane is a temporary dressing for a variety of wounds including ulcers, lacerations, and full-thickness burns. It may also be used on wounds that develop on donor sites—the areas from which healthy skin is transplanted to cover damaged skin. Made by Bertek Pharmaceuticals, Research Triangle Park, North Carolina, Biobrane uses an ultrathin silicone film and nylon fabric, which is partially imbedded into the film. The nylon material contains a gelatin derived from pig tissue that interacts with clotting factors in the wound. Biobrane is trimmed away as the wound heals or until autografting becomes possible.

Integra Dermal Regeneration Template was approved in 1996 to treat full-thickness and some partial-thickness burns. Made by Integra LifeSciences Corp., Plainsboro, New Jersey, Integra is a two-layer membrane. The bottom layer, made of shark cartilage and collagen from cow tendons, acts as a matrix onto which a person's own cells migrate over two to three weeks. The cells gradually absorb the cartilage and collagen to create a new dermis, or "neo-dermis." This bottom layer is a permanent cover. The top layer is a protective silicone sheet that is peeled off after several weeks. A very thin layer of the person's own skin is then grafted onto the neo-dermis.

Both Biobrane and Integra use animal tissue; the more recently approved cellular wound dressings are made with human tissue. One of these products is OrCel, made by Ortec International Inc. of New York. Approved by the FDA in 2001 to treat donor sites in burn patients, OrCel is made of living human skin cells grown on a cow collagen matrix. OrCel was also approved the same year to help treat epidermolysis bullosa, a rare skin condition in children.

TransCyte is made by Advanced Tissue Sciences Inc. of La Jolla, California, and was approved by the FDA in 1997. "TransCyte was the first product that FDA approved that delivered nonviable (dead) cellular material," says Rhodes. The product starts with living cells, but these cells die when frozen. TransCyte consists of human cells grown on nylon mesh, combined with a synthetic epidermal layer.

TransCyte is packaged and shipped in a frozen state to burn treatment facilities. The surgeon then thaws the product and stretches it over a burn site. In about one to two weeks, the TransCyte starts peeling off, not unlike a sunburn, and the surgeon trims it away as it peels.

TransCyte can be used as a temporary covering over full thickness and some partial-thickness burns until autografting is possible. It's also a temporary covering for some burn wounds that heal without autografting, as in Darren's case.

In addition to burn patients, people with chronic wounds can benefit from cellular wound dressings. Apligraf and Dermagraft are two products used for the treatment of diabetic foot ulcers. People with diabetes are particularly at risk for foot ulcers because of poor blood circulation in the legs and feet. If these ulcers do not heal, amputation of the foot may be required.

Apligraf, made by Organogenesis Inc., of Canton, Massachusetts, was approved by the FDA in 1998 for leg ulcers caused by blood flow problems and in 2000 for treating the hard-to-heal diabetic foot ulcers. Apligraf is a two-layer wound dressing that contains live human skin cells combined with cow collagen.

"Apligraf is unique in that it's the first product approval that delivered live cells from a different donor," says Rhodes. As with OrCel and TransCyte, the donor cells come from circumcised infant foreskin. One small patch of cells, about the size of a postage stamp, from a single donor can be grown in the laboratory to produce tens of thousands of pieces of Apligraf.

Dermagraft, approved by the FDA in 2001, is a product of Advanced Tissue Sciences. Dermagraft is made from human cells placed on a dissolvable mesh material. Once placed on the wound or ulcer, the mesh material is gradually absorbed and the human cells grow and replace the damaged skin.

## The Regulatory Challenge

Although the FDA has been regulating biological products for 100 years, the agency continues to adapt its experiences and regulatory approaches to the review of new technologies, such as cellular wound dressings. Some of these dressings use living cells and have a shelf life of only three days, says Rhodes. Some use a single donor to produce thousands of units of a product. These are just a few of the characteristics that require the agency to revise or adapt its existing regulatory approaches to these products, he says.

To help ensure the safety and quality of products such as cellular wound dressings, the FDA initiated a new regulatory system and issued a final rule, published in 2001, that requires all human cell, tissue, and cellular- and tissue-based product manufacturers to register and list their products with the FDA.

The FDA also issued other proposed rules under the regulatory system to ensure donor suitability and "good tissue practice." "The cells must be screened for a host of infectious agents and diseases," says Rhodes. And they must be handled properly to avoid viral contamination of tissue and cross-contamination that could occur if a donor cell is mixed up with another donor cell by accident in the laboratory.

"We're always walking this very delicate line between trying to be as safe as possible while also allowing progress to be made," says Noguchi. "It is very much of a dynamic balance. At FDA, we want to make sure that what we approve can be used in a way that is predictable for physicians to prescribe or to use in treatment, to the best of our ability, to the best of medicine's ability, and to the best of science's ability."

Despite the challenges of the evolving regulatory climate, the FDA is excited about these products, says Durfor. "We're attempting to set a very reasonable approach for getting cellular material grown up in tissue culture out in the commercial market, while ensuring the safety and effectiveness of every product."

## The Future of Wound Care

The technology of burn and wound care using cellular wound dressings and grafts continues to make tremendous strides forward. But most surgeons agree that nothing seems to work as well as a person's own skin.

Boyce of Shriners Burns Hospital and other researchers are experimenting with cultured skin grown from a burned person's own skin cells. With this method, cells are taken from a small patch of skin, grown in the laboratory, and combined with a collagen matrix. After this cultured skin is placed on the burned area, the matrix dissolves, and the transplanted cells reform skin tissue to heal the wound.

Boyce has found this method to be especially valuable for people who have burns over more than 50 percent of their bodies, which limits the amount of healthy skin available for grafting.

Boyce envisions other future efforts to be focused on improving cosmetic outcome after burn injury. "Smoothness and pliability may have been restored completely," says Boyce, "but better color matching to uninjured skin is needed." Also needed is new technology to make wound treatment faster, and to restore hair and glands of the skin that do not regenerate from grafts.

"Researchers continue to make advances, but the field is in its infancy," says Rhodes.

## Humanitarian Use of Cellular Wound Dressing

Children with a rare inherited, incurable disease called epidermolysis bullosa (EB) have a painful existence. In this disease, a genetic defect causes the skin to lack certain proteins that protect it from damage. Blisters and wounds develop easily on the fragile skin, particularly on fingers and toes. Life-threatening infections may set in when the wounds don't heal, and for those that do, they leave behind scar tissue. The scarring can make the fingers grow together into a gnarled fist that looks like a mitten, rendering it useless.

In 2001, the FDA approved OrCel, a cellular wound dressing, to help surgeons reconstruct the hands of people with EB. Once the fingers are surgically separated, OrCel is used to rebuild the "mitten hand."

OrCel is used on the fingers, thumb, and the palm of the hand, says Mark Eisenberg, M.D., developer of OrCel and co-founder of Ortec International, New York, the company that markets the product. It's also used on the wounds left after taking healthy skin from other parts of the body (donor sites) to help repair the hand. Depending on the severity of the disease, surgeons often must repeat the hand reconstruction, says Eisenberg. But OrCel significantly reduces the need for donor sites in these surgeries. Eisenberg originally developed the product and used it to treat his son, who had EB.

The FDA approved OrCel to help treat EB under a special program for humanitarian use devices (HUDs). A HUD is intended to benefit people with a disease or condition that affects fewer than 4,000 individuals in the United States each year. The regulations regarding HUDs exempt the product from extensive clinical studies while still requiring data to show evidence of safety. These reduced requirements help product developers offset their research and development costs for products that treat a relatively small population.

## Becoming a Skin Donor

On April 17, 2001, Health and Human Services Secretary Tommy G. Thompson launched a national organ donor initiative to encourage Americans to "Donate the Gift of Life." "Fifteen Americans die each day while waiting for an organ to become available," says Thompson. "More than 75,000 men, women, and children now wait for a transplant ... Every 16 minutes, another person joins the waiting list."

Many people don't realize that skin is an organ, but in fact it's the body's largest organ. And like other organ donations, skin donations are critically needed, says Phil Walters, director of the skin bank at Boston Shriners Hospital. Walters says the two most frequently asked questions he fields about skin donation are: is skin taken from a living donor, and can tissue surgically removed from a patient by procedures such as those performed to reduce obesity be donated? "The answer to both questions is no," says Walters. "Skin is procured from a deceased organ donor, just like any other donated organ."

No charge is made to the donor's family for donating organs. And it does not change the appearance of the donor's body or cause a delay in funeral arrangements.

For a downloadable donor card and brochure on organ and tissue donation, visit http://www.organdonor.gov, or call the Health Resources and Services Administration (HRSA) Information Center at 888-ASK-HRSA (888-275-4772).

## Cellular Wound Dressings and Terrorism

The Pentagon, headquarters for the American military and one of the world's largest office buildings, was one target of the terrorist attacks of September 11, 2001. A few miles from the Pentagon, at the Washington Hospital Center, surgeons worked around the clock to treat people who were severely burned from the Pentagon explosion.

Surgeons moved quickly to prevent infection by first removing burned tissue on each person, and then covering the open wounds using cadaver skin, pigskin, and two biosynthetic wound dressings approved by the FDA: Integra and TransCyte. All of the wound coverings were used temporarily to thwart bacterial infection until the burned person's body could heal itself or the person's own skin could be grafted. "They reduce the load of burned tissue, which has a poisonous effect to the body," says Marion Jordan, M.D., director of the Washington Hospital Center's burn center.

Jordan prefers to use skin donated from another person (known as cadaver skin, or human allograft). "Human allograft is still the best alternative to a person's own skin, but I rely on all of the products out there," says Jordan. "I believe each has a place [in the treatment of burns]."

The development of cellular wound dressings to treat burns and wounds is still in its infancy. "This is a small field, but it can have unusual, unexpected, and positive consequences," says Phillip Noguchi, M.D., director of the FDA's division of cellular and gene therapy. "We're committed to moving this area forward. Just as we move forward on many fronts, including fighting anthrax and smallpox, these other efforts will also have an impact on our ultimate response to terrorism."

# Chapter 57

# *Skin Grafts*

### *What is a skin graft?*

A skin graft consists of skin taken from another part of the body and applied to the site where skin is missing. This might follow surgical removal of a skin cancer or a burn. A skin graft is thus a skin transplant. Skin grafts are performed by surgeons (including plastic surgeons) and by some dermatologists.

### *Why do you need a skin graft?*

A skin graft is required when the area that has been cut out is too big to sew the edges together directly. The skin graft covers the wound and attaches itself to the cells beneath. If you didn't apply a skin graft, the area would be an open wound and take much longer to heal.

### *What is involved in having a skin graft?*

Your dermatologist will explain to you why the skin lesion needs excision and why a skin graft is required. He or she will explain the procedure involved. You may be asked to sign a consent form indicating that you agree to and understand the procedure. Tell your doctor

This information, from "Skin Grafting," is reprinted with the permission from DermNet, the website of the New Zealand Dermatological Society. Visit www .dermnet.org.nz for patient information on numerous skin conditions and their treatment. © 2006 New Zealand Dermatological Society.

if you are taking any medication (particularly aspirin or warfarin, which could make you bleed more), or if you have any allergies or medical conditions. Remember to tell your doctor if you take any herbal remedies as a number of these can also lead to abnormal bleeding.

The area to be excised is marked with a colored pen. Local anesthetic will then be injected which will sting briefly. The dermatologist will then cut around and under the lesion with a scalpel and sharp scissors so that it is completely removed (excision biopsy). The lesion will be microscopically examined by a pathologist.

There may be some bleeding in the area from where the lesion has been removed. The doctor may coagulate the blood vessels with diathermy. This can make a hissing sound and a burning smell.

The dermatologist will measure the area of the wound to know what size to make the skin graft. A piece of skin will be shaved or cut from another part of your body (leg or arm) that is large enough to cover the wound. When possible, skin of similar thickness and color will be selected.

The piece of skin (the graft) will be applied to the wound and secured in place with stitches. A special non stick dressing will be applied over the skin graft.

Usually this dressing is left in place for a few days until you see the dermatologist or nurse again. Make sure you have received instructions on how to care for the wound and when to get the stitches out.

### Will I have a scar?

It is impossible to cut the skin without scarring in some way, so some sort of scar is inevitable. Scarring depends on what sort of skin graft has been applied and the size of the graft. Your dermatologist will try to excise the lesion and apply the skin graft carefully, to keep scarring to a minimum. He or she will explain to you what the scar is likely to look like although this can be hard to predict for certain.

You will have two scars, the scar where the skin graft has been applied and the scar from where the skin graft was taken.

Some people have an abnormal response to skin healing resulting in larger scars than usual (keloid or hypertrophic scarring).

### What are the types of skin grafts?

**Split skin grafts:** This type of skin graft is taken by shaving the surface layers (epidermis and dermis) of the skin with a large knife called a dermatome. The shaved piece of skin is then applied to the wound. This type of skin graft is often taken from the leg. A split skin graft is often used after excision of a lesion on the lower leg.

**Full thickness skin grafts:** This type of skin graft is taken by removing all the layers of the skin with a scalpel (a Wolfe graft). It is done in a similar way to skin excision. The piece of skin is cut into the correct shape, then applied to the wound. This type of skin graft is often taken from the arm, neck, or behind the ear. It is often used after excisions on the hand or face.

## How do I look after the wound following skin grafting?

You will have two wounds, the site of the original lesion and the site where the skin graft was taken from.

Your wounds may be tender for an hour or two after the excision when the effect of the local anesthetic wears off.

Skin grafts are very fragile and great care must be taken when looking after them. Leave the dressing in place as advised by your dermatologist. Avoid strenuous exertion and stretching of the area until the stitches are removed and for some time afterwards.

If there is any bleeding, press on the wound firmly with a folded towel without looking at it for 20 minutes. If it is still bleeding after this time, seek medical attention. Do not rub the area as this may disturb the graft.

Keep the wounds dry until your dermatologist advises that you can wash them. If the wounds become red or very painful, consult your dermatologist: they could be infected.

## Does the skin graft always take?

Sometimes the skin graft doesn't stick to the wound underneath and falls off. This usually happens within the first two weeks after the procedure. It can happen for a variety of reasons including bleeding underneath the graft and wound infection. If this happens, your dermatologist will inform you what further treatment is required. It is quite normal for the graft to appear black and crusted on the surface when the dressings are removed. This does not necessarily mean it has failed.

# Chapter 58

# *Tissue Expansion*

Tissue expansion is a method of allowing the body to "grow" more skin so that a plastic surgeon can use the new skin to reconstruct or repair a part of the body that is injured or disfigured. A special balloon called a tissue expander is placed under the skin near the area of the body to be reconstructed. The tissue expander is gradually filled with sterile salt water over several weeks or months. The time involved in tissue expansion depends on the individual case and the size of the area to be repaired.

Tissue expansion is most commonly used for breast reconstruction, but it is also used to repair skin damaged by birth defects, accidents, or surgery, and in certain cosmetic procedures. It is especially useful in repairing or replacing areas of the scalp since the expanded tissue is able to continue to grow hair. Tissue expansion offers many advantages over other procedures such as skin graft and flap surgery. It offers a near-perfect match of color, texture, and hair-growing qualities. And because the skin remains connected to the donor area's blood and nerve supply, there is a smaller risk that it will die. Lastly, because the skin doesn't have to be moved from one area to another, there is often less scarring than with other procedures.

---

"Tissue Expansion," reprinted with permission from Metropolitan Institute for Plastic Surgery, Washington, DC, 202-785-4187, www.metplasticsurgery.com.

## Are You a Good Candidate for Tissue Expansion?

Almost anyone in need of additional skin can benefit from tissue expansion. In fact, the procedure has been performed on patients from infants to the elderly. Tissue expansion generally produces excellent results when reconstructing areas of the face and neck, the hand, arms, and legs. Expansion may be more difficult on the back, torso, or other areas where skin is thick. If the affected area is severely damaged or scarred, tissue expansion is probably not an option since healthy skin is the primary requirement.

Because tissue expansion often requires weeks or months to grow the necessary skin and can entail repeated visits to the doctor, you must feel comfortable with the time investment required. In addition, depending on the area of the body being expanded, tissue expansion can create a temporary unsightly bulge that can be quite noticeable in areas such as the scalp, face, hands, arms, or legs. Therefore, the inconvenience and obvious appearance of an expander are factors that you must consider when deciding to move forward with the procedure.

## Meeting with the Doctor

The first, and perhaps most important, step in tissue expansion is meeting at length with your doctor to discuss the options available and determine the best way to perform the procedure to meet your goals. During this meeting, the doctor will examine and evaluate your injury or disfigurement and explain in detail the possible tissue expansion procedures and their risks and results. The doctor and staff will also:

- Explain which type of anesthesia will be used, where the surgery will be performed, and if a hospital stay is required;

- Outline in detail how the tissue expansion surgery is performed and what you can expect before, during, and after the procedure;

- Discuss with you the current U.S. Food and Drug Administration (FDA) regulations governing the use of implants, if appropriate;

- Provide detailed cost, payment, and insurance information; and

- Answer all your questions.

You will be asked to provide the following information:

- Details about your medical history

- A list of all medications you currently take, including over the counter medications such as aspirin, vitamins, and herbal supplements

- Information regarding your tobacco and alcohol consumption

## How the Procedure Is Performed

Depending on the extent of your tissue expansion surgery, it will either be performed at an outpatient-based surgical facility or in a hospital if an overnight stay is required. The size and location of the expansion determines the type of anesthesia that will be used. Discuss with your doctor both where your surgery will be performed and the type of anesthesia to be used.

In most cases, the initial tissue expansion surgery takes between one to two hours to complete. The doctor makes a small incision next to the area of skin to be repaired. The doctor does everything possible to make the incision in the least visible location possible. The doctor then inserts the silicone balloon expander in a pocket created beneath the skin. The expander includes a tiny tube and a self-sealing valve that allows the doctor to gradually fill the expander with sterile saline solution. The valve is usually left just beneath the surface of the skin. Drains may be put in place to help drain fluid from the surgical area. The doctor then closes the incision with stitches and places a gauze dressing over the area.

Once your incision is healed, you will return to the doctor's office periodically so that the expander can be injected with saline solution. As the expander enlarges with saline solution, your skin stretches to accommodate the growing expander. When the skin has stretched enough to cover the affected area, you will have a second operation to remove the expander and reposition new tissue or an implant.

## What to Expect after Your Surgery

**Immediately after your surgery:** How you feel after surgery depends on the extent and complexity of your tissue expansion surgery. Most patients experience only mild discomfort after the procedure and this can be controlled with prescribed pain medication. You may also have some bruising, swelling, and numbness in the area of your surgery. In most cases, the procedure is performed on an outpatient basis and you are ready to go home shortly after your surgery. It is wise to have someone drive you home and to have someone stay with you for a few days.

**The first 24 to 48 hours after your surgery:** Any discomfort you experience will improve rapidly during the first 24 to 48 hours after your procedure. The doctor will prescribe pain medication to alleviate much of the discomfort. You may feel a bit tired from the anesthesia and have some soreness in the area of your incision.

You may also experience some minor bleeding or oozing in the area of your incision. This bleeding or oozing usually results in a slight staining of the gauze dressing placed over the surgical area. If more than a slight staining of the gauze occurs, call your doctor. If surgical drains were put in place during your surgery, they will most likely be removed within the first few days. Once they are removed, you can shower or bathe.

**The first two weeks after surgery:** You will notice a marked improvement in your discomfort and activity level during the first few weeks after your surgery. You should be able to return to work during this time and will, in most cases, have your stitches removed. Once your incision has healed, you will begin regular visits to the doctor's office to have saline solution injected into your expander. You may feel some minor discomfort each time the saline solution is injected into the expander. The discomfort generally lasts only a few hours and can usually be managed with over-the-counter pain medication.

## *Resuming Your Normal Routine*

Everyone heals at different rates and you are the best judge of when you are ready for certain activities, but the following are general guidelines:

**Table 58.1.** What to Expect after Your Surgery

| Activity | When |
| --- | --- |
| Drains removed | One to two days after surgery |
| Shower or bath | Once drains are removed |
| Back to work or school | One week after surgery |
| Driving | Usually within a week after surgery |
| Stitches removed | Ten to fourteen days after surgery |
| Strenuous activity | Three to six weeks after surgery |
| Fading of scars | Several months to one year |

- You can most likely return to work in about a week following your surgery to remove the expander and reposition the tissue or insert an implant.

- Most patients feel comfortable with their normal routine while the expander is in place. The only consideration is to be careful about bumping the area that holds the expander.

- Strenuous exercise can begin in about three to six weeks after surgery; the doctor will give you specific instructions on when to return to your exercise program and any post-surgery restrictions.

- The scars from your surgery should be protected from sunlight for at least a year after surgery.

- Most scars will fade substantially over time; though it may take one or two years for them to become much less visible.

## What Are The Possible Side Effects or Risks?

Like all surgical procedures, there are risks associated with tissue expansion surgery. During your pre-surgery consultation with your doctor, ask your doctor about your individual risks. As with any surgery, you can help reduce the risks associated with your surgery by closely following the instructions provided to you. Possible side effects include:

- Infection
- Leaking of the balloon expander
- Scarring

## How Long Will the Results of Your Tissue Expansion Surgery Last?

Tissue expansion surgery can begin the process of restoring and repairing injured or disfigured parts of the body. The results can be remarkable and are considered permanent.

### Questions You May Have

*Is there any risk that the balloon expander will leak or rupture?*

While expanders are rigorously tested and placed with care, leaks do occur. If the expander should leak, the sterile salt-water solution, also known as saline, will be harmlessly absorbed by the body. It is also worth noting that the tissue expander is filled with salt water and not with silicone, the type of fluid used for some breast implants.

### Will my insurance coverage pay for my tissue expansion surgery?

Generally, tissue expansion surgery is covered by insurance. As your doctor's office if they will work with you to obtain pre-approval from your insurance company.

### Are there alternatives to tissue expansion surgery?

In cases where the wound or disfigurement does not require extensive tissue or muscle, skin grafting may be suitable to correct the injury or disfigurement. Flap surgery is also an alternative. During your initial consultation, ask your doctor to go over any possible alternatives and their risks and benefits with you.

# Chapter 59

# *Burns Reconstruction*

The basic concerns in burns reconstruction are for function, comfort, and appearance. Normal and hypertrophic scarring, scar contracture, loss of parts of the body, and change in color and texture of injured skin are processes common to all seriously burnt patients and yet unique to each.

A realistic approach is necessary to harmonize patients' expectations (which are very high) with the probable outcomes of reconstructive surgery. Burn reconstruction starts when a patient is admitted with acute burns and lasts until the patient's expectations have been reached or there is nothing else to offer. However, even when this time has come, the patient-surgeon relationship may still continue and can last a lifetime.

Any surgeon undertaking burn reconstruction must have good understanding of wound healing and scar maturation to plan the time of reconstruction, and sound knowledge of all surgical techniques and all the aftercare required (usually in conjunction with a burn team). A strong patient-surgeon relationship is necessary in order to negotiate a master plan and agree on priorities.

## Time of Reconstruction

Definitive correction of burn scarring should generally be delayed for a year or more after scar healing. Unsightly scars mature over time, and, with the help of pressure and splints, many of them do not require surgery once the acute phase of scar maturation is over. Patience is often the best tool of a reconstructive surgeon. However, certain problems must be dealt with before scar maturation is complete. In burn reconstruction there are urgent procedures, others that are essential, and many that are desirable. It is for the last group that a good patient-surgeon relationship is necessary for negotiation on which procedures take priority.

**Urgent procedures:** Waiting for scar maturation is inappropriate when it is certain that an operation is needed to correct a deformity or if vital structures are exposed or can be severely damaged. Urgent procedures should be restricted to those needed to correct function for injuries that are not suitable for other treatments. Examples include an eyelid release to protect an exposed cornea, correction of distracted or entrapped neurovascular bundles, severe fourth degree contractures, and severe microstomia.

**Essential procedures:** Although they are not urgent since no important structure or the patient's overall health is challenged, essential procedures may, if performed early, improve the patient's final appearance and rehabilitation. Such procedures include operations for all burn scar contractures that do not respond to rehabilitation, and hypertrophic scarring and contractures that prevent a patient from eating, bathing, moving, or performing everyday activities.

**Desirable reconstructive procedures:** Most of the problems that patients may present fall in this category. These are often aesthetic problems and scars contractures that, although not prominent, produce great discomfort. For all desirable procedures, it is good practice to wait until all red and immature scars have disappeared before starting any kind of surgery. An early operation is often unnecessary in these circumstances.

### *Techniques for Use in Acute Phase of Scar Maturation to Diminish Reconstructive Needs*

- Use of darts in escharotomies when crossing joints

- Use sheet grafts when possible
- Use aesthetic units to face and hands with medium thickness split skin grafts
- Use of splints, face masks, and silicone inserts as soon as possible
- Place seams following skin tension lines
- Place grafts transversely over joints
- Early pressure therapy
- Early ambulation and exercise

### *Timing of Burn Reconstructive Surgery*

- Urgent procedures
  - Exposure of vital structures (such as eyelid releases)
  - Entrapment or compression of neurovascular bundles
  - Fourth degree contractures
  - Severe microstomia
- Essential procedures
  - Reconstruction of function (such as limited range of motion)
  - Progressive deformities not correctable by ordinary methods
- Desirable procedures
  - Reconstruction of passive areas
  - Aesthetics

## Patient-Surgeon Relationship

The relationship between a burns patients and a reconstructive burn surgeon is normally long lasting, often continuing for a lifetime. Patients not only require a surgeon's professional expertise, but also time, a good dose of optimism, and compassion.

The initial meeting is one of the most important events. The patient presents a set of problems, and the reconstructive surgeon has to evaluate these and the patient's motivation for surgery and psychological status. We have to remember, though, that the patient will also evaluate the surgeon's attitude and conduct.

Although deformities or chief complaints will often be apparent and ready for surgery, it is preferable to have further visits before surgery, to allow new queries to be addressed and unhurried preparation for surgery. Photographic workup is extremely important to assist in definitive preoperative planning and for documentation.

Patients need frequent reassurance. A reconstructive surgeon needs to know a patient's fears and feelings as the reconstructive plan goes on. A burn reconstruction project commonly requires more than 10 operations and many clinic visits over a long period before a final assessment is made. In the case of a small child, this may take more than 18 years. Patients' feelings and impressions must be addressed continuously, and any trouble, minor disappointment, or depression detected early and treated as needed.

### *Burn Reconstructive Visit*

One of the most important events during burn reconstruction is the burn reconstructive visit. At that time, a complete and accurate overview of the problems and possible solutions is performed in the following step wise manner:

- Obtain as complete a record of the acute hospitalization as possible.

- Take a thorough history and make a full physical examination.

- Make a complete record of all encountered problems. Note quality and color of the skin in the affected areas—abnormal scars, hyperpigmentation or hypopigmentation, contractures, atrophy, and open wounds.

- Consider function. Explore all affected joints and note ranges of motion. Outline any scar contracture extending beyond joints.

- Consider skeletal deformities. Scar contractures may distract joints and the body maintains an abnormal position to overcome the deformity. This is particularly true in children; the effect of traction on a growing joint and bone can create long term deformities.

- Consider needs for physiotherapy, occupational therapy, and pressure garments. If any of these devices will be needed after surgery the patient must be referred to the rehabilitation department for consideration.

- Make an inventory of all possible sites for donor tissue.

Once a patient has voiced all his or her chief complaints and a thorough examination of the patient has been done, a master plan is developed. All reconstructive possibilities are discussed with the patient, and the timing and order of such procedures are outlined.

### *Essentials of Burn Reconstruction*

- Strong patient-surgeon relationship

- Psychological support

- Clarify expectations

- Explain priorities

- Note all available donor sites

- Start with a "winner" (easy and quick operation)

- As many surgeries as possible in preschool years

- Offer multiple, simultaneous procedures

- Reassure and support patient

## *Surgical Procedures*

Burn reconstructive surgery has advanced in recent decades, though not as dramatically as in other areas of plastic surgery. For many years, burn reconstructive surgery comprised incisional or excisional releases of scars and skin autografting. Nowadays, however, the first approach that should be considered is use of local or regional flaps. These provide new and vascularized tissue to the area, they grow in children, and they give the best functional and cosmetic results. Such flaps can be raised either with normal skin or with burn scar. Even though burnt tissue generally has a high tendency to congestion, ischemia, and necrosis, it can be used as a reliable flap if extreme care is taken while raising the flap and the injured skin is left attached to the underlying tissues.

When planning surgery for a burn patient, a surgeon must consider what is the patient's primary complaint, what tissues are left, what parts are missing, and what sort of donor sites are available. This will help to determine the techniques available for burn reconstruction. The patient's chief complaint or complaints need to be carefully evaluated. If immature scars or an increasing deformity is present, and no urgent or essential procedure is required, pressure garments and occupational and physical therapy are indicated. If the deformity is stable and there is a need for reconstruction, an inventory of donor sites and priorities should be made.

### Dealing with Deficiency of Tissue

At this point, the burn injury must be assessed for deficiency in tissue. If there is no deficiency and local tissues can be easily mobilized, excision and direct closure or Z-plasties can be performed.

If, however, there is a deficiency in tissue, the problem of how to reconstruct underlying structures must be addressed. If the deformity affects the skin and subcutaneous tissues, skin autografting, Z-plasties, and all the modifications of them (such as trident flaps) are advised. When reconstruction of underlying structures is necessary, flaps should be considered, including direct cutaneous, musculocutaneous, perforator based, and expanded flaps and microvascular transfer of tissues (free flaps). The precise choice is made on an individual basis.

In addition, composite grafts and bone or cartilage grafts are often necessary in order to perform a complete reconstruction. The use of alloplastic materials in these circumstances is not advisable because of their tendency to extrusion.

### Techniques for Burn Reconstruction

- Without deficiency of tissue
  - Excision and primary closure
  - Z-plasty
- With deficiency of tissue
  - Simple reconstruction
  - Skin graft
  - Dermal templates and skin grafts; transposition flaps (Z-plasty and modifications)
  - Reconstruction of skin and underlying tissues: axial and random flaps; myocutaneous flaps; tissue expansion
  - Free flaps
  - Prefabricated flaps

### Summary

Even though incisional or excisional release and skin autografting (with or without use of dermal templates) are still the main techniques used in burn reconstruction, flaps should be used when possible (remember that Z-plasty and its modifications are transposition flaps). The burn reconstruction plan needs to be tailored to the individual patient and the patient's chief complaint, since certain anatomical areas are better suited to some techniques than others.

## *Further Reading*

Herndon DN, ed. *Total burn care*. 2nd ed. London: WB Saunders, 2002.

Engrav LH, Donelan MB. *Operative techniques in plastic and reconstructive surgery. Face burns: acute care and reconstruction*. London: WB Saunders, 1997.

Achauer BM. *Burn reconstruction*. New York: Thiene, 1991.

Barret JP, Herndon DN. *Color atlas of burn care*. London: WB Saunders, 2001.

Brou JA, Robson MC, McCauley RL. Inventory of potential reconstructive needs in the patient with burns. *J Burn Care Rehabil* 1989;10: 555–60.

# Chapter 60

# *Eyebrow and Eyelash Restoration*

Eyebrows and eyelashes make an important contribution to facial symmetry and presentation of self to others. A person without eyebrows or eyelashes may feel very self-conscious about his/her appearance. Transplantation or reconstructive surgery can often restore eyebrows and eyelashes.

Eyebrows and eyelashes are lost in a variety of ways:

- Physical trauma—auto accident, thermal, chemical or electrical burns

- Systemic or local disease that causes loss of eyebrow or eyelashes

- Congenital inability to grow eyebrows or eyelashes

- Plucking (to reshape the eyebrow) that results in permanent loss of eyebrows

- Self-inflicted obsessive plucking or eyebrows or eyelashes (trichotillomania)

- Medical or surgical treatments that result in eyebrow or eyelash loss—radiation therapy, chemotherapy, surgical removal of tumor

The cause of eyebrow/eyelash loss is evaluated in medical history and examination prior to consideration of hair restoration:

- Systemic or local disease that causes hair loss must be under control to assure that hair restoration can succeed.

- Obsessive-compulsive plucking (trichotillomania) must be treated to assure that restored hair will not be plucked out.

- Trauma, burns or surgery may have resulted in formation of scar tissue; reconstructive surgery may be necessary before eyebrow/eyelash restoration. The degree of eyebrow loss may vary from complete to partial; the degree of loss may be a consideration in selection of the restoration procedure.

- Some patients have no eyebrow/eyelash loss, but seek eyebrow/eyelash enhancement for cosmetic reasons.

## Eyebrow Hair Restoration

A number of procedures are available for restoration of all or part of the eyebrow:

Transplantation of micrografts or single hairs from a donor area to the eyebrow, and a reconstructive flap or graft procedure that brings a strip of hair from another site to the eyebrow.

The patient and surgeon must agree on the procedure best suited to the needs of the patient. Eyebrow and eyelash restoration procedures are usually performed in an outpatient setting. Postoperative complications are usually limited to minor pain and swelling.

Reconstructive surgery has been used for many years to restore missing eyebrows or to repair partially missing eyebrows. Technical considerations and the needs of the patient determine which reconstructive procedure is used:

**Transplants:** A strip of hair-bearing skin and subcutaneous tissue is removed from a donor area on the scalp and grafted into the surgically-prepared eyebrow site. The transplant procedure is performed by selecting a hair-bearing area of scalp with hair that is of appropriate texture and orientation to serve as eyebrow hair. Micrografts of one to two hairs placed into incisions should be used for eyebrow reconstruction.

**Scalp-to-eyebrow pedicle flaps:** (Less commonly used) A strip of hair-bearing skin and subcutaneous tissue is raised from the temple area just in front of the ear, with its blood supply (a branch of the superficial temporal artery and vein) attached. This type of donor graft attached to a blood supply is called a pedicle flap. After the pedicle flap

442

is raised, the recipient area (the eyebrow) is prepared to receive the flap. A subcutaneous "tunnel" is created from the base of the pedicle flap to the eyebrow recipient site; the flap is pulled through the tunnel and secured to the recipient site with stitches. The pedicle flap's blood supply nourishes the grafted tissue until the grafted tissue develops its own blood supply from surrounding tissue. Hairs grown from grafts and pedicles may have to be "trained" with gel or wax to lay flat to the skin like eyebrow hair; grafted hair also may have to be trimmed occasionally.

**Transplantation to correct eyebrow loss:** A purpose of transplantation of hair to the eyebrow is to recreate the eyebrow in a natural contour. Patient and physician must work together to outline the eyebrow area to conform to the natural symmetry of the patient's face. Depending on the size of the area to be transplanted, more than one transplant session may be required; two or more sessions several months apart are common.

Donor hair for the transplant is taken from a site that furnishes finer rather than coarser hair; finer hair is a better "match" for eyebrow hair. Donor hair is transplanted as micrografts of one to two hairs. Each graft is placed into an incision prepared for it. The use of single hairs or micrografts permits meticulous adherence to the eyebrow contour for a natural appearance.

As the transplanted hairs grow in their new position they may require occasional trimming as well as "training" with gel or wax.

## Eyelash Hair Restoration

Transplantation is the only procedure used to restore eyelash hair. This is a very specialized procedure that is performed by just a few surgeons. As is the case for eyebrows, donor hair for transplantation must be finer rather than coarser. All grafts are single hairs meticulously placed into the lid. As few as six hairs per lid may be adequate to create a natural effect.

Itching is a common and troublesome postoperative complication. If the patient gives in to temptation and scratches, there is risk for dislodging the hair grafts and initiating infection. Eyeglasses may be worn to deter scratching. The dermatologist can prescribe medications to relieve itching.

Training of transplanted hairs into eyelash conformation is accomplished by use of lash oil and an eyelash curler.

# Part Seven

# Additional Help and Information

# Chapter 61

# *Cosmetic and Reconstructive Surgery: Terms You Should Know*

**allograft:** A graft transplanted between genetically nonidentical individuals of the same species.[3]

**ambulatory phlebectomy:** Removal of undesired varicose and spider leg veins through a series of tiny incisions along the path of an enlarged vein.[1]

**anesthesia:** Loss of physical sensation from sedation. General: affecting the entire body and accompanied by loss of consciousness; Regional: affecting a region of the body; Local: affecting a limited and usually superficial area of the body[1]

**anesthetic:** Drugs that cause the loss of feeling or sensation.[2]

**autograft:** Tissue or organ transferred into a new position in the body of the same individual.[3]

**blepharoplasty:** Upper and lower eyelid surgery to remove loose skin and excess fatty tissue.[1]

**botulinum toxin (Botox®):** Botulinum toxin injections are used primarily to paralyze certain facial muscles which cause frown lines,

---

Terms in this chapter marked [1] are excerpted from "Glossary of Terms," reprinted with permission from the American Society for Dermatologic Surgery, http://asds-net.org. © 2005. All rights reserved; terms marked [2] are excerpted from "Liposuction Information: Glossary," U.S. Food and Drug Administration, August 2002; terms marked [3] are from *Stedman's Medical Dictionary, 27th Edition*, copyright © 2000 Lippincott Williams & Wilkins. All rights reserved.

crows feet, and other wrinkles. It works by relaxing the underlying facial muscles that help form wrinkles, an effect that lasts for 3–4 months. It also is used to improve neck lines and control excessive sweating. [1]

**cannula (or canula):** A hollow pen-like instrument or tube used to draw off fluid. [2]

**chemical peeling:** Application of a chemical solution to remove the outer layer of skin to treat fine lines, wrinkles, mild scarring, acne, skin discoloration, and pre-cancerous growths. [1]

**composite graft:** A graft composed of several tissues, such as skin and cartilage or a full-thickness segment of the ear. [3]

**contracture:** Static muscle shortening due to tonic spasm or fibrosis, to loss of muscular balance, the antagonists being paralyzed or to a loss of motion of the adjacent joint. [3]

**cosmeceuticals:** Topically applied products containing ingredients that influence the biological function of the skin; they improve appearance by delivering nutrients for healthier skin. [1]

**cosmetic surgery:** Aesthetic procedures to improve and rejuvenate the appearance of the skin: laser resurfacing, wrinkle fillers, liposuction, chemical peeling. [1]

**cryosurgery:** Freezing the skin tissue with liquid nitrogen to remove skin growths. [1]

**curettage and desiccation:** Use of a sharp instrument to scrape away skin tissue, followed by application of a heated electric needle to destroy skin growths. [1]

**cutaneous:** Relating to the skin. [3]

**dermabrasion:** Surgical sanding or planing of the outer layer of skin to improve acne and other scars, remove tattoos, and minimize age spots, wrinkles, and certain types of skin growths. [1]

**dermal filler injections:** Filler substances are generally used to "plump up" and minimize wrinkles, furrows and hollows in the face, correct depressions and scars, and enhance the definition of the lips. Filler substances include collagen, one's own fat, hyaluronic acid (Restylane® and Hylaform®), plastic microbeads, and liquid silicone. [1]

**edema:** Swelling caused by large amount of fluid in cells or tissues. [2]

**emboli:** Something that blocks a blood vessel. See embolism. [2]

**embolism:** The blocking of a blood vessel or organ by pieces of matter such as fat. [2]

**emulsify:** To break up into small pieces. [2]

**epinephrine:** A drug injected before liposuction to reduce bleeding during the procedure. [2]

**escharotomy:** Surgical incision in an eschar (necrotic dermis) to lessen constriction, especially after a circumferential third degree burn of an extremity or the thorax. [3]

**excision and closure:** Cutting into the skin to remove a growth and then closing the wound with stitches. [1]

**flap surgery:** Transfer of adjacent skin tissue, often used to move hair-bearing skin to cover balding areas of the scalp. [1]

**free flap:** Flap in which the donor vessels are severed, the tissue is transported to another area, and the flap is revascularized by anastomosis (connecting) of vessels in the recipient bed to the artery and vein(s) of the flap. [3]

**grafting:** Surgical transplantation of skin to repair a defect. [1]

**hair restoration surgery:** A variety of techniques, such as punch transplanting, mini- and micro-grafts, scalp reduction, and skin flaps, to correct baldness and restore a person's natural hairline. [1]

**hyperpigmentation:** An excess of pigment in a tissue or part. [3]

**incision:** A cut; a surgical wound; a division of the soft parts usually made with a knife. [3]

**infection:** Invasion by and multiplication of bacteria or microorganisms that can produce tissue injury. [2]

**laser hair removal:** Various laser and light-based systems are utilized for efficient and long-lasting hair removal. The laser light energy causes thermal damage to the hair follicle, thus stunting regrowth. [1]

**laser therapy:** A beam of laser or light directed at a site to cut, seal, or vaporize skin tissue and blood vessels. Laser therapy is used to rejuvenate aging and sun-damaged skin by resurfacing wrinkles and lines; selectively eliminate tissue abnormalities such as vascular and pigmented skin lesions and tattoos; improve scars and stretch marks; erase spider veins and birthmarks; remove unwanted facial and body hair.[1]

**lidocaine:** An anesthetic that may be injected in large amounts of liquid during liposuction. [2]

**lipoatrophy:** Loss of or redistribution of subcutaneous fat in the body resulting in changes in bodily conformation. [1]

**lipoplasty:** Another name for liposuction. [2]

**liposuction:** Liposuction is the removal of excess fat with a cannula, a small, straw-like instrument, attached to a suction machine. The use of tumescent (local anesthesia) liposuction allows dermasurgeons to safely and effectively remove deep and superficial layers of undesired fat in an office facility with relatively little discomfort, virtually no complications, and improved cosmetic results. [1]

**microdermabrasion:** A non-invasive facial rejuvenation treatment that uses micro-particles to abrade and rub off the top skin layer, vacuuming out the particles of dead skin. [1]

**microlipoinjection:** A form of soft tissue augmentation using one's own fat to fill and contour wrinkles, folds, and depressions resulting from aging, sun-damage, injury, or surgery. [1]

**micropigmentation:** A permanent method of implanting pigment into the skin to add color for the treatment of vitiligo, skin grafts, or burn scars and for cosmetic purposes. [1]

**microstomia:** Smallness of the oral aperture (mouth opening).[3]

**Mohs surgery:** Precise removal of skin cancer, layer by layer, with the aid of a microscope. [1]

**musculocutaneous:** Relating to both muscle and skin.[3]

**nail surgery:** Removal or repair of a nail abnormality for the purposes of diagnosis or treatment. [1]

**necrosis:** Pathologic death of one or more cells, or of a portion of tissue or organ, resulting from irreversible damage.[3]

**necrotizing fasciitis:** A bacterial infection in which bacteria infect and kill the skin and underlying tissues. [2]

**neurovascular:** Relating to both nervous and vascular systems; relating to the nerves supplying the walls of the blood vessels, the vasomotor nerves.[3]

**nonablative skin rejuvenation:** Non-wounding laser, intense pulsed light, and other technologies work beneath the surface skin layer to stimulate collagen production, tone and tighten skin, and improve mild to moderate skin damage. [1]

**paresthesia:** A change in feelings or sensation. May be an increase in feeling (pain) or a decrease in feeling (numbness). [2]

**pedicle flap:** In surgery, a flap which remains joined at one side, to an adjacent position and suturing the free end.

**probe:** See cannula. [2]

**pulmonary embolism:** Pieces of fat may find their way into the blood stream and get stuck in the lungs during liposuction. This causes shortness of breath or trouble breathing. [2]

**resurfacing:** Using techniques such as chemical peels, laser therapy, or microdermabrasion, resurfacing procedures are designed to remove or buff the top layers of aged, discolored, or irregular skin. Fresh skin is then generated, which is typically smoother, has less wrinkles, and is more even in color. [1]

**sclerotherapy:** Injection of a solution to remove unwanted varicose and spider leg veins. [1]

**sedative:** A drug which helps a person to relax and may make them feel sleepy. [2]

**seroma:** A collection of fluid from the blood that has pooled at the liposuction site. [2]

**skin necrosis:** Skin or underlying tissue dies and falls off. [2]

**soft tissue fillers:** Filler substances are generally used to "plump up" and minimize wrinkles, furrows and hollows in the face, giving the skin a smoother and more pleasing appearance. Fillers such as bovine collagen and related materials, one's own fat, and polymer implants are effective for contouring specific facial sites and correcting depressions and scars. [1]

**suction assisted liposuction:** See liposuction. [2]

**thrombophlebitis:** Inflammation of a vein caused by a blood clot. [2]

**tissue expansion:** A technique used to close large surgical wounds and aid in reconstructive surgery.[1]

**topical treatments:** Skin care products that contain drugs, such as retinoids, alpha or beta hydroxyl, or other active ingredients that have a biologic effect on living tissue. [1]

**toxic shock syndrome:** An infection caused by bacteria that release toxins into the body. This type of infection can occur after surgery if bacteria are accidentally introduced during the surgery. [2]

**ultrasound assisted liposuction:** A type of liposuction in which fat is first loosened by using an ultrasonic probe and then removed by means of suction. [2]

**vein treatment:** Procedures used to minimize or remove varicose and spider veins, most typically on the face or legs. Procedures include lasers, sclerotherapy (injection of a solution to collapse the vein), and ambulatory phlebectomy (vein is removed through a series of tiny incisions along the path of the enlarged vein).[1]

**visceral perforations:** Organs may be punctured accidentally with the liposuction probe or cannula during liposuction. [2]

**xenograft:** A graft transferred from an animal of one species to one of another species.[3]

**z-plasty:** Technique to elongate a contracted scar or to rotate tension 90°; the middle line of a Z-shaped incision is made along the line of greatest tension or contraction, and triangular flaps are raised on opposite sides of the two ends and transposed.[3]

# Chapter 62

# Resources for More Information about Plastic Surgery

**Accreditation Association for Ambulatory Health Care, Inc.**
5250 Old Orchard Road
Suite 200
Skokie, IL 60077
Phone: 847-853-6060
Fax: 847-853-9028
Website: http://www.aaahc.org
E-mail: info@aaahc.org

**American Academy of Cosmetic Surgery**
737 North Michigan Avenue,
Suite 2100
Chicago, IL 60611-5405
Phone: 312-981-6760
Fax: 312-981-6787
Website: http://
www.cosmeticsurgery.org
E-mail: info@cosmeticsurgery.org

**American Academy of Dermatology**
P.O. Box 4014
Schaumburg, IL 60168-4014
Toll-Free: 888-462-3376 or
866-503-SKIN (7546)
Phone: 847-240-1280
Fax: 847-240-1859 (to order products)
Website: http://www.aad.org
E-mail: MRC@aad.org

————

Information in this chapter was compiled from many sources deemed reliable; inclusion does not constitute endorsement and omission does not imply objection. All contact information was updated and verified in March 2007.

**American Academy of Facial Plastic and Reconstructive Surgery**
310 South Henry Street
Alexandria, VA 22314
Toll-Free: 800-332-3223
(800-332-FACE)
Phone: 703-299-9291
Fax: 703-299-8898
Website: http://www.aafprs.org
or http://facial-plastic-surgery
.org
E-mail: info@aafprs.org

**American Academy of Family Physicians**
P.O. Box 11210
Shawnee Mission, KS 66207-1210
Toll-Free: 800-274-2237
Phone: 913-906-6000
Website: http://www.aafp.org or
http://www.familydoctor.org

**American Academy of Micropigmentation**
2709 Medical Office Place
Goldsboro, NC 27534
Toll Free: 800-441-2515
Fax: 919-735-3701
Website: http://
www.micropigmentation.org

**American Academy of Orthopedic Surgery**
6300 North River Road
Rosemont, IL 60018-4262
Toll-Free: 800-346-AAOS
(346-2267)
Phone: 847-823-7186
Fax: 847-823-8125
Website: http://www.aaos.org

**American Academy of Otolaryngology-Head and Neck Surgery**
One Prince St.
Alexandria, VA 22314-3357
Phone: 703-836-4444
Website: http://www.entnet.org

**American Anaplastology Association**
6060 Sunrise Vista Drive
Suite 1300
Citrus Heights, CA 95610
Phone: 916-726-2910
Fax: 916-722-8149
Website: http://
www.anaplastology.org
E-mail: aaa@anaplastology.org

**American Association for Accreditation of Ambulatory Surgery Facilities**
5101 Washington Street,
Suite #2F
Gumee, IL 60031
Toll-Free: 888-545-5222
Fax: 847-775-1985
Website: http://www.aaaasf.org

**American Association of Nurse Anesthetists**
222 S. Prospect Avenue
Park Ridge, IL 60068
Phone: 847-692-7050
Fax: 847-692-6968
Website: http://www.aana.com
E-mail: info@aana.com

**American Association of Oral and Maxillofacial Surgeons**
9700 West Bryn Mawr Ave.
Rosemont, IL 60018-5701
Toll-Free: 800-822-6637
Phone: 847-678-6200
Fax: 847-678-6286
Website: http://www.aaoms.org

**American Association of Plastic Surgeons**
900 Cummings Center
Suite 211-U
Beverly, MA 01915
Phone: 978-927-8330
Fax: 978-524-8890
Website: http://
www.aaps1921.org

**American Board of Cosmetic Surgery**
Website: http://www
.americanboardcosmeticsurgery
.org

**American Board of Plastic Surgery**
Seven Penn Center, Suite 400
1635 Market Street
Philadelphia, PA 19103-2204
Phone: 215-587-9322
Fax: 215-587-9622
Website: http://
www.abplsurg.org
E-mail: info@abplsurg.org

**American Cleft Palate-Craniofacial Association**
1504 East Franklin Street
Suite 102
Chapel Hill, NC 27514-2820
Phone: 919-933-9044
Fax: 919-933-9604
Website: http://www.cleftline.org
E-mail: info@cleftline.org

**American College of Mohs Micrographic Surgery and Cutaneous Oncology**
555 East Wells Street, Suite 1100
Milwaukee, WI 53202-3823
Toll-Free: 800-500-7224
Phone: 414-347-1103
Fax: 414-276-2146
Website: http://
www.mohscollege.org
E-mail: info@mohscollege.org

**American College of Phlebology**
100 Webster Street, Suite 101
Oakland, CA 94607-3724
Phone: 510-834-6500
Fax: 510-832-7300
Website: http://
www.phlebology.org
E-mail: acp@amsinc.org

**American Osteopathic College of Dermatology**
1501 East Illinois Street
P.O. Box 7525
Kirksville, MO 63501
Toll-Free: 800-449-2623
Phone: 660-665-2184
Fax: 660-627-2623
Website: http://www.aocd.org
E-mail: info@aocd.org

**American Psychological Association**
750 First Street NE
Washington, DC 20002-4242
Toll-Free: 800-374-2721
Phone: 202-336-5500
TDD/TTY: 202-336-6123
Website: http://www.apa.org

**American Society for Aesthetic Plastic Surgery**
11081 Winners Circle
Los Alamitos, CA 90720
Toll-Free: 888-272-7711
Website: http://www.surgery.org

**American Society for Bariatric Surgery**
100 SW 75th Street, Suite 201
Gainesville, FL 32607
Phone: 352-331-4900
Fax: 352-331-4975
Website: http://www.asbs.org
E-mail: info@asbs.org

**American Society for Dermatologic Surgery**
5550 Meadowbrook Drive
Suite 120
Rolling Meadows, IL 60008
Toll-Free: 800-441-2737
Phone: 847-956-0900
Fax: 847-956-0999
Website: http://www.asds.net
E-mail: info@asds.net

**American Society for Laser Medicine and Surgery, Inc.**
2100 Stewart Ave, Suite 240
Wausau, WI 54401
Phone: 715-845-9283
Fax: 715-848-2493
Website: http://www.aslms.org
E-mail: information@aslms.org

**American Society for Surgery of the Hand**
6300 North River Road
Suite 600
Rosemont, IL 60018-4256
Phone: 847-384-8300
Fax: 847-384-1435
Website: http://www.assh.org
E-mail: info@assh.org

**American Society of Anesthesiologists**
520 N. Northwest Hwy.
Park Ridge, IL 60068
Phone: 847-825-5586
Fax: 847-825-1692
Website: http://www.ASAhq.org
E-mail: mail@ASAhq.org

**American Society of Maxillofacial Surgeons**
Website: http://www.maxface.org

**American Society of Ophthalmic Plastic and Reconstructive Surgery**
5841 Cedar Lake Rd., Suite 204
Minneapolis, MN 55416
Phone: 952-646-2038
Website: http://www.asoprs.org

**American Society of Plastic and Reconstructive Surgeons**
444 E. Algonquin Road
Arlington Heights, IL 60005
Toll-Free: 800-635-0635
Referral Service: 888-475-2784
(888-4-PLASTIC)
Phone: 847-228-9900
Website: http://
www.plasticsurgery.org

**BreastCancer.org**
111 Forrest Avenue 1R
Narberth, PA 19072
Website: http://
www.breastcancer.org

**Burn Survivor Resource Center**
Website: http://
www.burnsurvivor.com

**Canadian Academy of Facial Plastic and Reconstructive Surgery**
Mount Sinai Hospital
600 University Avenue
Suite 401
Toronto, ON M5G 1X5
Canada
Phone: 905-569-6965
Website: http://
www.facialcosmeticsurgery.org

**Canadian Association for Accreditation of Ambulatory Surgery Facilities, Inc.**
2334 Heska Road
Pickering, ON L1V 2P9
Canada
Phone: 905-831-5804
Fax: 905-831-7248
Website: http://www.caaasf.org

**Canadian Laser Aesthetic Surgery Society**
2334 Heska Road
Pickering, ON L1V 2P9
Canada
Fax: 905-831-7248
Website: http://www.class.ca
E-mail: info@class.ca

**Canadian Society for Aesthetic Plastic Surgery**
Website: http://www.csaps.ca

**Canadian Society of Otolaryngology–Head and Neck Surgery**
221 Millford Cres.
Elora, ON N0B 1S0
Toll-Free: 800-655-9533
Phone: 519-846-0630
Fax: 519-846-9529
Website: http://
www.entcanada.org
E-mail: cso.hns@symatico.ca

**Changes Plastic Surgery**
11515 El Camino Real
Suite 150
San Diego, CA 92130
Phone: 858-720-1440
Fax: 858-509-7738
Website: http://www
.changesplasticsurgery.com
E-mail:
info@changesplasticsurgery.com

**Children's Craniofacial Association**
Toll-Free: 800-535-3643
Website: http://
www.CCAkids.org
E-mail:
contactCCA@ccakids.com

**Children's Hospital of Wisconsin**
9000 W. Wisconsin Ave.
P.O. Box 1997
Milwaukee, WI 53201-1997
Website: http://www.chw.org

**Cleft Palate Foundation**
Website: http://www.cleft.com

**Cleveland Clinic**
Department of Plastic Surgery
9500 Euclid Avenue
Cleveland, OH 44195
Toll-Free: 800-223-2273
Website: http://
www.clevelandclinic.org/plastics

**Columbia Presbyterian Medical Center**
Website: http://
www.entcolumbia.org

**Columbia University Department of Surgery**
Center for Specialty Care
622 W. 168th Street
New York, NY 10032
Toll-Free: 800-227-2762
Phone: 201-346-7001
Fax: 201-346-7010
Website: http://
www.columbiasurgery.org/
divisions/plastic

**Cosmetic Surgery Guide**
Website: http://
www.cosmeticsurgeryguide.ca

**Facial Plastic Surgery Network**
Toll-Free: 800-533-2906
Website: http://
www.facialplasticsurgery.net

**Great Ormond Street Hospital for Children**
Great Ormond Street
London WC1N 3JH
UK
Phone: 44 (0)20 7405 9200
Phone: 44 (0)20 7829 8643
Website: http://
www.ich.ucl.ac.uk

**Hand University**
3010 N. Circle Dr. #200
Colorado Springs, CO 80909
Phone: 719-471-2980
Website: http://
www.handuniversity.com
E-mail:
info@handuniversity.com

### Imaginis Corporation
P.O. Box 27018
Greenville, South Carolina 29616
Website: http://www.imaginis.com
E-mail: learnmore@imaginis.com

### International Society of Aesthetic Plastic Surgery
Lyme Road, Suite 304
Hanover, NH 03755
Phone: 603-643-2325
Fax: 603-643-1444
Website: http://www.isaps.org
E-mail: isaps@sover.net

### International Society of Hair Restoration Surgery
13 South 2nd Street
Geneva, IL 60134
Toll-Free: 800-444-2737
Phone: 630-262-5399
Fax: 630-262-1520
Website: http://www.ishrs.org
E-mail: info@ishrs.org

### Johns Hopkins Cosmetic Center
10755 Falls Road
Pavilion I, Suite 350
Lutherville, MD 21093
Phone: 410-847-3767
Website: http://
www.hopkinscosmetic.com

### Metropolitan Institute for Plastic Surgery
1145 19th Street NW, Suite 717
Washington, DC 20036
Phone: 202-785-4187
Website:
www.metplasticsurgery.com

### National Institute of Arthritis and Musculoskeletal and Skin Diseases
1 AMS Circle
Bethesda, MD 20892-3675
Toll-Free: 877-22-NIAMS
Phone: 301-495-4484
TTY: 301-565-2966
Fax: 301-718-6366
Website: www.niams.nih.gov
E-mail: niamsinfo@mail.nih.gov

### National Institute of Dental and Craniofacial Research
Bethesda, MD 20892-2190
Phone: 301-496-4261
Website: www.nidcr.nih.gov
E-mail: nidcrinfo@mail.nih.gov

### National Skin Cancer Foundation
149 Madison Avenue, Suite 901
New York, NY 10016
Toll-Free: 800-754-6490
(800-SKIN-490)
Phone: 212-725-5176
Website: http://
www.skincancer.org
E-mail: info@skincancer.org

### National Women's Health Information Center
8270 Willow Oaks Corporate Dr.
Fairfax, VA 22031
Toll-Free: 800-994-9662
TTY: 888-220-5446
Website: http://
www.womenshealth.gov

**National Women's Health Network**
514 10th Street NW, Suite 400
Washington DC 20004
Phone: 202-347-1140
Woman's Health Voice:
202-628-7814
Fax: 202-347-1168
Website: http://www.nwhn.org
E-mail for general inquiries:
nwhn@nwhn.org
E-mail for health information
requests:
healthquestions@nwhn.org

**National Women's Health Resource Center**
157 Broad Street, Suite 315
Red Bank, NJ 07701
Toll-Free: 877-986-9472
Fax: 732-530-3347
Website: http://
www.healthywomen.org
E-mail: info@healthywomen.org

**New England Society of Plastic and Reconstructive Surgeons**
Phone: 603-880-4385
Website: http://
www.neplasticsurgery.com

**New York-Presbyterian Hospital**
New York-Presbyterian/Columbia
Main Campus
622 West 168th Street
New York, NY 10032
Toll-Free: 877-697-9355
(877-NYP-WELL)
Phone: 212-305-2500
Website: http://www.nyp.org

**New Zealand Dermatological Society**
Website: http://
www.dermnetnz.org

**Oculoplastic Surgery Service**
Eye and Ear Infirmary
1855 W. Taylor Street, Room 3158
Chicago IL 60612
Phone: 312-996-9120
Fax: 312-413-7895
Website: http://www.uic.edu/
com/eye
E-mail: eyeweb@uic.edu

**T.J. Samson Community Hospital**
Website: http://
tjsamson.client.web-health.com
E-mail: tjsamson@tjsamson.org

**Skin Care Guide**
Skincareguide.com Ltd.
1107–750 West Pender St.
Vancouver, BC V6C 2T8
Canada
Fax: 604-688-9171
Website: http://
www.skincareguide.com

**Smart Plastic Surgery**
Website: http://
www.smartplasticsurgery.com
E-mail:
info@smartplasticsurgery.com

### Society of Permanent Cosmetic Professionals

SPCP Membership Office
Membership Services
69 North Broadway
Des Plaines, IL  60016
Phone: 847-635-1330
Fax: 847-635-1326
Website: http://www.spcp.org

### U.S. Food and Drug Administration

Office of Consumer Affairs
5600 Fishers Lane
HFE-50
Rockville, Maryland 20857
Toll-Free: 888-463-6332
(888-INFO-FDA)
Phone: 301-827-4420
Fax: 301-443-9767
Website: http://www.fda.gov

### University of Chicago Hospitals

5841 S. Maryland Avenue
Chicago, IL 60637
Phone: 773-702-1000
Website: http://
www.uchospitals.edu/specialties/
plastic-surgery

### University of Michigan Kellogg Eye Center

1000 Wall Street
Ann Arbor, MI 48105
Phone: 734-763-8122
Website: http://
www.kellogg.umich.edu

### University of Missouri Children's Hospital

1 Hospital Dr.
Columbia, MO 65212
Phone: 573-882-4176
Website: http://
www.surgery.missouri.edu

### University of Washington Medical Center

1959 NE Pacific
Seattle, WA 98195
Phone: 206-598-3300
TTY: 206-598-4002
Website: http://
www.uwmedicine.org

### Washington University School of Medicine

Facial Plastic Surgery Center
605 Old Ballas Road, Suite 100
St. Louis, MO 63141
Phone: 314-432-7760
Website: http://
facialplasticsurgery.wustl.edu

### Your Plastic Surgery Guide

Access Media Group, LLC
7590 Fay Avenue, Suite 302
La Jolla, CA 92037
Phone: 858-454-2145
Fax: 858-454-5668
Website: http://
www.yourplasticsurgeryguide.com

# *Index*

# Index

Page numbers followed by 'n' indicate a footnote. Page numbers in *italics* indicate a table or illustration.

## A

## O

## P

479

# Health Reference Series

## COMPLETE CATALOG

List price $87 per volume. **School and library price $78 per volume.**

## Adolescent Health Sourcebook, 2nd Edition

*Basic Consumer Health Information about the Physical, Mental, and Emotional Growth and Development of Adolescents, Including Medical Care, Nutritional and Physical Activity Requirements, Puberty, Sexual Activity, Acne, Tanning, Body Piercing, Common Physical Illnesses and Disorders, Eating Disorders, Attention Deficit Hyperactivity Disorder, Depression, Bullying, Hazing, and Adolescent Injuries Related to Sports, Driving, and Work*

*Along with Substance Abuse Information about Nicotine, Alcohol, and Drug Use, a Glossary, and Directory of Additional Resources*

Edited by Joyce Brennfleck Shannon. 683 pages. 2006. 978-0-7808-0943-7.

"It is written in clear, nontechnical language aimed at general readers. . . . Recommended for public libraries, community colleges, and other agencies serving health care consumers."
— *American Reference Books Annual, 2003*

"Recommended for school and public libraries. Parents and professionals dealing with teens will appreciate the easy-to-follow format and the clearly written text. This could become a 'must have' for every high school teacher." — *E-Streams, Jan '03*

"A good starting point for information related to common medical, mental, and emotional concerns of adolescents." — *School Library Journal, Nov '02*

"This book provides accurate information in an easy to access format. It addresses topics that parents and caregivers might not be aware of and provides practical, useable information."
— *Doody's Health Sciences Book Review Journal, Sep-Oct '02*

"Recommended reference source."
— *Booklist, American Library Association, Sep '02*

## AIDS Sourcebook, 3rd Edition

*Basic Consumer Health Information about Acquired Immune Deficiency Syndrome (AIDS) and Human Immunodeficiency Virus (HIV) Infection, Including Facts about Transmission, Prevention, Diagnosis, Treatment, Opportunistic Infections, and Other Complications, with a Section for Women and Children, Including Details about Associated Gynecological Concerns, Pregnancy, and Pediatric Care*

*Along with Updated Statistical Information, Reports on Current Research Initiatives, a Glossary, and Directories of Internet, Hotline, and Other Resources*

Edited by Dawn D. Matthews. 664 pages. 2003. 978-0-7808-0631-3.

"The 3rd edition of the *AIDS Sourcebook*, part of Omnigraphics' *Health Reference Series*, is a welcome update. . . . This resource is highly recommended for academic and public libraries."
— *American Reference Books Annual, 2004*

"Excellent sourcebook. This continues to be a highly recommended book. There is no other book that provides as much information as this book provides."
— *AIDS Book Review Journal, Dec-Jan '00*

"Recommended reference source."
— *Booklist, American Library Association, Dec '99*

## Alcoholism Sourcebook, 2nd Edition

*Basic Consumer Health Information about Alcohol Use, Abuse, and Dependence, Featuring Facts about the Physical, Mental, and Social Health Effects of Alcohol Addiction, Including Alcoholic Liver Disease, Pancreatic Disease, Cardiovascular Disease, Neurological Disorders, and the Effects of Drinking during Pregnancy*

*Along with Information about Alcohol Treatment, Medications, and Recovery Programs, in Addition to Tips for Reducing the Prevalence of Underage Drinking, Statistics about Alcohol Use, a Glossary of Related Terms, and Directories of Resources for More Help and Information*

Edited by Amy L. Sutton. 653 pages. 2006. 978-0-7808-0942-0.

"This title is one of the few reference works on alcoholism for general readers. For some readers this will be a welcome complement to the many self-help books on the market. Recommended for collections serving general readers and consumer health collections."
— *E-Streams, Mar '01*

"This book is an excellent choice for public and academic libraries."
— *American Reference Books Annual, 2001*

"Recommended reference source."
— *Booklist, American Library Association, Dec '00*

"Presents a wealth of information on alcohol use and abuse and its effects on the body and mind, treatment, and prevention." — *SciTech Book News, Dec '00*

"Important new health guide which packs in the latest consumer information about the problems of alcoholism." — *Reviewer's Bookwatch, Nov '00*

*SEE ALSO Drug Abuse Sourcebook*

# Allergies Sourcebook, 3rd Edition

*Basic Consumer Health Information about Allergic Disorders, Such as Anaphylaxis, Hives, Eczema, Rhinitis, Sinusitis, and Conjunctivitis, and Their Triggers, Including Pollen, Mold, Dust Mites, Animal Dander, Insects, Chemicals, Food, Food Additives, and Medications;*

*Along with Advice about the Diagnosis and Treatment of Allergy Symptoms, a Glossary of Related Terms, a Directory of Resources for Help and Information, and Suggestions for Additional Reading*

Edited by Amy L. Sutton. 616 pages. 2007. 978-0-7808-0950-5.

"This book brings a great deal of useful material together. . . . This is an excellent addition to public and consumer health library collections."
— *American Reference Books Annual, 2003*

"This second edition would be useful to laypersons with little or advanced knowledge of the subject matter. This book would also serve as a resource for nursing and other health care professions students. It would be useful in public, academic, and hospital libraries with consumer health collections." — *E-Streams, Jul '02*

■

# Alternative Medicine Sourcebook

*SEE Complementary & Alternative Medicine Sourcebook*

■

# Alzheimer's Disease Sourcebook, 3rd Edition

*Basic Consumer Health Information about Alzheimer's Disease, Other Dementias, and Related Disorders, Including Multi-Infarct Dementia, AIDS Dementia Complex, Dementia with Lewy Bodies, Huntington's Disease, Wernicke-Korsakoff Syndrome (Alcohol-Related Dementia), Delirium, and Confusional States*

*Along with Information for People Newly Diagnosed with Alzheimer's Disease and Caregivers, Reports Detailing Current Research Efforts in Prevention, Diagnosis, and Treatment, Facts about Long-Term Care Issues, and Listings of Sources for Additional Information*

Edited by Karen Bellenir. 645 pages. 2003. 978-0-7808-0666-5.

"This very informative and valuable tool will be a great addition to any library serving consumers, students and health care workers."
— *American Reference Books Annual, 2004*

"This is a valuable resource for people affected by dementias such as Alzheimer's. It is easy to navigate and includes important information and resources."
— *Doody's Review Service, Feb '04*

"Recommended reference source."
— *Booklist, American Library Association, Oct '99*

*SEE ALSO Brain Disorders Sourcebook*

# Arthritis Sourcebook, 2nd Edition

*Basic Consumer Health Information about Osteoarthritis, Rheumatoid Arthritis, Other Rheumatic Disorders, Infectious Forms of Arthritis, and Diseases with Symptoms Linked to Arthritis, Featuring Facts about Diagnosis, Pain Management, and Surgical Therapies*

*Along with Coping Strategies, Research Updates, a Glossary, and Resources for Additional Help and Information*

Edited by Amy L. Sutton. 593 pages. 2004. 978-0-7808-0667-2.

"This easy-to-read volume is recommended for consumer health collections within public or academic libraries." — *E-Streams, May '05*

"As expected, this updated edition continues the excellent reputation of this series in providing sound, usable health information. . . . Highly recommended."
— *American Reference Books Annual, 2005*

"Excellent reference." — *The Bookwatch, Jan '05*

■

# Asthma Sourcebook, 2nd Edition

*Basic Consumer Health Information about the Causes, Symptoms, Diagnosis, and Treatment of Asthma in Infants, Children, Teenagers, and Adults, Including Facts about Different Types of Asthma, Common Co-Occurring Conditions, Asthma Management Plans, Triggers, Medications, and Medication Delivery Devices*

*Along with Asthma Statistics, Research Updates, a Glossary, a Directory of Asthma-Related Resources, and More*

Edited by Karen Bellenir. 609 pages. 2006. 978-0-7808-0866-9.

"A worthwhile reference acquisition for public libraries and academic medical libraries whose readers desire a quick introduction to the wide range of asthma information." — *Choice, Association of College & Research Libraries, Jun '01*

"Recommended reference source."
— *Booklist, American Library Association, Feb '01*

"Highly recommended." — *The Bookwatch, Jan '01*

"There is much good information for patients and their families who deal with asthma daily."
— *American Medical Writers Association Journal, Winter '01*

"This informative text is recommended for consumer health collections in public, secondary school, and community college libraries and the libraries of universities with a large undergraduate population."
— *American Reference Books Annual, 2001*

■

# Attention Deficit Disorder Sourcebook

*Basic Consumer Health Information about Attention Deficit/Hyperactivity Disorder in Children and Adults,*

*Including Facts about Causes, Symptoms, Diagnostic Criteria, and Treatment Options Such as Medications, Behavior Therapy, Coaching, and Homeopathy*

*Along with Reports on Current Research Initiatives, Legal Issues, and Government Regulations, and Featuring a Glossary of Related Terms, Internet Resources, and a List of Additional Reading Material*

Edited by Dawn D. Matthews. 470 pages. 2002. 978-0-7808-0624-5.

"Recommended reference source."
— *Booklist, American Library Association, Jan '03*

"This book is recommended for all school libraries and the reference or consumer health sections of public libraries." — *American Reference Books Annual, 2003*

■

# Back & Neck Sourcebook, 2nd Edition

*Basic Consumer Health Information about Spinal Pain, Spinal Cord Injuries, and Related Disorders, Such as Degenerative Disk Disease, Osteoarthritis, Scoliosis, Sciatica, Spina Bifida, and Spinal Stenosis, and Featuring Facts about Maintaining Spinal Health, Self-Care, Pain Management, Rehabilitative Care, Chiropractic Care, Spinal Surgeries, and Complementary Therapies*

*Along with Suggestions for Preventing Back and Neck Pain, a Glossary of Related Terms, and a Directory of Resources*

Edited by Amy L. Sutton. 633 pages. 2004. 978-0-7808-0738-9.

"Recommended . . . an easy to use, comprehensive medical reference book." — *E-Streams, Sep '05*

"The strength of this work is its basic, easy-to-read format. Recommended." — *Reference and User Services Quarterly, American Library Association, Winter '97*

■

# Blood & Circulatory Disorders Sourcebook, 2nd Edition

*Basic Consumer Health Information about the Blood and Circulatory System and Related Disorders, Such as Anemia and Other Hemoglobin Diseases, Cancer of the Blood and Associated Bone Marrow Disorders, Clotting and Bleeding Problems, and Conditions That Affect the Veins, Blood Vessels, and Arteries, Including Facts about the Donation and Transplantation of Bone Marrow, Stem Cells, and Blood and Tips for Keeping the Blood and Circulatory System Healthy*

*Along with a Glossary of Related Terms and Resources for Additional Help and Information*

Edited by Amy L. Sutton. 659 pages. 2005. 978-0-7808-0746-4.

"Highly recommended pick for basic consumer health reference holdings at all levels."
— *The Bookwatch, Aug '05*

"Recommended reference source."
— *Booklist, American Library Association, Feb '99*

"An important reference sourcebook written in simple language for everyday, non-technical users. "
— *Reviewer's Bookwatch, Jan '99*

■

# Brain Disorders Sourcebook, 2nd Edition

*Basic Consumer Health Information about Acquired and Traumatic Brain Injuries, Infections of the Brain, Epilepsy and Seizure Disorders, Cerebral Palsy, and Degenerative Neurological Disorders, Including Amyotrophic Lateral Sclerosis (ALS), Dementias, Multiple Sclerosis, and More*

*Along with Information on the Brain's Structure and Function, Treatment and Rehabilitation Options, Reports on Current Research Initiatives, a Glossary of Terms Related to Brain Disorders and Injuries, and a Directory of Sources for Further Help and Information*

Edited by Sandra J. Judd. 625 pages. 2005. 978-0-7808-0744-0.

"Highly recommended pick for basic consumer health reference holdings at all levels."
— *The Bookwatch, Aug '05*

"Belongs on the shelves of any library with a consumer health collection." — *E-Streams, Mar '00*

"Recommended reference source."
— *Booklist, American Library Association, Oct '99*

*SEE ALSO Alzheimer's Disease Sourcebook*

■

# Breast Cancer Sourcebook, 2nd Edition

*Basic Consumer Health Information about Breast Cancer, Including Facts about Risk Factors, Prevention, Screening and Diagnostic Methods, Treatment Options, Complementary and Alternative Therapies, Post-Treatment Concerns, Clinical Trials, Special Risk Populations, and New Developments in Breast Cancer Research*

*Along with Breast Cancer Statistics, a Glossary of Related Terms, and a Directory of Resources for Additional Help and Information*

Edited by Sandra J. Judd. 595 pages. 2004. 978-0-7808-0668-9.

"This book will be an excellent addition to public, community college, medical, and academic libraries."
— *American Reference Books Annual, 2006*

"It would be a useful reference book in a library or on loan to women in a support group."
— *Cancer Forum, Mar '03*

"Recommended reference source."
— *Booklist, American Library Association, Jan '02*

"This reference source is highly recommended. It is quite informative, comprehensive and detailed in nature, and yet it offers practical advice in easy-to-read language. It could be thought of as the 'bible' of breast cancer for the consumer." —E-Streams, Jan '02

"From the pros and cons of different screening methods and results to treatment options, *Breast Cancer Sourcebook* provides the latest information on the subject."
—Library Bookwatch, Dec '01

"This thoroughgoing, very readable reference covers all aspects of breast health and cancer. . . . Readers will find much to consider here. Recommended for all public and patient health collections."
—Library Journal, Sep '01

**SEE ALSO** *Cancer Sourcebook for Women, Women's Health Concerns Sourcebook*

■

# Breastfeeding Sourcebook

*Basic Consumer Health Information about the Benefits of Breastmilk, Preparing to Breastfeed, Breastfeeding as a Baby Grows, Nutrition, and More, Including Information on Special Situations and Concerns Such as Mastitis, Illness, Medications, Allergies, Multiple Births, Prematurity, Special Needs, and Adoption*

*Along with a Glossary and Resources for Additional Help and Information*

Edited by Jenni Lynn Colson. 388 pages. 2002. 978-0-7808-0332-9.

"Particularly useful is the information about professional lactation services and chapters on breastfeeding when returning to work. . . . *Breastfeeding Sourcebook* will be useful for public libraries, consumer health libraries, and technical schools offering nurse assistant training, especially in areas where Internet access is problematic."
—American Reference Books Annual, 2003

**SEE ALSO** *Pregnancy & Birth Sourcebook*

■

# Burns Sourcebook

*Basic Consumer Health Information about Various Types of Burns and Scalds, Including Flame, Heat, Cold, Electrical, Chemical, and Sun Burns*

*Along with Information on Short-Term and Long-Term Treatments, Tissue Reconstruction, Plastic Surgery, Prevention Suggestions, and First Aid*

Edited by Allan R. Cook. 604 pages. 1999. 978-0-7808-0204-9.

"This is an exceptional addition to the series and is highly recommended for all consumer health collections, hospital libraries, and academic medical centers."
—E-Streams, Mar '00

"This key reference guide is an invaluable addition to all health care and public libraries in confronting this ongoing health issue."
—American Reference Books Annual, 2000

"Recommended reference source."
—Booklist, American Library Association, Dec '99

**SEE ALSO** *Dermatological Disorders Sourcebook*

# Cancer Sourcebook, 5th Edition

*Basic Consumer Health Information about Major Forms and Stages of Cancer, Featuring Facts about Head and Neck Cancers, Lung Cancers, Gastrointestinal Cancers, Genitourinary Cancers, Lymphomas, Blood Cell Cancers, Endocrine Cancers, Skin Cancers, Bone Cancers, Metastatic Cancers, and More*

*Along with Facts about Cancer Treatments, Cancer Risks and Prevention, a Glossary of Related Terms, Statistical Data, and a Directory of Resources for Additional Information*

Edited by Karen Bellenir. 1,133 pages. 2007. 978-0-7808-0947-5.

"With cancer being the second leading cause of death for Americans, a prodigious work such as this one, which locates centrally so much cancer-related information, is clearly an asset to this nation's citizens and others."
—Journal of the National Medical Association, 2004

"This title is recommended for health sciences and public libraries with consumer health collections."
—E-Streams, Feb '01

". . . can be effectively used by cancer patients and their families who are looking for answers in a language they can understand. Public and hospital libraries should have it on their shelves."
—American Reference Books Annual, 2001

"Recommended reference source."
—Booklist, American Library Association, Dec '00

**SEE ALSO** *Breast Cancer Sourcebook, Cancer Sourcebook for Women, Pediatric Cancer Sourcebook, Prostate Cancer Sourcebook*

■

# Cancer Sourcebook for Women, 3rd Edition

*Basic Consumer Health Information about Leading Causes of Cancer in Women, Featuring Facts about Gynecologic Cancers and Related Concerns, Such as Breast Cancer, Cervical Cancer, Endometrial Cancer, Uterine Sarcoma, Vaginal Cancer, Vulvar Cancer, and Common Non-Cancerous Gynecologic Conditions, in Addition to Facts about Lung Cancer, Colorectal Cancer, and Thyroid Cancer in Women*

*Along with Information about Cancer Risk Factors, Screening and Prevention, Treatment Options, and Tips on Coping with Life after Cancer Treatment, a Glossary of Cancer Terms, and a Directory of Resources for Additional Help and Information*

Edited by Amy L. Sutton. 715 pages. 2006. 978-0-7808-0867-6.

"An excellent addition to collections in public, consumer health, and women's health libraries."
—American Reference Books Annual, 2003

"Overall, the information is excellent, and complex topics are clearly explained. As a reference book for the consumer it is a valuable resource to assist them to make informed decisions about cancer and its treatments." —Cancer Forum, Nov '02

"Highly recommended for academic and medical reference collections." — *Library Bookwatch, Sep '02*

"This is a highly recommended book for any public or consumer library, being reader friendly and containing accurate and helpful information."
— *E-Streams, Aug '02*

"Recommended reference source."
—*Booklist, American Library Association, Jul '02*

**SEE ALSO** *Breast Cancer Sourcebook, Women's Health Concerns Sourcebook*

# Cancer Survivorship Sourcebook

*Basic Consumer Health Information about the Physical, Educational, Emotional, Social, and Financial Needs of Cancer Patients from Diagnosis, through Cancer Treatment, and Beyond, Including Facts about Researching Specific Types of Cancer and Learning about Clinical Trials and Treatment Options, and Featuring Tips for Coping with the Side Effects of Cancer Treatments and Adjusting to Life after Cancer Treatment Concludes*

*Along with Suggestions for Caregivers, Friends, and Family Members of Cancer Patients, a Glossary of Cancer Care Terms, and Directories of Related Resources*

Edited by Karen Bellenir. 6561 pages. 2007. 978-0-7808-0985-7.

# Cardiovascular Diseases & Disorders Sourcebook, 3rd Edition

*Basic Consumer Health Information about Heart and Vascular Diseases and Disorders, Such as Angina, Heart Attacks, Arrhythmias, Cardiomyopathy, Valve Disease, Atherosclerosis, and Aneurysms, with Information about Managing Cardiovascular Risk Factors and Maintaining Heart Health, Medications and Procedures Used to Treat Cardiovascular Disorders, and Concerns of Special Significance to Women*

*Along with Reports on Current Research Initiatives, a Glossary of Related Medical Terms, and a Directory of Sources for Further Help and Information*

Edited by Sandra J. Judd. 713 pages. 2005. 978-0-7808-0739-6.

"This updated sourcebook is still the best first stop for comprehensive introductory information on cardiovascular diseases."
— *American Reference Books Annual, 2006*

"Recommended for public libraries and libraries supporting health care professionals."
— *E-Streams, Sep '05*

"This should be a standard health library reference."
—*The Bookwatch, Jun '05*

"Recommended reference source."
—*Booklist, American Library Association, Dec '00*

"... comprehensive format provides an extensive overview on this subject."
—*Choice, Association of College & Research Libraries*

# Caregiving Sourcebook

*Basic Consumer Health Information for Caregivers, Including a Profile of Caregivers, Caregiving Responsibilities and Concerns, Tips for Specific Conditions, Care Environments, and the Effects of Caregiving*

*Along with Facts about Legal Issues, Financial Information, and Future Planning, a Glossary, and a Listing of Additional Resources*

Edited by Joyce Brennfleck Shannon. 600 pages. 2001. 978-0-7808-0331-2.

"Essential for most collections."
— *Library Journal, Apr 1, 2002*

"An ideal addition to the reference collection of any public library. Health sciences information professionals may also want to acquire the *Caregiving Sourcebook* for their hospital or academic library for use as a ready reference tool by health care workers interested in aging and caregiving." — *E-Streams, Jan '02*

"Recommended reference source."
—*Booklist, American Library Association, Oct '01*

# Child Abuse Sourcebook

*Basic Consumer Health Information about the Physical, Sexual, and Emotional Abuse of Children, with Additional Facts about Neglect, Munchausen Syndrome by Proxy (MSBP), Shaken Baby Syndrome, and Controversial Issues Related to Child Abuse, Such as Withholding Medical Care, Corporal Punishment, and Child Maltreatment in Youth Sports, and Featuring Facts about Child Protective Services, Foster Care, Adoption, Parenting Challenges, and Other Abuse Prevention Efforts*

*Along with a Glossary of Related Terms and Resources for Additional Help and Information*

Edited by Dawn D. Matthews. 620 pages. 2004. 978-0-7808-0705-1.

"A valuable and highly recommended resource for school, academic and public libraries whether used on its own or as a starting point for more in-depth research." — *E-Streams, Apr '05*

"Every week the news brings cases of child abuse or neglect, so it is useful to have a source that supplies so much helpful information. . . . Recommended. Public and academic libraries, and child welfare offices."
—*Choice, Association of College & Research Libraries, Mar '05*

"Packed with insights on all kinds of issues, from foster care and adoption to parenting and abuse prevention."
—*The Bookwatch, Nov '04*

**SEE ALSO:** *Domestic Violence Sourcebook*

## Childhood Diseases & Disorders Sourcebook

*Basic Consumer Health Information about Medical Problems Often Encountered in Pre-Adolescent Children, Including Respiratory Tract Ailments, Ear Infections, Sore Throats, Disorders of the Skin and Scalp, Digestive and Genitourinary Diseases, Infectious Diseases, Inflammatory Disorders, Chronic Physical and Developmental Disorders, Allergies, and More*

*Along with Information about Diagnostic Tests, Common Childhood Surgeries, and Frequently Used Medications, with a Glossary of Important Terms and Resource Directory*

Edited by Chad T. Kimball. 662 pages. 2003. 978-0-7808-0458-6.

**"This is an excellent book for new parents and should be included in all health care and public libraries."**
*—American Reference Books Annual, 2004*

*SEE ALSO: Healthy Children Sourcebook*

■

## Colds, Flu & Other Common Ailments Sourcebook

*Basic Consumer Health Information about Common Ailments and Injuries, Including Colds, Coughs, the Flu, Sinus Problems, Headaches, Fever, Nausea and Vomiting, Menstrual Cramps, Diarrhea, Constipation, Hemorrhoids, Back Pain, Dandruff, Dry and Itchy Skin, Cuts, Scrapes, Sprains, Bruises, and More*

*Along with Information about Prevention, Self-Care, Choosing a Doctor, Over-the-Counter Medications, Folk Remedies, and Alternative Therapies, and Including a Glossary of Important Terms and a Directory of Resources for Further Help and Information*

Edited by Chad T. Kimball. 638 pages. 2001. 978-0-7808-0435-7.

**"A good starting point for research on common illnesses. It will be a useful addition to public and consumer health library collections."**
*— American Reference Books Annual, 2002*

**"Will prove valuable to any library seeking to maintain a current, comprehensive reference collection of health resources. . . . Excellent reference."**
*— The Bookwatch, Aug '01*

**"Recommended reference source."**
*— Booklist, American Library Association, Jul '01*

■

## Communication Disorders Sourcebook

*Basic Information about Deafness and Hearing Loss, Speech and Language Disorders, Voice Disorders, Balance and Vestibular Disorders, and Disorders of Smell, Taste, and Touch*

Edited by Linda M. Ross. 533 pages. 1996. 978-0-7808-0077-9.

**"This is skillfully edited and is a welcome resource for the layperson. It should be found in every public and medical library."** *— Booklist Health Sciences Supplement, American Library Association, Oct '97*

■

## Complementary & Alternative Medicine Sourcebook, 3rd Edition

*Basic Consumer Health Information about Complementary and Alternative Medical Therapies, Including Acupuncture, Ayurveda, Traditional Chinese Medicine, Herbal Medicine, Homeopathy, Naturopathy, Biofeedback, Hypnotherapy, Yoga, Art Therapy, Aromatherapy, Clinical Nutrition, Vitamin and Mineral Supplements, Chiropractic, Massage, Reflexology, Crystal Therapy, Therapeutic Touch, and More*

*Along with Facts about Alternative and Complementary Treatments for Specific Conditions Such as Cancer, Diabetes, Osteoarthritis, Chronic Pain, Menopause, Gastrointestinal Disorders, Headaches, and Mental Illness, a Glossary, and a Resource List for Additional Help and Information*

Edited by Sandra J. Judd. 657 pages. 2006. 978-0-7808-0864-5.

**"Recommended for public, high school, and academic libraries that have consumer health collections. Hospital libraries that also serve the public will find this to be a useful resource."** *— E-Streams, Feb '03*

**"Recommended reference source."**
*—Booklist, American Library Association, Jan '03*

**"An important alternate health reference."**
*— MBR Bookwatch, Oct '02*

**"A great addition to the reference collection of every type of library."** *— American Reference Books Annual, 2000*

■

## Congenital Disorders Sourcebook, 2nd Edition

*Basic Consumer Health Information about Nonhereditary Birth Defects and Disorders Related to Prematurity, Gestational Injuries, Congenital Infections, and Birth Complications, Including Heart Defects, Hydrocephalus, Spina Bifida, Cleft Lip and Palate, Cerebral Palsy, and More*

*Along with Facts about the Prevention of Birth Defects, Fetal Surgery and Other Treatment Options, Research Initiatives, a Glossary of Related Terms, and Resources for Additional Information and Support*

Edited by Sandra J. Judd. 647 pages. 2006. 978-0-7808-0945-1.

**"Recommended reference source."**
*— Booklist, American Library Association, Oct '97*

*SEE ALSO Pregnancy & Birth Sourcebook*

■

## Contagious Diseases Sourcebook

*Basic Consumer Health Information about Infectious Diseases Spread by Person-to-Person Contact through*

Direct Touch, Airborne Transmission, Sexual Contact, or Contact with Blood or Other Body Fluids, Including Hepatitis, Herpes, Influenza, Lice, Measles, Mumps, Pinworm, Ringworm, Severe Acute Respiratory Syndrome (SARS), Streptococcal Infections, Tuberculosis, and Others

Along with Facts about Disease Transmission, Antimicrobial Resistance, and Vaccines, with a Glossary and Directories of Resources for More Information

Edited by Karen Bellenir. 643 pages. 2004. 978-0-7808-0736-5.

"This easy-to-read volume is recommended for consumer health collections within public or academic libraries." — E-Streams, May '05

"This informative book is highly recommended for public libraries, consumer health collections, and secondary schools and undergraduate libraries." — American Reference Books Annual, 2005

"Excellent reference." — The Bookwatch, Jan '05

---

# Death & Dying Sourcebook, 2nd Edition

Basic Consumer Health Information about End-of-Life Care and Related Perspectives and Ethical Issues, Including End-of-Life Symptoms and Treatments, Pain Management, Quality-of-Life Concerns, the Use of Life Support, Patients' Rights and Privacy Issues, Advance Directives, Physician-Assisted Suicide, Caregiving, Organ and Tissue Donation, Autopsies, Funeral Arrangements, and Grief

Along with Statistical Data, Information about the Leading Causes of Death, a Glossary, and Directories of Support Groups and Other Resources

Edited by Joyce Brennfleck Shannon. 653 pages. 2006. 978-0-7808-0871-3.

"Public libraries, medical libraries, and academic libraries will all find this sourcebook a useful addition to their collections." — American Reference Books Annual, 2001

"An extremely useful resource for those concerned with death and dying in the United States." — Respiratory Care, Nov '00

"Recommended reference source." — Booklist, American Library Association, Aug '00

"This book is a definite must for all those involved in end-of-life care." — Doody's Review Service, 2000

---

# Dental Care & Oral Health Sourcebook, 2nd Edition

Basic Consumer Health Information about Dental Care, Including Oral Hygiene, Dental Visits, Pain Management, Cavities, Crowns, Bridges, Dental Implants, and Fillings, and Other Oral Health Concerns, Such as Gum Disease, Bad Breath, Dry Mouth, Genetic and Developmental Abnormalities, Oral Cancers, Orthodontics, and Temporomandibular Disorders

Along with Updates on Current Research in Oral Health, a Glossary, a Directory of Dental and Oral Health Organizations, and Resources for People with Dental and Oral Health Disorders

Edited by Amy L. Sutton. 609 pages. 2003. 978-0-7808-0634-4.

"This book could serve as a turning point in the battle to educate consumers in issues concerning oral health." — American Reference Books Annual, 2004

"Unique source which will fill a gap in dental sources for patients and the lay public. A valuable reference tool even in a library with thousands of books on dentistry. Comprehensive, clear, inexpensive, and easy to read and use. It fills an enormous gap in the health care literature." — Reference & User Services Quarterly, American Library Association, Summer '98

"Recommended reference source." — Booklist, American Library Association, Dec '97

---

# Depression Sourcebook

Basic Consumer Health Information about Unipolar Depression, Bipolar Disorder, Postpartum Depression, Seasonal Affective Disorder, and Other Types of Depression in Children, Adolescents, Women, Men, the Elderly, and Other Selected Populations

Along with Facts about Causes, Risk Factors, Diagnostic Criteria, Treatment Options, Coping Strategies, Suicide Prevention, a Glossary, and a Directory of Sources for Additional Help and Information

Edited by Karen Bellenir. 602 pages. 2002. 978-0-7808-0611-5.

"Depression Sourcebook is of a very high standard. Its purpose, which is to serve as a reference source to the lay reader, is very well served." — Journal of the National Medical Association, 2004

"Invaluable reference for public and school library collections alike." — Library Bookwatch, Apr '03

"Recommended for purchase." — American Reference Books Annual, 2003

---

# Dermatological Disorders Sourcebook, 2nd Edition

Basic Consumer Health Information about Conditions and Disorders Affecting the Skin, Hair, and Nails, Such as Acne, Rosacea, Rashes, Dermatitis, Pigmentation Disorders, Birthmarks, Skin Cancer, Skin Injuries, Psoriasis, Scleroderma, and Hair Loss, Including Facts about Medications and Treatments for Dermatological Disorders and Tips for Maintaining Healthy Skin, Hair, and Nails

Along with Information about How Aging Affects the Skin, a Glossary of Related Terms, and a Directory of Resources for Additional Help and Information

Edited by Amy L. Sutton. 645 pages. 2005. 978-0-7808-0795-2.

"... comprehensive, easily read reference book."
—*Doody's Health Sciences Book Reviews, Oct '97*

**SEE ALSO** *Burns Sourcebook*

■

# Diabetes Sourcebook, 3rd Edition

*Basic Consumer Health Information about Type 1 Diabetes (Insulin-Dependent or Juvenile-Onset Diabetes), Type 2 Diabetes (Noninsulin-Dependent or Adult-Onset Diabetes), Gestational Diabetes, Impaired Glucose Tolerance (IGT), and Related Complications, Such as Amputation, Eye Disease, Gum Disease, Nerve Damage, and End-Stage Renal Disease, Including Facts about Insulin, Oral Diabetes Medications, Blood Sugar Testing, and the Role of Exercise and Nutrition in the Control of Diabetes*

*Along with a Glossary and Resources for Further Help and Information*

Edited by Dawn D. Matthews. 622 pages. 2003. 978-0-7808-0629-0.

"This edition is even more helpful than earlier versions. . . . It is a truly valuable tool for anyone seeking readable and authoritative information on diabetes."
— *American Reference Books Annual, 2004*

"An invaluable reference." — *Library Journal, May '00*

Selected as one of the 250 "Best Health Sciences Books of 1999." — *Doody's Rating Service, Mar-Apr '00*

"Provides useful information for the general public."
— *Healthlines, University of Michigan Health Management Research Center, Sep/Oct '99*

"... provides reliable mainstream medical information ... belongs on the shelves of any library with a consumer health collection." — *E-Streams, Sep '99*

"Recommended reference source."
— *Booklist, American Library Association, Feb '99*

■

# Diet & Nutrition Sourcebook, 3rd Edition

*Basic Consumer Health Information about Dietary Guidelines and the Food Guidance System, Recommended Daily Nutrient Intakes, Serving Proportions, Weight Control, Vitamins and Supplements, Nutrition Issues for Different Life Stages and Lifestyles, and the Needs of People with Specific Medical Concerns, Including Cancer, Celiac Disease, Diabetes, Eating Disorders, Food Allergies, and Cardiovascular Disease*

*Along with Facts about Federal Nutrition Support Programs, a Glossary of Nutrition and Dietary Terms, and Directories of Additional Resources for More Information about Nutrition*

Edited by Joyce Brennfleck Shannon. 633 pages. 2006. 978-0-7808-0800-3.

"This book is an excellent source of basic diet and nutrition information." — *Booklist Health Sciences Supplement, American Library Association, Dec '00*

"This reference document should be in any public library, but it would be a very good guide for beginning students in the health sciences. If the other books in this publisher's series are as good as this, they should all be in the health sciences collections."
— *American Reference Books Annual, 2000*

"This book is an excellent general nutrition reference for consumers who desire to take an active role in their health care for prevention. Consumers of all ages who select this book can feel confident they are receiving current and accurate information." — *Journal of Nutrition for the Elderly, Vol. 19, No. 4, 2000*

**SEE ALSO** *Digestive Diseases & Disorders Sourcebook, Eating Disorders Sourcebook, Gastrointestinal Diseases & Disorders Sourcebook, Vegetarian Sourcebook*

■

# Digestive Diseases & Disorders Sourcebook

*Basic Consumer Health Information about Diseases and Disorders that Impact the Upper and Lower Digestive System, Including Celiac Disease, Constipation, Crohn's Disease, Cyclic Vomiting Syndrome, Diarrhea, Diverticulosis and Diverticulitis, Gallstones, Heartburn, Hemorrhoids, Hernias, Indigestion (Dyspepsia), Irritable Bowel Syndrome, Lactose Intolerance, Ulcers, and More*

*Along with Information about Medications and Other Treatments, Tips for Maintaining a Healthy Digestive Tract, a Glossary, and Directory of Digestive Diseases Organizations*

Edited by Karen Bellenir. 335 pages. 2000. 978-0-7808-0327-5.

"This title would be an excellent addition to all public or patient-research libraries."
— *American Reference Books Annual, 2001*

"This title is recommended for public, hospital, and health sciences libraries with consumer health collections." — *E-Streams, Jul-Aug '00*

"Recommended reference source."
— *Booklist, American Library Association, May '00*

**SEE ALSO** *Eating Disorders Sourcebook, Gastrointestinal Diseases & Disorders Sourcebook*

■

# Disabilities Sourcebook

*Basic Consumer Health Information about Physical and Psychiatric Disabilities, Including Descriptions of Major Causes of Disability, Assistive and Adaptive Aids, Workplace Issues, and Accessibility Concerns*

*Along with Information about the Americans with Disabilities Act, a Glossary, and Resources for Additional Help and Information*

Edited by Dawn D. Matthews. 616 pages. 2000. 978-0-7808-0389-3.

"It is a must for libraries with a consumer health section." — *American Reference Books Annual, 2002*

"A much needed addition to the Omnigraphics *Health Reference Series*. A current reference work to provide people with disabilities, their families, caregivers or those who work with them, a broad range of information in one volume, has not been available until now. . . . It is recommended for all public and academic library reference collections."    —*E-Streams, May '01*

"An excellent source book in easy-to-read format covering many current topics; highly recommended for all libraries."    —*Choice, Association of College & Research Libraries, Jan '01*

"Recommended reference source."
—*Booklist, American Library Association, Jul '00*

■

# Domestic Violence Sourcebook, 2nd Edition

*Basic Consumer Health Information about the Causes and Consequences of Abusive Relationships, Including Physical Violence, Sexual Assault, Battery, Stalking, and Emotional Abuse, and Facts about the Effects of Violence on Women, Men, Young Adults, and the Elderly, with Reports about Domestic Violence in Selected Populations, and Featuring Facts about Medical Care, Victim Assistance and Protection, Prevention Strategies, Mental Health Services, and Legal Issues*

*Along with a Glossary of Related Terms and Resources for Additional Help and Information*

Edited by Dawn D. Matthews. 628 pages. 2004. 978-0-7808-0669-6.

"Educators, clergy, medical professionals, police, and victims and their families will benefit from this realistic and easy-to-understand resource."
—*American Reference Books Annual, 2005*

"Recommended for all collections supporting consumer health information. It should also be considered for any collection needing general, readable information on domestic violence."    —*E-Streams, Jan '05*

"This sourcebook complements other books in its field, providing a one-stop resource . . . Recommended."
—*Choice, Association of College & Research Libraries, Jan '05*

"Interested lay persons should find the book extremely beneficial. . . . A copy of *Domestic Violence and Child Abuse Sourcebook* should be in every public library in the United States."
—*Social Science & Medicine, No. 56, 2003*

"This is important information. The Web has many resources but this sourcebook fills an important societal need. I am not aware of any other resources of this type."    —*Doody's Review Service, Sep '01*

"Recommended reference source."
—*Booklist, American Library Association, Apr '01*

"Important pick for college-level health reference libraries."    —*The Bookwatch, Mar '01*

"Because this problem is so widespread and because this book includes a lot of issues within one volume, this work is recommended for all public libraries."
—*American Reference Books Annual, 2001*

**SEE ALSO** *Child Abuse Sourcebook*

■

# Drug Abuse Sourcebook, 2nd Edition

*Basic Consumer Health Information about Illicit Substances of Abuse and the Misuse of Prescription and Over-the-Counter Medications, Including Depressants, Hallucinogens, Inhalants, Marijuana, Stimulants, and Anabolic Steroids*

*Along with Facts about Related Health Risks, Treatment Programs, Prevention Programs, a Glossary of Abuse and Addiction Terms, a Glossary of Drug-Related Street Terms, and a Directory of Resources for More Information*

Edited by Catherine Ginther. 607 pages. 2004. 978-0-7808-0740-2.

"Commendable for organizing useful, normally scattered government and association-produced data into a logical sequence."
—*American Reference Books Annual, 2006*

"This easy-to-read volume is recommended for consumer health collections within public or academic libraries."    —*E-Streams, Sep '05*

"An excellent library reference."
—*The Bookwatch, May '05*

"Containing a wealth of information, this book will be useful to the college student just beginning to explore the topic of substance abuse. This resource belongs in libraries that serve a lower-division undergraduate or community college clientele as well as the general public."    —*Choice, Association of College & Research Libraries, Jun '01*

"Recommended reference source."
—*Booklist, American Library Association, Feb '01*

**SEE ALSO** *Alcoholism Sourcebook*

■

# Ear, Nose & Throat Disorders Sourcebook, 2nd Edition

*Basic Consumer Health Information about Disorders of the Ears, Hearing Loss, Vestibular Disorders, Nasal and Sinus Problems, Throat and Vocal Cord Disorders, and Otolaryngologic Cancers, Including Facts about Ear Infections and Injuries, Genetic and Congenital Deafness, Sensorineural Hearing Disorders, Tinnitus, Vertigo, Ménière Disease, Rhinitis, Sinusitis, Snoring, Sore Throats, Hoarseness, and More*

*Along with Reports on Current Research Initiatives, a Glossary of Related Medical Terms, and a Directory of Sources for Further Help and Information*

Edited by Sandra J. Judd. 659 pages. 2006. 978-0-7808-0872-0.

"Overall, this sourcebook is helpful for the consumer seeking information on ENT issues. It is recommended for public libraries."
— *American Reference Books Annual, 1999*

"Recommended reference source."
— *Booklist, American Library Association, Dec '98*

<hr>

# Eating Disorders Sourcebook, 2nd Edition

*Basic Consumer Health Information about Anorexia Nervosa, Bulimia Nervosa, Binge Eating, Compulsive Exercise, Female Athlete Triad, and Other Eating Disorders, Including Facts about Body Image and Other Cultural and Age-Related Risk Factors, Prevention Efforts, Adverse Health Effects, Treatment Options, and the Recovery Process*

*Along with Guidelines for Healthy Weight Control, a Glossary, and Directories of Additional Resources*

Edited by Joyce Brennfleck Shannon. 585 pages. 2007. 978-0-7808-0948-2.

"Recommended for health science libraries that are open to the public, as well as hospital libraries. This book is a good resource for the consumer who is concerned about eating disorders."   — *E-Streams, Mar '02*

"This volume is another convenient collection of excerpted articles. Recommended for school and public library patrons; lower-division undergraduates; and two-year technical program students."
— *Choice, Association of College & Research Libraries, Jan '02*

"Recommended reference source."
— *Booklist, American Library Association, Oct '01*

**SEE ALSO** *Diet & Nutrition Sourcebook, Digestive Diseases & Disorders Sourcebook, Gastrointestinal Diseases & Disorders Sourcebook*

<hr>

# Emergency Medical Services Sourcebook

*Basic Consumer Health Information about Preventing, Preparing for, and Managing Emergency Situations, When and Who to Call for Help, What to Expect in the Emergency Room, the Emergency Medical Team, Patient Issues, and Current Topics in Emergency Medicine*

*Along with Statistical Data, a Glossary, and Sources of Additional Help and Information*

Edited by Jenni Lynn Colson. 494 pages. 2002. 978-0-7808-0420-3.

"Handy and convenient for home, public, school, and college libraries. Recommended."
— *Choice, Association of College & Research Libraries, Apr '03*

"This reference can provide the consumer with answers to most questions about emergency care in the United States, or it will direct them to a resource where the answer can be found."
— *American Reference Books Annual, 2003*

"Recommended reference source."
— *Booklist, American Library Association, Feb '03*

<hr>

# Endocrine & Metabolic Disorders Sourcebook

*Basic Information for the Layperson about Pancreatic and Insulin-Related Disorders Such as Pancreatitis, Diabetes, and Hypoglycemia; Adrenal Gland Disorders Such as Cushing's Syndrome, Addison's Disease, and Congenital Adrenal Hyperplasia; Pituitary Gland Disorders Such as Growth Hormone Deficiency, Acromegaly, and Pituitary Tumors; Thyroid Disorders Such as Hypothyroidism, Graves' Disease, Hashimoto's Disease, and Goiter; Hyperparathyroidism; and Other Diseases and Syndromes of Hormone Imbalance or Metabolic Dysfunction*

*Along with Reports on Current Research Initiatives*

Edited by Linda M. Shin. 574 pages. 1998. 978-0-7808-0207-0.

"Omnigraphics has produced another needed resource for health information consumers."
— *American Reference Books Annual, 2000*

"Recommended reference source."
— *Booklist, American Library Association, Dec '98*

<hr>

# Environmental Health Sourcebook, 2nd Edition

*Basic Consumer Health Information about the Environment and Its Effect on Human Health, Including the Effects of Air Pollution, Water Pollution, Hazardous Chemicals, Food Hazards, Radiation Hazards, Biological Agents, Household Hazards, Such as Radon, Asbestos, Carbon Monoxide, and Mold, and Information about Associated Diseases and Disorders, Including Cancer, Allergies, Respiratory Problems, and Skin Disorders*

*Along with Information about Environmental Concerns for Specific Populations, a Glossary of Related Terms, and Resources for Further Help and Information*

Edited by Dawn D. Matthews. 673 pages. 2003. 978-0-7808-0632-0.

"This recently updated edition continues the level of quality and the reputation of the numerous other volumes in Omnigraphics' *Health Reference Series*."
— *American Reference Books Annual, 2004*

"An excellent updated edition."
— *The Bookwatch, Oct '03*

"Recommended reference source."
— *Booklist, American Library Association, Sep '98*

"This book will be a useful addition to anyone's library."   — *Choice Health Sciences Supplement, Association of College & Research Libraries, May '98*

". . . a good survey of numerous environmentally induced physical disorders . . . a useful addition to anyone's library."
— *Doody's Health Sciences Book Reviews, Jan '98*

# Ethnic Diseases Sourcebook

*Basic Consumer Health Information for Ethnic and Racial Minority Groups in the United States, Including General Health Indicators and Behaviors, Ethnic Diseases, Genetic Testing, the Impact of Chronic Diseases, Women's Health, Mental Health Issues, and Preventive Health Care Services*

*Along with a Glossary and a Listing of Additional Resources*

Edited by Joyce Brennfleck Shannon. 664 pages. 2001. 978-0-7808-0336-7.

"Recommended for health sciences libraries where public health programs are a priority."
— *E-Streams, Jan '02*

"Not many books have been written on this topic to date, and the *Ethnic Diseases Sourcebook* is a strong addition to the list. It will be an important introductory resource for health consumers, students, health care personnel, and social scientists. It is recommended for public, academic, and large hospital libraries."
— *American Reference Books Annual, 2002*

"Recommended reference source."
— *Booklist, American Library Association, Oct '01*

"Will prove valuable to any library seeking to maintain a current, comprehensive reference collection of health resources. . . . An excellent source of health information about genetic disorders which affect particular ethnic and racial minorities in the U.S."
— *The Bookwatch, Aug '01*

---

# Eye Care Sourcebook, 2nd Edition

*Basic Consumer Health Information about Eye Care and Eye Disorders, Including Facts about the Diagnosis, Prevention, and Treatment of Common Refractive Problems Such as Myopia, Hyperopia, Astigmatism, and Presbyopia, and Eye Diseases, Including Glaucoma, Cataract, Age-Related Macular Degeneration, and Diabetic Retinopathy*

*Along with a Section on Vision Correction and Refractive Surgeries, Including LASIK and LASEK, a Glossary, and Directories of Resources for Additional Help and Information*

Edited by Amy L. Sutton. 543 pages. 2003. 978-0-7808-0635-1.

". . . a solid reference tool for eye care and a valuable addition to a collection."
— *American Reference Books Annual, 2004*

---

# Family Planning Sourcebook

*Basic Consumer Health Information about Planning for Pregnancy and Contraception, Including Traditional Methods, Barrier Methods, Hormonal Methods, Permanent Methods, Future Methods, Emergency Contraception, and Birth Control Choices for Women at Each Stage of Life*

*Along with Statistics, a Glossary, and Sources of Additional Information*

Edited by Amy Marcaccio Keyzer. 520 pages. 2001. 978-0-7808-0379-4.

"Recommended for public, health, and undergraduate libraries as part of the circulating collection."
— *E-Streams, Mar '02*

"Information is presented in an unbiased, readable manner, and the sourcebook will certainly be a necessary addition to those public and high school libraries where Internet access is restricted or otherwise problematic." — *American Reference Books Annual, 2002*

"Recommended reference source."
— *Booklist, American Library Association, Oct '01*

"Will prove valuable to any library seeking to maintain a current, comprehensive reference collection of health resources. . . . Excellent reference."
— *The Bookwatch, Aug '01*

**SEE ALSO** *Pregnancy & Birth Sourcebook*

---

# Fitness & Exercise Sourcebook, 3rd Edition

*Basic Consumer Health Information about the Physical and Mental Benefits of Fitness, Including Cardiorespiratory Endurance, Muscular Strength, Muscular Endurance, and Flexibility, with Facts about Sports Nutrition and Exercise-Related Injuries and Tips about Physical Activity and Exercises for People of All Ages and for People with Health Concerns*

*Along with Advice on Selecting and Using Exercise Equipment, Maintaining Exercise Motivation, a Glossary of Related Terms, and a Directory of Resources for More Help and Information*

Edited by Amy L. Sutton. 663 pages. 2007. 978-0-7808-0946-8.

"This work is recommended for all general reference collections."
— *American Reference Books Annual, 2002*

"Highly recommended for public, consumer, and school grades fourth through college." — *E-Streams, Nov '01*

"Recommended reference source."
— *Booklist, American Library Association, Oct '01*

"The information appears quite comprehensive and is considered reliable. . . . This second edition is a welcomed addition to the series."
— *Doody's Review Service, Sep '01*

---

# Food Safety Sourcebook

*Basic Consumer Health Information about the Safe Handling of Meat, Poultry, Seafood, Eggs, Fruit Juices, and Other Food Items, and Facts about Pesticides, Drinking Water, Food Safety Overseas, and the Onset, Duration, and Symptoms of Foodborne Illnesses, Including Types of Pathogenic Bacteria, Parasitic Protozoa, Worms, Viruses, and Natural Toxins*

Along with the Role of the Consumer, the Food Handler, and the Government in Food Safety; a Glossary, and Resources for Additional Help and Information

Edited by Dawn D. Matthews. 339 pages. 1999. 978-0-7808-0326-8.

"This book is recommended for public libraries and universities with home economic and food science programs." — *E-Streams, Nov '00*

"Recommended reference source."
— *Booklist, American Library Association, May '00*

"This book takes the complex issues of food safety and foodborne pathogens and presents them in an easily understood manner. [It does] an excellent job of covering a large and often confusing topic."
— *American Reference Books Annual, 2000*

---

# Forensic Medicine Sourcebook

*Basic Consumer Information for the Layperson about Forensic Medicine, Including Crime Scene Investigation, Evidence Collection and Analysis, Expert Testimony, Computer-Aided Criminal Identification, Digital Imaging in the Courtroom, DNA Profiling, Accident Reconstruction, Autopsies, Ballistics, Drugs and Explosives Detection, Latent Fingerprints, Product Tampering, and Questioned Document Examination*

*Along with Statistical Data, a Glossary of Forensics Terminology, and Listings of Sources for Further Help and Information*

Edited by Annemarie S. Muth. 574 pages. 1999. 978-0-7808-0232-2.

"Given the expected widespread interest in its content and its easy to read style, this book is recommended for most public and all college and university libraries."
— *E-Streams, Feb '01*

"Recommended for public libraries."
— *Reference & User Services Quarterly, American Library Association, Spring 2000*

"Recommended reference source."
— *Booklist, American Library Association, Feb '00*

"A wealth of information, useful statistics, references are up-to-date and extremely complete. This wonderful collection of data will help students who are interested in a career in any type of forensic field. It is a great resource for attorneys who need information about types of expert witnesses needed in a particular case. It also offers useful information for fiction and nonfiction writers whose work involves a crime. A fascinating compilation. All levels."
— *Choice, Association of College & Research Libraries, Jan '00*

"There are several items that make this book attractive to consumers who are seeking certain forensic data. . . . This is a useful current source for those seeking general forensic medical answers."
— *American Reference Books Annual, 2000*

# Gastrointestinal Diseases & Disorders Sourcebook, 2nd Edition

*Basic Consumer Health Information about the Upper and Lower Gastrointestinal (GI) Tract, Including the Esophagus, Stomach, Intestines, Rectum, Liver, and Pancreas, with Facts about Gastroesophageal Reflux Disease, Gastritis, Hernias, Ulcers, Celiac Disease, Diverticulitis, Irritable Bowel Syndrome, Hemorrhoids, Gastrointestinal Cancers, and Other Diseases and Disorders Related to the Digestive Process*

*Along with Information about Commonly Used Diagnostic and Surgical Procedures, Statistics, Reports on Current Research Initiatives and Clinical Trials, a Glossary, and Resources for Additional Help and Information*

Edited by Sandra J. Judd. 681 pages. 2006. 978-0-7808-0798-3.

". . . very readable form. The successful editorial work that brought this material together into a useful and understandable reference makes accessible to all readers information that can help them more effectively understand and obtain help for digestive tract problems."
— *Choice, Association of College & Research Libraries, Feb '97*

SEE ALSO *Diet & Nutrition Sourcebook, Digestive Diseases & Disorders Sourcebook, Eating Disorders Sourcebook*

---

# Genetic Disorders Sourcebook, 3rd Edition

*Basic Consumer Health Information about Hereditary Diseases and Disorders, Including Facts about the Human Genome, Genetic Inheritance Patterns, Disorders Associated with Specific Genes, Such as Sickle Cell Disease, Hemophilia, and Cystic Fibrosis, Chromosome Disorders, Such as Down Syndrome, Fragile X Syndrome, and Turner Syndrome, and Complex Diseases and Disorders Resulting from the Interaction of Environmental and Genetic Factors, Such as Allergies, Cancer, and Obesity*

*Along with Facts about Genetic Testing, Suggestions for Parents of Children with Special Needs, Reports on Current Research Initiatives, a Glossary of Genetic Terminology, and Resources for Additional Help and Information*

Edited by Karen Bellenir. 777 pages. 2004. 978-0-7808-0742-6.

"This text is recommended for any library with an interest in providing consumer health resources."
— *E-Streams, Aug '05*

"This is a valuable resource for anyone wishing to have an understandable description of any of the topics or disorders included. The editor succeeds in making complex genetic issues understandable."
— *Doody's Book Review Service, May '05*

"A good acquisition for public libraries."
— *American Reference Books Annual, 2005*

# Head Trauma Sourcebook

*Basic Information for the Layperson about Open-Head and Closed-Head Injuries, Treatment Advances, Recovery, and Rehabilitation*

*Along with Reports on Current Research Initiatives*

Edited by Karen Bellenir. 414 pages. 1997. 978-0-7808-0208-7.

# Headache Sourcebook

*Basic Consumer Health Information about Migraine, Tension, Cluster, Rebound and Other Types of Headaches, with Facts about the Cause and Prevention of Headaches, the Effects of Stress and the Environment, Headaches during Pregnancy and Menopause, and Childhood Headaches*

*Along with a Glossary and Other Resources for Additional Help and Information*

Edited by Dawn D. Matthews. 362 pages. 2002. 978-0-7808-0337-4.

# Healthy Aging Sourcebook

*Basic Consumer Health Information about Maintaining Health through the Aging Process, Including Advice on Nutrition, Exercise, and Sleep, Help in Making Decisions about Midlife Issues and Retirement, and Guidance Concerning Practical and Informed Choices in Health Consumerism*

*Along with Data Concerning the Theories of Aging, Different Experiences in Aging by Minority Groups, and Facts about Aging Now and Aging in the Future; and Featuring a Glossary, a Guide to Consumer Help, Additional Suggested Reading, and Practical Resource Directory*

Edited by Jenifer Swanson. 536 pages. 1999. 978-0-7808-0390-9.

***SEE ALSO*** *Physical & Mental Issues in Aging Sourcebook*

# Healthy Children Sourcebook

*Basic Consumer Health Information about the Physical and Mental Development of Children between the Ages of 3 and 12, Including Routine Health Care, Preventative Health Services, Safety and First Aid,*

*Healthy Sleep, Dental Care, Nutrition, and Fitness, and Featuring Parenting Tips on Such Topics as Bedwetting, Choosing Day Care, Monitoring TV and Other Media, and Establishing a Foundation for Substance Abuse Prevention*

*Along with a Glossary of Commonly Used Pediatric Terms and Resources for Additional Help and Information.*

Edited by Chad T. Kimball. 647 pages. 2003. 978-0-7808-0247-6.

***SEE ALSO*** *Childhood Diseases & Disorders Sourcebook*

# Healthy Heart Sourcebook for Women

*Basic Consumer Health Information about Cardiac Issues Specific to Women, Including Facts about Major Risk Factors and Prevention, Treatment and Control Strategies, and Important Dietary Issues*

*Along with a Special Section Regarding the Pros and Cons of Hormone Replacement Therapy and Its Impact on Heart Health, and Additional Help, Including Recipes, a Glossary, and a Directory of Resources*

Edited by Dawn D. Matthews. 336 pages. 2000. 978-0-7808-0329-9.

***SEE ALSO*** *Cardiovascular Diseases & Disorders Sourcebook, Women's Health Concerns Sourcebook*

# Hepatitis Sourcebook

*Basic Consumer Health Information about Hepatitis A, Hepatitis B, Hepatitis C, and Other Forms of Hepatitis, Including Autoimmune Hepatitis, Alcoholic Hepatitis, Nonalcoholic Steatohepatitis, and Toxic Hepatitis, with*

*Facts about Risk Factors, Screening Methods, Diagnostic Tests, and Treatment Options*

*Along with Information on Liver Health, Tips for People Living with Chronic Hepatitis, Reports on Current Research Initiatives, a Glossary of Terms Related to Hepatitis, and a Directory of Sources for Further Help and Information*

Edited by Sandra J. Judd. 597 pages. 2005. 978-0-7808-0749-5.

**"Highly recommended."**
— *American Reference Books Annual, 2006*

▪

# Household Safety Sourcebook

*Basic Consumer Health Information about Household Safety, Including Information about Poisons, Chemicals, Fire, and Water Hazards in the Home*

*Along with Advice about the Safe Use of Home Maintenance Equipment, Choosing Toys and Nursery Furniture, Holiday and Recreation Safety, a Glossary, and Resources for Further Help and Information*

Edited by Dawn D. Matthews. 606 pages. 2002. 978-0-7808-0338-1.

**"This work will be useful in public libraries with large consumer health and wellness departments."**
— *American Reference Books Annual, 2003*

**"As a sourcebook on household safety this book meets its mark. It is encyclopedic in scope and covers a wide range of safety issues that are commonly seen in the home."** — *E-Streams, Jul '02*

▪

# Hypertension Sourcebook

*Basic Consumer Health Information about the Causes, Diagnosis, and Treatment of High Blood Pressure, with Facts about Consequences, Complications, and Co-Occurring Disorders, Such as Coronary Heart Disease, Diabetes, Stroke, Kidney Disease, and Hypertensive Retinopathy, and Issues in Blood Pressure Control, Including Dietary Choices, Stress Management, and Medications*

*Along with Reports on Current Research Initiatives and Clinical Trials, a Glossary, and Resources for Additional Help and Information*

Edited by Dawn D. Matthews and Karen Bellenir. 613 pages. 2004. 978-0-7808-0674-0.

**"Academic, public, and medical libraries will want to add the *Hypertension Sourcebook* to their collections."**
— *E-Streams, Aug '05*

**"The strength of this source is the wide range of information given about hypertension."**
— *American Reference Books Annual, 2005*

▪

# Immune System Disorders Sourcebook, 2nd Edition

*Basic Consumer Health Information about Disorders of the Immune System, Including Immune System Function and Response, Diagnosis of Immune Disorders, Information about Inherited Immune Disease, Acquired Immune Disease, and Autoimmune Diseases, Including Primary Immune Deficiency, Acquired Immunodeficiency Syndrome (AIDS), Lupus, Multiple Sclerosis, Type 1 Diabetes, Rheumatoid Arthritis, and Graves' Disease*

*Along with Treatments, Tips for Coping with Immune Disorders, a Glossary, and a Directory of Additional Resources.*

Edited by Joyce Brennfleck Shannon. 671 pages. 2005. 978-0-7808-0748-8.

**"Highly recommended for academic and public libraries."** — *American Reference Books Annual, 2006*

**"The updated second edition is a 'must' for any consumer health library seeking a solid resource covering the treatments, symptoms, and options for immune disorder sufferers. . . . An excellent guide."**
— *MBR Bookwatch, Jan '06*

▪

# Infant & Toddler Health Sourcebook

*Basic Consumer Health Information about the Physical and Mental Development of Newborns, Infants, and Toddlers, Including Neonatal Concerns, Nutrition Recommendations, Immunization Schedules, Common Pediatric Disorders, Assessments and Milestones, Safety Tips, and Advice for Parents and Other Caregivers*

*Along with a Glossary of Terms and Resource Listings for Additional Help*

Edited by Jenifer Swanson. 585 pages. 2000. 978-0-7808-0246-9.

**"As a reference for the general public, this would be useful in any library."** — *E-Streams, May '01*

**"Recommended reference source."**
— *Booklist, American Library Association, Feb '01*

**"This is a good source for general use."**
— *American Reference Books Annual, 2001*

▪

# Infectious Diseases Sourcebook

*Basic Consumer Health Information about Non-Contagious Bacterial, Viral, Prion, Fungal, and Parasitic Diseases Spread by Food and Water, Insects and Animals, or Environmental Contact, Including Botulism, E. Coli, Encephalitis, Legionnaires' Disease, Lyme Disease, Malaria, Plague, Rabies, Salmonella, Tetanus, and Others, and Facts about Newly Emerging Diseases, Such as Hantavirus, Mad Cow Disease, Monkeypox, and West Nile Virus*

*Along with Information about Preventing Disease Transmission, the Threat of Bioterrorism, and Current Research Initiatives, with a Glossary and Directory of Resources for More Information*

Edited by Karen Bellenir. 634 pages. 2004. 978-0-7808-0675-7.

"This reference continues the excellent tradition of the *Health Reference Series* in consolidating a wealth of information on a selected topic into a format that is easy to use and accessible to the general public."
— *American Reference Books Annual, 2005*

"Recommended for public and academic libraries."
— *E-Streams, Jan '05*

■

# Injury & Trauma Sourcebook

*Basic Consumer Health Information about the Impact of Injury, the Diagnosis and Treatment of Common and Traumatic Injuries, Emergency Care, and Specific Injuries Related to Home, Community, Workplace, Transportation, and Recreation*

*Along with Guidelines for Injury Prevention, a Glossary, and a Directory of Additional Resources*

Edited by Joyce Brennfleck Shannon. 696 pages. 2002. 978-0-7808-0421-0.

"This publication is the most comprehensive work of its kind about injury and trauma."
— *American Reference Books Annual, 2003*

"This sourcebook provides concise, easily readable, basic health information about injuries. . . . This book is well organized and an easy to use reference resource suitable for hospital, health sciences and public libraries with consumer health collections."
— *E-Streams, Nov '02*

"Practitioners should be aware of guides such as this in order to facilitate their use by patients and their families."
— *Doody's Health Sciences Book Review Journal, Sep-Oct '02*

"Recommended reference source."
— *Booklist, American Library Association, Sep '02*

"Highly recommended for academic and medical reference collections."
— *Library Bookwatch, Sep '02*

■

# Kidney & Urinary Tract Diseases & Disorders Sourcebook

*SEE Urinary Tract & Kidney Diseases & Disorders Sourcebook*

■

# Learning Disabilities Sourcebook, 2nd Edition

*Basic Consumer Health Information about Learning Disabilities, Including Dyslexia, Developmental Speech and Language Disabilities, Non-Verbal Learning Disorders, Developmental Arithmetic Disorder, Developmental Writing Disorder, and Other Conditions That Impede Learning Such as Attention Deficit/Hyperactivity Disorder, Brain Injury, Hearing Impairment, Klinefelter Syndrome, Dyspraxia, and Tourette's Syndrome*

*Along with Facts about Educational Issues and Assistive Technology, Coping Strategies, a Glossary of Related Terms, and Resources for Further Help and Information*

Edited by Dawn D. Matthews. 621 pages. 2003. 978-0-7808-0626-9.

"The second edition of Learning Disabilities Sourcebook far surpasses the earlier edition in that it is more focused on information that will be useful as a consumer health resource."
— *American Reference Books Annual, 2004*

"Teachers as well as consumers will find this an essential guide to understanding various syndromes and their latest treatments. [An] invaluable reference for public and school library collections alike."
— *Library Bookwatch, Apr '03*

Named "Outstanding Reference Book of 1999."
— *New York Public Library, Feb '00*

"An excellent candidate for inclusion in a public library reference section. It's a great source of information. Teachers will also find the book useful. Definitely worth reading."
— *Journal of Adolescent & Adult Literacy, Feb 2000*

"Readable . . . provides a solid base of information regarding successful techniques used with individuals who have learning disabilities, as well as practical suggestions for educators and family members. Clear language, concise descriptions, and pertinent information for contacting multiple resources add to the strength of this book as a useful tool." — *Choice, Association of College & Research Libraries, Feb '99*

"Recommended reference source."
— *Booklist, American Library Association, Sep '98*

"A useful resource for libraries and for those who don't have the time to identify and locate the individual publications." — *Disability Resources Monthly, Sep '98*

■

# Leukemia Sourcebook

*Basic Consumer Health Information about Adult and Childhood Leukemias, Including Acute Lymphocytic Leukemia (ALL), Chronic Lymphocytic Leukemia (CLL), Acute Myelogenous Leukemia (AML), Chronic Myelogenous Leukemia (CML), and Hairy Cell Leukemia, and Treatments Such as Chemotherapy, Radiation Therapy, Peripheral Blood Stem Cell and Marrow Transplantation, and Immunotherapy*

*Along with Tips for Life During and After Treatment, a Glossary, and Directories of Additional Resources*

Edited by Joyce Brennfleck Shannon. 587 pages. 2003. 978-0-7808-0627-6.

"Unlike other medical books for the layperson, . . . the language does not talk down to the reader. . . . This volume is highly recommended for all libraries."
— *American Reference Books Annual, 2004*

". . . a fine title which ranges from diagnosis to alternative treatments, staging, and tips for life during and after diagnosis." — *The Bookwatch, Dec '03*

# Liver Disorders Sourcebook

*Basic Consumer Health Information about the Liver and How It Works; Liver Diseases, Including Cancer, Cirrhosis, Hepatitis, and Toxic and Drug Related Diseases; Tips for Maintaining a Healthy Liver; Laboratory Tests, Radiology Tests, and Facts about Liver Transplantation*

*Along with a Section on Support Groups, a Glossary, and Resource Listings*

Edited by Joyce Brennfleck Shannon. 591 pages. 2000. 978-0-7808-0383-1.

**"A valuable resource."**
*—American Reference Books Annual, 2001*

**"This title is recommended for health sciences and public libraries with consumer health collections."**
*—E-Streams, Oct '00*

**"Recommended reference source."**
*—Booklist, American Library Association, Jun '00*

■

# Lung Disorders Sourcebook

*Basic Consumer Health Information about Emphysema, Pneumonia, Tuberculosis, Asthma, Cystic Fibrosis, and Other Lung Disorders, Including Facts about Diagnostic Procedures, Treatment Strategies, Disease Prevention Efforts, and Such Risk Factors as Smoking, Air Pollution, and Exposure to Asbestos, Radon, and Other Agents*

*Along with a Glossary and Resources for Additional Help and Information*

Edited by Dawn D. Matthews. 678 pages. 2002. 978-0-7808-0339-8.

**"This title is a great addition for public and school libraries because it provides concise health information on the lungs."**
*—American Reference Books Annual, 2003*

**"Highly recommended for academic and medical reference collections."** *—Library Bookwatch, Sep '02*

**SEE ALSO** *Respiratory Diseases & Disorders Sourcebook*

■

# Medical Tests Sourcebook, 2nd Edition

*Basic Consumer Health Information about Medical Tests, Including Age-Specific Health Tests, Important Health Screenings and Exams, Home-Use Tests, Blood and Specimen Tests, Electrical Tests, Scope Tests, Genetic Testing, and Imaging Tests, Such as X-Rays, Ultrasound, Computed Tomography, Magnetic Resonance Imaging, Angiography, and Nuclear Medicine*

*Along with a Glossary and Directory of Additional Resources*

Edited by Joyce Brennfleck Shannon. 654 pages. 2004. 978-0-7808-0670-2.

**"Recommended for hospital and health sciences**

libraries with consumer health collections."**
*—E-Streams, Mar '00*

**"This is an overall excellent reference with a wealth of general knowledge that may aid those who are reluctant to get vital tests performed."**
*—Today's Librarian, Jan '00*

**"A valuable reference guide."**
*—American Reference Books Annual, 2000*

■

# Men's Health Concerns Sourcebook, 2nd Edition

*Basic Consumer Health Information about the Medical and Mental Concerns of Men, Including Theories about the Shorter Male Lifespan, the Leading Causes of Death and Disability, Physical Concerns of Special Significance to Men, Reproductive and Sexual Concerns, Sexually Transmitted Diseases, Men's Mental and Emotional Health, and Lifestyle Choices That Affect Wellness, Such as Nutrition, Fitness, and Substance Use*

*Along with a Glossary of Related Terms and a Directory of Organizational Resources in Men's Health*

Edited by Robert Aquinas McNally. 644 pages. 2004. 978-0-7808-0671-9.

**"A very accessible reference for non-specialist general readers and consumers."** *—The Bookwatch, Jun '04*

**"This comprehensive resource and the series are highly recommended."**
*—American Reference Books Annual, 2000*

**"Recommended reference source."**
*—Booklist, American Library Association, Dec '98*

■

# Mental Health Disorders Sourcebook, 3rd Edition

*Basic Consumer Health Information about Mental and Emotional Health and Mental Illness, Including Facts about Depression, Bipolar Disorder, and Other Mood Disorders, Phobias, Post-Traumatic Stress Disorder (PTSD), Obsessive-Compulsive Disorder, and Other Anxiety Disorders, Impulse Control Disorders, Eating Disorders, Personality Disorders, and Psychotic Disorders, Including Schizophrenia and Dissociative Disorders*

*Along with Statistical Information, a Special Section Concerning Mental Health Issues in Children and Adolescents, a Glossary, and Directories of Resources for Additional Help and Information*

Edited by Karen Bellenir. 661 pages. 2005. 978-0-7808-0747-1.

**"Recommended for public libraries and academic libraries with an undergraduate program in psychology."**
*—American Reference Books Annual, 2006*

**"Recommended reference source."**
*—Booklist, American Library Association, Jun '00*

## Mental Retardation Sourcebook

*Basic Consumer Health Information about Mental Retardation and Its Causes, Including Down Syndrome, Fetal Alcohol Syndrome, Fragile X Syndrome, Genetic Conditions, Injury, and Environmental Sources*

*Along with Preventive Strategies, Parenting Issues, Educational Implications, Health Care Needs, Employment and Economic Matters, Legal Issues, a Glossary, and a Resource Listing for Additional Help and Information*

Edited by Joyce Brennfleck Shannon. 642 pages. 2000. 978-0-7808-0377-0.

**"Public libraries will find the book useful for reference and as a beginning research point for students, parents, and caregivers."**
*— American Reference Books Annual, 2001*

**"The strength of this work is that it compiles many basic fact sheets and addresses for further information in one volume. It is intended and suitable for the general public. This sourcebook is relevant to any collection providing health information to the general public."**
*— E-Streams, Nov '00*

**"From preventing retardation to parenting and family challenges, this covers health, social and legal issues and will prove an invaluable overview."**
*— Reviewer's Bookwatch, Jul '00*

■

## Movement Disorders Sourcebook

*Basic Consumer Health Information about Neurological Movement Disorders, Including Essential Tremor, Parkinson's Disease, Dystonia, Cerebral Palsy, Huntington's Disease, Myasthenia Gravis, Multiple Sclerosis, and Other Early-Onset and Adult-Onset Movement Disorders, Their Symptoms and Causes, Diagnostic Tests, and Treatments*

*Along with Mobility and Assistive Technology Information, a Glossary, and a Directory of Additional Resources*

Edited by Joyce Brennfleck Shannon. 655 pages. 2003. 978-0-7808-0628-3.

**". . . a good resource for consumers and recommended for public, community college and undergraduate libraries."** *— American Reference Books Annual, 2004*

■

## Muscular Dystrophy Sourcebook

*Basic Consumer Health Information about Congenital, Childhood-Onset, and Adult-Onset Forms of Muscular Dystrophy, Such as Duchenne, Becker, Emery-Dreifuss, Distal, Limb-Girdle, Facioscapulohumeral (FSHD), Myotonic, and Ophthalmoplegic Muscular Dystrophies, Including Facts about Diagnostic Tests, Medical and Physical Therapies, Management of Co-Occurring Conditions, and Parenting Guidelines*

*Along with Practical Tips for Home Care, a Glossary, and Directories of Additional Resources*

Edited by Joyce Brennfleck Shannon. 577 pages. 2004. 978-0-7808-0676-4.

**"This book is highly recommended for public and academic libraries as well as health care offices that support the information needs of patients and their families."**
*— E-Streams, Apr '05*

**"Excellent reference."** *— The Bookwatch, Jan '05*

■

## Obesity Sourcebook

*Basic Consumer Health Information about Diseases and Other Problems Associated with Obesity, and Including Facts about Risk Factors, Prevention Issues, and Management Approaches*

*Along with Statistical and Demographic Data, Information about Special Populations, Research Updates, a Glossary, and Source Listings for Further Help and Information*

Edited by Wilma Caldwell and Chad T. Kimball. 376 pages. 2001. 978-0-7808-0333-6.

**"The book synthesizes the reliable medical literature on obesity into one easy-to-read and useful resource for the general public."**
*— American Reference Books Annual, 2002*

**"This is a very useful resource book for the lay public."**
*— Doody's Review Service, Nov '01*

**"Well suited for the health reference collection of a public library or an academic health science library that serves the general population."** *— E-Streams, Sep '01*

**"Recommended reference source."**
*— Booklist, American Library Association, Apr '01*

**"Recommended pick both for specialty health library collections and any general consumer health reference collection."** *— The Bookwatch, Apr '01*

■

## Oral Health Sourcebook

*SEE Dental Care & Oral Health Sourcebook*

■

## Osteoporosis Sourcebook

*Basic Consumer Health Information about Primary and Secondary Osteoporosis and Juvenile Osteoporosis and Related Conditions, Including Fibrous Dysplasia, Gaucher Disease, Hyperthyroidism, Hypophosphatasia, Myeloma, Osteopetrosis, Osteogenesis Imperfecta, and Paget's Disease*

*Along with Information about Risk Factors, Treatments, Traditional and Non-Traditional Pain Management, a Glossary of Related Terms, and a Directory of Resources*

Edited by Allan R. Cook. 584 pages. 2001. 978-0-7808-0239-1.

**"This would be a book to be kept in a staff or patient library. The targeted audience is the layperson, but the therapist who needs a quick bit of information on a particular topic will also find the book useful."**
*— Physical Therapy, Jan '02*

"This resource is recommended as a great reference source for public, health, and academic libraries, and is another triumph for the editors of Omnigraphics."
— *American Reference Books Annual, 2002*

"Recommended for all public libraries and general health collections, especially those supporting patient education or consumer health programs."
— *E-Streams, Nov '01*

"Will prove valuable to any library seeking to maintain a current, comprehensive reference collection of health resources. . . . From prevention to treatment and associated conditions, this provides an excellent survey."
— *The Bookwatch, Aug '01*

"Recommended reference source."
— *Booklist, American Library Association, Jul '01*

**SEE ALSO** *Healthy Aging Sourcebook, Physical & Mental Issues in Aging Sourcebook, Women's Health Concerns Sourcebook*

■

## Pain Sourcebook, 2nd Edition

*Basic Consumer Health Information about Specific Forms of Acute and Chronic Pain, Including Muscle and Skeletal Pain, Nerve Pain, Cancer Pain, and Disorders Characterized by Pain, Such as Fibromyalgia, Shingles, Angina, Arthritis, and Headaches*

*Along with Information about Pain Medications and Management Techniques, Complementary and Alternative Pain Relief Options, Tips for People Living with Chronic Pain, a Glossary, and a Directory of Sources for Further Information*

Edited by Karen Bellenir. 670 pages. 2002. 978-0-7808-0612-2.

"A source of valuable information. . . . This book offers help to nonmedical people who need information about pain and pain management. It is also an excellent reference for those who participate in patient education."
— *Doody's Review Service, Sep '02*

"Highly recommended for academic and medical reference collections." — *Library Bookwatch, Sep '02*

"The text is readable, easily understood, and well indexed. This excellent volume belongs in all patient education libraries, consumer health sections of public libraries, and many personal collections."
— *American Reference Books Annual, 1999*

"The information is basic in terms of scholarship and is appropriate for general readers. Written in journalistic style . . . intended for non-professionals. Quite thorough in its coverage of different pain conditions and summarizes the latest clinical information regarding pain treatment." — *Choice, Association of College and Research Libraries, Jun '98*

"Recommended reference source."
— *Booklist, American Library Association, Mar '98*

■

## Pediatric Cancer Sourcebook

*Basic Consumer Health Information about Leukemias, Brain Tumors, Sarcomas, Lymphomas, and Other Cancers in Infants, Children, and Adolescents, Including Descriptions of Cancers, Treatments, and Coping Strategies*

*Along with Suggestions for Parents, Caregivers, and Concerned Relatives, a Glossary of Cancer Terms, and Resource Listings*

Edited by Edward J. Prucha. 587 pages. 1999. 978-0-7808-0245-2.

"An excellent source of information. Recommended for public, hospital, and health science libraries with consumer health collections." — *E-Streams, Jun '00*

"Recommended reference source."
— *Booklist, American Library Association, Feb '00*

"A valuable addition to all libraries specializing in health services and many public libraries."
— *American Reference Books Annual, 2000*

**SEE ALSO** *Childhood Diseases & Disorders Sourcebook, Healthy Children Sourcebook*

■

## Physical & Mental Issues in Aging Sourcebook

*Basic Consumer Health Information on Physical and Mental Disorders Associated with the Aging Process, Including Concerns about Cardiovascular Disease, Pulmonary Disease, Oral Health, Digestive Disorders, Musculoskeletal and Skin Disorders, Metabolic Changes, Sexual and Reproductive Issues, and Changes in Vision, Hearing, and Other Senses*

*Along with Data about Longevity and Causes of Death, Information on Acute and Chronic Pain, Descriptions of Mental Concerns, a Glossary of Terms, and Resource Listings for Additional Help*

Edited by Jenifer Swanson. 660 pages. 1999. 978-0-7808-0233-9.

"This is a treasure of health information for the layperson." — *Choice Health Sciences Supplement, Association of College & Research Libraries, May '00*

"Recommended for public libraries."
— *American Reference Books Annual, 2000*

"Recommended reference source."
— *Booklist, American Library Association, Oct '99*

**SEE ALSO** *Healthy Aging Sourcebook*

■

## Podiatry Sourcebook, 2nd Edition

*Basic Consumer Health Information about Disorders, Diseases, Deformities, and Injuries that Affect the Foot and Ankle, Including Sprains, Corns, Calluses, Bunions, Plantar Warts, Plantar Fasciitis, Neuromas, Clubfoot, Flat Feet, Achilles Tendonitis, and Much More*

*Along with Information about Selecting a Foot Care Specialist, Foot Fitness, Shoes and Socks, Diagnostic Tests and Corrective Procedures, Financial Assistance for Corrective Devices, a Glossary of Related Terms, and a Directory of Resources for Additional Help and Information*

Edited by Ivy L. Alexander. 543 pages. 2007. 978-0-7808-0944-4.

"**Recommended reference source.**"
*— Booklist, American Library Association, Feb '02*

"**There is a lot of information presented here on a topic that is usually only covered sparingly in most larger comprehensive medical encyclopedias.**"
*— American Reference Books Annual, 2002*

■

# Pregnancy & Birth Sourcebook, 2nd Edition

*Basic Consumer Health Information about Conception and Pregnancy, Including Facts about Fertility, Infertility, Pregnancy Symptoms and Complications, Fetal Growth and Development, Labor, Delivery, and the Postpartum Period, as Well as Information about Maintaining Health and Wellness during Pregnancy and Caring for a Newborn*

*Along with Information about Public Health Assistance for Low-Income Pregnant Women, a Glossary, and Directories of Agencies and Organizations Providing Help and Support*

Edited by Amy L. Sutton. 626 pages. 2004. 978-0-7808-0672-6.

"**Will appeal to public and school reference collections strong in medicine and women's health. . . . Deserves a spot on any medical reference shelf.**"
*— The Bookwatch, Jul '04*

"**A well-organized handbook. Recommended.**"
*— Choice, Association of College & Research Libraries, Apr '98*

"**Recommended reference source.**"
*— Booklist, American Library Association, Mar '98*

"**Recommended for public libraries.**"
*— American Reference Books Annual, 1998*

***SEE ALSO*** *Breastfeeding Sourcebook, Congenital Disorders Sourcebook, Family Planning Sourcebook*

■

# Prostate & Urological Disorders Sourcebook

*Basic Consumer Health Information about Urogenital and Sexual Disorders in Men, Including Prostate and Other Andrological Cancers, Prostatitis, Benign Prostatic Hyperplasia, Testicular and Penile Trauma, Cryptorchidism, Peyronie Disease, Erectile Dysfunction, and Male Factor Infertility, and Facts about Commonly Used Tests and Procedures, Such as Prostatectomy, Vasectomy, Vasectomy Reversal, Penile Implants, and Semen Analysis*

*Along with a Glossary of Andrological Terms and a Directory of Resources for Additional Information*

Edited by Karen Bellenir. 631 pages. 2005. 978-0-7808-0797-6.

# Prostate Cancer Sourcebook

*Basic Consumer Health Information about Prostate Cancer, Including Information about the Associated Risk Factors, Detection, Diagnosis, and Treatment of Prostate Cancer*

*Along with Information on Non-Malignant Prostate Conditions, and Featuring a Section Listing Support and Treatment Centers and a Glossary of Related Terms*

Edited by Dawn D. Matthews. 358 pages. 2001. 978-0-7808-0324-4.

"**Recommended reference source.**"
*— Booklist, American Library Association, Jan '02*

"**A valuable resource for health care consumers seeking information on the subject. . . . All text is written in a clear, easy-to-understand language that avoids technical jargon. Any library that collects consumer health resources would strengthen their collection with the addition of the *Prostate Cancer Sourcebook*.**"
*— American Reference Books Annual, 2002*

***SEE ALSO*** *Men's Health Concerns Sourcebook*

■

# Reconstructive & Cosmetic Surgery Sourcebook

*Basic Consumer Health Information on Cosmetic and Reconstructive Plastic Surgery, Including Statistical Information about Different Surgical Procedures, Things to Consider Prior to Surgery, Plastic Surgery Techniques and Tools, Emotional and Psychological Considerations, and Procedure-Specific Information*

*Along with a Glossary of Terms and a Listing of Resources for Additional Help and Information*

Edited by M. Lisa Weatherford. 374 pages. 2001. 978-0-7808-0214-8.

"**An excellent reference that addresses cosmetic and medically necessary reconstructive surgeries. . . . The style of the prose is calm and reassuring, discussing the many positive outcomes now available due to advances in surgical techniques.**"
*— American Reference Books Annual, 2002*

"**Recommended for health science libraries that are open to the public, as well as hospital libraries that are open to the patients. This book is a good resource for the consumer interested in plastic surgery.**"
*— E-Streams, Dec '01*

"**Recommended reference source.**"
*— Booklist, American Library Association, Jul '01*

■

# Rehabilitation Sourcebook

*Basic Consumer Health Information about Rehabilitation for People Recovering from Heart Surgery, Spinal Cord Injury, Stroke, Orthopedic Impairments, Amputation, Pulmonary Impairments, Traumatic Injury, and More, Including Physical Therapy, Occupational Therapy, Speech/Language Therapy, Massage Therapy, Dance Therapy, Art Therapy, and Recreational Therapy*

Along with Information on Assistive and Adaptive Devices, a Glossary, and Resources for Additional Help and Information

Edited by Dawn D. Matthews. 531 pages. 1999. 978-0-7808-0236-0.

"This is an excellent resource for public library reference and health collections."
— American Reference Books Annual, 2001

"Recommended reference source."
— Booklist, American Library Association, May '00

■

# Respiratory Diseases & Disorders Sourcebook

Basic Information about Respiratory Diseases and Disorders, Including Asthma, Cystic Fibrosis, Pneumonia, the Common Cold, Influenza, and Others, Featuring Facts about the Respiratory System, Statistical and Demographic Data, Treatments, Self-Help Management Suggestions, and Current Research Initiatives

Edited by Allan R. Cook and Peter D. Dresser. 771 pages. 1995. 978-0-7808-0037-3.

"Designed for the layperson and for patients and their families coping with respiratory illness. . . . an extensive array of information on diagnosis, treatment, management, and prevention of respiratory illnesses for the general reader." — Choice, Association of College & Research Libraries, Jun '96

"A highly recommended text for all collections. It is a comforting reminder of the power of knowledge that good books carry between their covers."
— Academic Library Book Review, Spring '96

"A comprehensive collection of authoritative information presented in a nontechnical, humanitarian style for patients, families, and caregivers."
— Association of Operating Room Nurses, Sep/Oct '95

SEE ALSO Lung Disorders Sourcebook

■

# Sexually Transmitted Diseases Sourcebook, 3rd Edition

Basic Consumer Health Information about Chlamydial Infections, Gonorrhea, Hepatitis, Herpes, HIV/AIDS, Human Papillomavirus, Pubic Lice, Scabies, Syphilis, Trichomoniasis, Vaginal Infections, and Other Sexually Transmitted Diseases, Including Facts about Risk Factors, Symptoms, Diagnosis, Treatment, and the Prevention of Sexually Transmitted Infections

Along with Updates on Current Research Initiatives, a Glossary of Related Terms, and Resources for Additional Help and Information

Edited by Amy L. Sutton. 629 pages. 2006. 978-0-7808-0824-9.

"Recommended for consumer health collections in public libraries, and secondary school and community college libraries."
— American Reference Books Annual, 2002

"Every school and public library should have a copy of this comprehensive and user-friendly reference book."
— Choice, Association of College & Research Libraries, Sep '01

"This is a highly recommended book. This is an especially important book for all school and public libraries."
— AIDS Book Review Journal, Jul-Aug '01

"Recommended reference source."
— Booklist, American Library Association, Apr '01

■

# Sleep Disorders Sourcebook, 2nd Edition

Basic Consumer Health Information about Sleep and Sleep Disorders, Including Insomnia, Sleep Apnea, Restless Legs Syndrome, Narcolepsy, Parasomnias, and Other Health Problems That Affect Sleep, Plus Facts about Diagnostic Procedures, Treatment Strategies, Sleep Medications, and Tips for Improving Sleep Quality

Along with a Glossary of Related Terms and Resources for Additional Help and Information

Edited by Amy L. Sutton. 567 pages. 2005. 978-0-7808-0743-3.

"This book will be useful for just about everybody, especially the 40 million Americans with sleep disorders."
— American Reference Books Annual, 2006

"Recommended for public libraries and libraries supporting health care professionals." — E-Streams, Sep '05

". . . key medical library acquisition."
— The Bookwatch, Jun '05

■

# Smoking Concerns Sourcebook

Basic Consumer Health Information about Nicotine Addiction and Smoking Cessation, Featuring Facts about the Health Effects of Tobacco Use, Including Lung and Other Cancers, Heart Disease, Stroke, and Respiratory Disorders, Such as Emphysema and Chronic Bronchitis

Along with Information about Smoking Prevention Programs, Suggestions for Achieving and Maintaining a Smoke-Free Lifestyle, Statistics about Tobacco Use, Reports on Current Research Initiatives, a Glossary of Related Terms, and Directories of Resources for Additional Help and Information

Edited by Karen Bellenir. 621 pages. 2004. 978-0-7808-0323-7.

"Provides everything needed for the student or general reader seeking practical details on the effects of tobacco use." — The Bookwatch, Mar '05

"Public libraries and consumer health care libraries will find this work useful."
— American Reference Books Annual, 2005

# Sports Injuries Sourcebook, 3rd Edition

*Basic Consumer Health Information about Sprains and Strains, Fractures, Growth Plate Injuries, Overtraining Injuries, and Injuries to the Head, Face, Shoulders, Elbows, Hands, Spinal Column, Knees, Ankles, and Feet, and with Facts about Heat-Related Illness, Steroids and Sport Supplements, Protective Equipment, Diagnostic Procedures, Treatment Options, and Rehabilitation*

*Along with a Glossary of Related Terms and a Directory of Resources for Additional Help and Information*

Edited by Sandra J. Judd. 651 pages. 2007. 978-0-7808-0949-9.

"This is an excellent reference for consumers and it is recommended for public, community college, and undergraduate libraries."
— *American Reference Books Annual, 2003*

"Recommended reference source."
— *Booklist, American Library Association, Feb '03*

■

# Stress-Related Disorders Sourcebook

*Basic Consumer Health Information about Stress and Stress-Related Disorders, Including Stress Origins and Signals, Environmental Stress at Work and Home, Mental and Emotional Stress Associated with Depression, Post-Traumatic Stress Disorder, Panic Disorder, Suicide, and the Physical Effects of Stress on the Cardiovascular, Immune, and Nervous Systems*

*Along with Stress Management Techniques, a Glossary, and a Listing of Additional Resources*

Edited by Joyce Brennfleck Shannon. 610 pages. 2002. 978-0-7808-0560-6.

"Well written for a general readership, the *Stress-Related Disorders Sourcebook* is a useful addition to the health reference literature."
— *American Reference Books Annual, 2003*

"I am impressed by the amount of information. It offers a thorough overview of the causes and consequences of stress for the layperson. . . . A well-done and thorough reference guide for professionals and nonprofessionals alike." — *Doody's Review Service, Dec '02*

■

# Stroke Sourcebook

*Basic Consumer Health Information about Stroke, Including Ischemic, Hemorrhagic, Transient Ischemic Attack (TIA), and Pediatric Stroke, Stroke Triggers and Risks, Diagnostic Tests, Treatments, and Rehabilitation Information*

*Along with Stroke Prevention Guidelines, Legal and Financial Information, a Glossary, and a Directory of Additional Resources*

Edited by Joyce Brennfleck Shannon. 606 pages. 2003. 978-0-7808-0630-6.

"This volume is highly recommended and should be in every medical, hospital, and public library."
— *American Reference Books Annual, 2004*

"Highly recommended for the amount and variety of topics and information covered." — *Choice, Nov '03*

■

# Surgery Sourcebook

*Basic Consumer Health Information about Inpatient and Outpatient Surgeries, Including Cardiac, Vascular, Orthopedic, Ocular, Reconstructive, Cosmetic, Gynecologic, and Ear, Nose, and Throat Procedures and More*

*Along with Information about Operating Room Policies and Instruments, Laser Surgery Techniques, Hospital Errors, Statistical Data, a Glossary, and Listings of Sources for Further Help and Information*

Edited by Annemarie S. Muth and Karen Bellenir. 596 pages. 2002. 978-0-7808-0380-0.

"Large public libraries and medical libraries would benefit from this material in their reference collections."
— *American Reference Books Annual, 2004*

"Invaluable reference for public and school library collections alike." — *Library Bookwatch, Apr '03*

■

# Thyroid Disorders Sourcebook

*Basic Consumer Health Information about Disorders of the Thyroid and Parathyroid Glands, Including Hypothyroidism, Hyperthyroidism, Graves Disease, Hashimoto Thyroiditis, Thyroid Cancer, and Parathyroid Disorders, Featuring Facts about Symptoms, Risk Factors, Tests, and Treatments*

*Along with Information about the Effects of Thyroid Imbalance on Other Body Systems, Environmental Factors That Affect the Thyroid Gland, a Glossary, and a Directory of Additional Resources*

Edited by Joyce Brennfleck Shannon. 599 pages. 2005. 978-0-7808-0745-7.

"Recommended for consumer health collections."
— *American Reference Books Annual, 2006*

"Highly recommended pick for basic consumer health reference holdings at all levels."
— *The Bookwatch, Aug '05*

■

# Transplantation Sourcebook

*Basic Consumer Health Information about Organ and Tissue Transplantation, Including Physical and Financial Preparations, Procedures and Issues Relating to Specific Solid Organ and Tissue Transplants, Rehabilitation, Pediatric Transplant Information, the Future of Transplantation, and Organ and Tissue Donation*

*Along with a Glossary and Listings of Additional Resources*

Edited by Joyce Brennfleck Shannon. 628 pages. 2002. 978-0-7808-0322-0.

"Along with these advances [in transplantation technology] have come a number of daunting questions for potential transplant patients, their families, and their health care providers. This reference text is the best single tool to address many of these questions. . . . It will be a much-needed addition to the reference collections in health care, academic, and large public libraries."
— *American Reference Books Annual, 2003*

"Recommended for libraries with an interest in offering consumer health information." — *E-Streams, Jul '02*

"This is a unique and valuable resource for patients facing transplantation and their families."
— *Doody's Review Service, Jun '02*

## Traveler's Health Sourcebook

*Basic Consumer Health Information for Travelers, Including Physical and Medical Preparations, Transportation Health and Safety, Essential Information about Food and Water, Sun Exposure, Insect and Snake Bites, Camping and Wilderness Medicine, and Travel with Physical or Medical Disabilities*

*Along with International Travel Tips, Vaccination Recommendations, Geographical Health Issues, Disease Risks, a Glossary, and a Listing of Additional Resources*

Edited by Joyce Brennfleck Shannon. 613 pages. 2000. 978-0-7808-0384-8.

"Recommended reference source."
— *Booklist, American Library Association, Feb '01*

"This book is recommended for any public library, any travel collection, and especially any collection for the physically disabled."
— *American Reference Books Annual, 2001*

*SEE ALSO* Worldwide Health Sourcebook

## Urinary Tract & Kidney Diseases & Disorders Sourcebook, 2nd Edition

*Basic Consumer Health Information about the Urinary System, Including the Bladder, Urethra, Ureters, and Kidneys, with Facts about Urinary Tract Infections, Incontinence, Congenital Disorders, Kidney Stones, Cancers of the Urinary Tract and Kidneys, Kidney Failure, Dialysis, and Kidney Transplantation*

*Along with Statistical and Demographic Information, Reports on Current Research in Kidney and Urologic Health, a Summary of Commonly Used Diagnostic Tests, a Glossary of Related Terms, and a Directory of Resources for Additional Help and Information*

Edited by Ivy L. Alexander. 649 pages. 2005. 978-0-7808-0750-1.

"A good choice for a consumer health information library or for a medical library needing information to refer to their patients."
— *American Reference Books Annual, 2006*

## Vegetarian Sourcebook

*Basic Consumer Health Information about Vegetarian Diets, Lifestyle, and Philosophy, Including Definitions of Vegetarianism and Veganism, Tips about Adopting Vegetarianism, Creating a Vegetarian Pantry, and Meeting Nutritional Needs of Vegetarians, with Facts Regarding Vegetarianism's Effect on Pregnant and Lactating Women, Children, Athletes, and Senior Citizens*

*Along with a Glossary of Commonly Used Vegetarian Terms and Resources for Additional Help and Information*

Edited by Chad T. Kimball. 360 pages. 2002. 978-0-7808-0439-5.

"Organizes into one concise volume the answers to the most common questions concerning vegetarian diets and lifestyles. This title is recommended for public and secondary school libraries." — *E-Streams, Apr '03*

"Invaluable reference for public and school library collections alike." — *Library Bookwatch, Apr '03*

"The articles in this volume are easy to read and come from authoritative sources. The book does not necessarily support the vegetarian diet but instead provides the pros and cons of this important decision. The Vegetarian Sourcebook is recommended for public libraries and consumer health libraries."
— *American Reference Books Annual, 2003*

*SEE ALSO* Diet & Nutrition Sourcebook

## Women's Health Concerns Sourcebook, 2nd Edition

*Basic Consumer Health Information about the Medical and Mental Concerns of Women, Including Maintaining Health and Wellness, Gynecological Concerns, Breast Health, Sexuality and Reproductive Issues, Menopause, Cancer in Women, Leading Causes of Death and Disability among Women, Physical Concerns of Special Significance to Women, and Women's Mental and Emotional Health*

*Along with a Glossary of Related Terms and Directories of Resources for Additional Help and Information*

Edited by Amy L. Sutton. 746 pages. 2004. 978-0-7808-0673-3.

"This is a useful reference book, which makes the reader knowledgeable about several issues that concern women's health. It is recommended for public libraries and home library collections." — *E-Streams, May '05*

"A useful addition to public and consumer health library collections."
— *American Reference Books Annual, 2005*

"A highly recommended title."
— *The Bookwatch, May '04*

"Handy compilation. There is an impressive range of diseases, devices, disorders, procedures, and other physical and emotional issues covered . . . well organized, illustrated, and indexed." — *Choice, Association of College & Research Libraries, Jan '98*

SEE ALSO *Breast Cancer Sourcebook, Cancer Sourcebook for Women, Healthy Heart Sourcebook for Women, Osteoporosis Sourcebook*

# Workplace Health & Safety Sourcebook

*Basic Consumer Health Information about Workplace Health and Safety, Including the Effect of Workplace Hazards on the Lungs, Skin, Heart, Ears, Eyes, Brain, Reproductive Organs, Musculoskeletal System, and Other Organs and Body Parts*

*Along with Information about Occupational Cancer, Personal Protective Equipment, Toxic and Hazardous Chemicals, Child Labor, Stress, and Workplace Violence*

Edited by Chad T. Kimball. 626 pages. 2000. 978-0-7808-0231-5.

"As a reference for the general public, this would be useful in any library." — *E-Streams, Jun '01*

"Provides helpful information for primary care physicians and other caregivers interested in occupational medicine. . . . General readers; professionals."
— *Choice, Association of College & Research Libraries, May '01*

"Recommended reference source."
— *Booklist, American Library Association, Feb '01*

"Highly recommended." — *The Bookwatch, Jan '01*

# Worldwide Health Sourcebook

*Basic Information about Global Health Issues, Including Malnutrition, Reproductive Health, Disease Dispersion and Prevention, Emerging Diseases, Risky Health Behaviors, and the Leading Causes of Death*

*Along with Global Health Concerns for Children, Women, and the Elderly, Mental Health Issues, Research and Technology Advancements, and Economic, Environmental, and Political Health Implications, a Glossary, and a Resource Listing for Additional Help and Information*

Edited by Joyce Brennfleck Shannon. 614 pages. 2001. 978-0-7808-0330-5.

"Named an Outstanding Academic Title."
— *Choice, Association of College & Research Libraries, Jan '02*

"Yet another handy but also unique compilation in the extensive *Health Reference Series,* this is a useful work because many of the international publications reprinted or excerpted are not readily available. Highly recommended." — *Choice, Association of College & Research Libraries, Nov '01*

"Recommended reference source."
— *Booklist, American Library Association, Oct '01*

SEE ALSO *Traveler's Health Sourcebook*

507

# Teen Health Series
## Helping Young Adults Understand, Manage, and Avoid Serious Illness

List price $65 per volume. **School and library price $58 per volume.**

## Alcohol Information for Teens
### Health Tips about Alcohol and Alcoholism

*Including Facts about Underage Drinking, Preventing Teen Alcohol Use, Alcohol's Effects on the Brain and the Body, Alcohol Abuse Treatment, Help for Children of Alcoholics, and More*

Edited by Joyce Brennfleck Shannon. 370 pages. 2005. 978-0-7808-0741-9.

**"Boxed facts and tips add visual interest to the well-researched and clearly written text."**
— *Curriculum Connection, Apr '06*

■

## Allergy Information for Teens
### Health Tips about Allergic Reactions Such as Anaphylaxis, Respiratory Problems, and Rashes

*Including Facts about Identifying and Managing Allergies to Food, Pollen, Mold, Animals, Chemicals, Drugs, and Other Substances*

Edited by Karen Bellenir. 410 pages. 2006. 978-0-7808-0799-0.

■

## Asthma Information for Teens
### Health Tips about Managing Asthma and Related Concerns

*Including Facts about Asthma Causes, Triggers, Symptoms, Diagnosis, and Treatment*

Edited by Karen Bellenir. 386 pages. 2005. 978-0-7808-0770-9.

**"Highly recommended for medical libraries, public school libraries, and public libraries."**
— *American Reference Books Annual, 2006*

**"It is so clearly written and well organized that even hesitant readers will be able to find the facts they need, whether for reports or personal information. . . . A succinct but complete resource."**
— *School Library Journal, Sep '05*

■

## Body Information for Teens
### Health Tips about Maintaining Well-Being for a Lifetime

*Including Facts about the Development and Functioning of the Body's Systems, Organs, and Structures and the Health Impact of Lifestyle Choices*

Edited by Sandra Augustyn Lawton. 458 pages. 2007. 978-0-7808-0443-2.

■

## Cancer Information for Teens
### Health Tips about Cancer Awareness, Prevention, Diagnosis, and Treatment

*Including Facts about Frequently Occurring Cancers, Cancer Risk Factors, and Coping Strategies for Teens Fighting Cancer or Dealing with Cancer in Friends or Family Members*

Edited by Wilma R. Caldwell. 428 pages. 2004. 978-0-7808-0678-8.

**"Recommended for school libraries, or consumer libraries that see a lot of use by teens."**
— *E-Streams, May '05*

**"A valuable educational tool."**
— *American Reference Books Annual, 2005*

**"Young adults and their parents alike will find this new addition to the *Teen Health Series* an important reference to cancer in teens."**
— *Children's Bookwatch, Feb '05*

■

## Complementary and Alternative Medicine Information for Teens
### Health Tips about Non-Traditional and Non-Western Medical Practices

*Including Information about Acupuncture, Chiropractic Medicine, Dietary and Herbal Supplements, Hypnosis, Massage Therapy, Prayer and Spirituality, Reflexology, Yoga, and More*

Edited by Sandra Augustyn Lawton. 405 pages. 2006. 978-0-7808-0966-6.

■

## Diabetes Information for Teens
### Health Tips about Managing Diabetes and Preventing Related Complications

*Including Information about Insulin, Glucose Control, Healthy Eating, Physical Activity, and Learning to Live with Diabetes*

Edited by Sandra Augustyn Lawton. 410 pages. 2006. 978-0-7808-0811-9.

# Diet Information for Teens, 2nd Edition

### Health Tips about Diet and Nutrition

*Including Facts about Dietary Guidelines, Food Groups, Nutrients, Healthy Meals, Snacks, Weight Control, Medical Concerns Related to Diet, and More*

Edited by Karen Bellenir. 432 pages. 2006. 978-0-7808-0820-1.

"Full of helpful insights and facts throughout the book. . . . An excellent resource to be placed in public libraries or even in personal collections."
— *American Reference Books Annual, 2002*

"Recommended for middle and high school libraries and media centers as well as academic libraries that educate future teachers of teenagers. It is also a suitable addition to health science libraries that serve patrons who are interested in teen health promotion and education."
— *E-Streams, Oct '01*

"This comprehensive book would be beneficial to collections that need information about nutrition, dietary guidelines, meal planning, and weight control. . . . This reference is so easy to use that its purchase is recommended."
— *The Book Report, Sep-Oct '01*

"This book is written in an easy to understand format describing issues that many teens face every day, and then provides thoughtful explanations so that teens can make informed decisions. This is an interesting book that provides important facts and information for today's teens."
— *Doody's Health Sciences Book Review Journal, Jul-Aug '01*

"A comprehensive compendium of diet and nutrition. The information is presented in a straightforward, plain-spoken manner. This title will be useful to those working on reports on a variety of topics, as well as to general readers concerned about their dietary health."
— *School Library Journal, Jun '01*

# Drug Information for Teens, 2nd Edition

### Health Tips about the Physical and Mental Effects of Substance Abuse

*Including Information about Marijuana, Inhalants, Club Drugs, Stimulants, Hallucinogens, Opiates, Prescription and Over-the-Counter Drugs, Herbal Products, Tobacco, Alcohol, and More*

Edited by Sandra Augustyn Lawton. 468 pages. 2006. 978-0-7808-0862-1.

"A clearly written resource for general readers and researchers alike."
— *School Library Journal*

"This book is well-balanced. . . . a must for public and school libraries."
— *VOYA: Voice of Youth Advocates, Dec '03*

"The chapters are quick to make a connection to their teenage reading audience. The prose is straightforward and the book lends itself to spot reading. It should be useful both for practical information and for research, and it is suitable for public and school libraries."
— *American Reference Books Annual, 2003*

"Recommended reference source."
— *Booklist, American Library Association, Feb '03*

"This is an excellent resource for teens and their parents. Education about drugs and substances is key to discouraging teen drug abuse and this book provides this much needed information in a way that is interesting and factual."
— *Doody's Review Service, Dec '02*

# Eating Disorders Information for Teens

### Health Tips about Anorexia, Bulimia, Binge Eating, and Other Eating Disorders

*Including Information on the Causes, Prevention, and Treatment of Eating Disorders, and Such Other Issues as Maintaining Healthy Eating and Exercise Habits*

Edited by Sandra Augustyn Lawton. 337 pages. 2005. 978-0-7808-0783-9.

"An excellent resource for teens and those who work with them."
— *VOYA: Voice of Youth Advocates, Apr '06*

"A welcome addition to high school and undergraduate libraries." — *American Reference Books Annual, 2006*

"This book covers the topic in a lucid manner but delves deeper into every aspect of an eating disorder. A solid addition for any nonfiction or reference collection."
— *School Library Journal, Dec '05*

# Fitness Information for Teens

### Health Tips about Exercise, Physical Well-Being, and Health Maintenance

*Including Facts about Aerobic and Anaerobic Conditioning, Stretching, Body Shape and Body Image, Sports Training, Nutrition, and Activities for Non-Athletes*

Edited by Karen Bellenir. 425 pages. 2004. 978-0-7808-0679-5.

"Another excellent offering from Omnigraphics in their *Teen Health Series*. . . . This book will be a great addition to any public, junior high, senior high, or secondary school library."
— *American Reference Books Annual, 2005*

# Learning Disabilities Information for Teens

### Health Tips about Academic Skills Disorders and Other Disabilities That Affect Learning

*Including Information about Common Signs of Learning Disabilities, School Issues, Learning to Live with a Learning Disability, and Other Related Issues*

Edited by Sandra Augustyn Lawton. 337 pages. 2005. 978-0-7808-0796-9.

"This book provides a wealth of information for any reader interested in the signs, causes, and consequences of learning disabilities, as well as related legal rights and educational interventions. . . . Public and academic libraries should want this title for both students and general readers."

— *American Reference Books Annual, 2006*

■

# Mental Health Information for Teens, 2nd Edition

**Health Tips about Mental Wellness and Mental Illness**

*Including Facts about Mental and Emotional Health, Depression and Other Mood Disorders, Anxiety Disorders, Behavior Disorders, Self-Injury, Psychosis, Schizophrenia, and More*

Edited by Karen Bellenir. 400 pages. 2006. 978-0-7808-0863-8.

"In both language and approach, this user-friendly entry in the *Teen Health Series* is on target for teens needing information on mental health concerns."
— *Booklist, American Library Association, Jan '02*

"Readers will find the material accessible and informative, with the shaded notes, facts, and embedded glossary insets adding appropriately to the already interesting and succinct presentation."
— *School Library Journal, Jan '02*

"This title is highly recommended for any library that serves adolescents and parents/caregivers of adolescents." — *E-Streams, Jan '02*

"Recommended for high school libraries and young adult collections in public libraries. Both health professionals and teenagers will find this book useful."
— *American Reference Books Annual, 2002*

"This is a nice book written to enlighten the society, primarily teenagers, about common teen mental health issues. It is highly recommended to teachers and parents as well as adolescents."
— *Doody's Review Service, Dec '01*

■

# Pregnancy Information for Teens

**Health Tips about Teen Pregnancy and Teen Parenting**

*Including Facts about Prenatal Care, Pregnancy Complications, Labor and Delivery, Postpartum Care, Pregnancy-Related Lifestyle Concerns, and More*

Edited by Robert Aquinas McNally. 425 pages. 2007. 978-0-7808-0984-0.

■

# Sexual Health Information for Teens

**Health Tips about Sexual Development, Human Reproduction, and Sexually Transmitted Diseases**

*Including Facts about Puberty, Reproductive Health, Chlamydia, Human Papillomavirus, Pelvic Inflam-*

*matory Disease, Herpes, AIDS, Contraception, Pregnancy, and More*

Edited by Deborah A. Stanley. 391 pages. 2003. 978-0-7808-0445-6.

"This work should be included in all high school libraries and many larger public libraries. . . . highly recommended."
— *American Reference Books Annual, 2004*

"*Sexual Health* approaches its subject with appropriate seriousness and offers easily accessible advice and information." — *School Library Journal, Feb '04*

# Skin Health Information for Teens

**Health Tips about Dermatological Concerns and Skin Cancer Risks**

*Including Facts about Acne, Warts, Hives, and Other Conditions and Lifestyle Choices, Such as Tanning, Tattooing, and Piercing, That Affect the Skin, Nails, Scalp, and Hair*

Edited by Robert Aquinas McNally. 429 pages. 2003. 978-0-7808-0446-3.

"This volume, as with others in the series, will be a useful addition to school and public library collections." — *American Reference Books Annual, 2004*

"There is no doubt that this reference tool is valuable."
— *VOYA: Voice of Youth Advocates, Feb '04*

"This volume serves as a one-stop source and should be a necessity for any health collection."
— *Library Media Connection*

■

# Sports Injuries Information for Teens

**Health Tips about Sports Injuries and Injury Protection**

*Including Facts about Specific Injuries, Emergency Treatment, Rehabilitation, Sports Safety, Competition Stress, Fitness, Sports Nutrition, Steroid Risks, and More*

Edited by Joyce Brennfleck Shannon. 405 pages. 2003. 978-0-7808-0447-0.

"This work will be useful in the young adult collections of public libraries as well as high school libraries."
— *American Reference Books Annual, 2004*

■

# Suicide Information for Teens

**Health Tips about Suicide Causes and Prevention**

*Including Facts about Depression, Risk Factors, Getting Help, Survivor Support, and More*

Edited by Joyce Brennfleck Shannon. 368 pages. 2005. 978-0-7808-0737-2.

# Tobacco Information for Teens

**Health Tips about the Hazards of Using Cigarettes, Smokeless Tobacco, and Other Nicotine Products**

*Including Facts about Nicotine Addiction, Immediate and Long-Term Health Effects of Tobacco Use, Related Cancers, Smoking Cessation, Tobacco Use Prevention, and Tobacco Use Statistics*

Edited by Karen Bellenir. 440 pages. 2007. 978-0-7808-0976-5.

# Health Reference Series